A Practical Approach to Transesophageal Echocardiography

A Practical Approach to Transesophageal Echocardiography

Editors

Albert C. Perrino, Jr., M.D.

Associate Professor
Department of Anesthesiology
Yale University School of Medicine
Chief, Anesthesiology Service
VA-Connecticut Healthcare System
New Haven, Connecticut

Scott T. Reeves, M.D., M.B.A., F.A.C.C.

Professor
Department of Anesthesiology and Perioperative Medicine
Medical University of South Carolina
Charleston, South Carolina

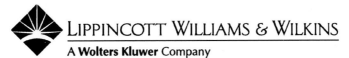

LIPPINCOTT WILLIAMS & WILKINS
A **Wolters Kluwer** Company

Philadelphia • Baltimore • New York • London
Buenos Aires • Hong Kong • Sydney • Tokyo

Acquisitions Editor: R. Craig Percy
Developmental Editor: Sonya Seigafuse
Project Editor: Sheila Higgins
Manufacturing Manager: Benjamin Rivera
Cover Designer: Wendolyn Hill and David Levy
Compositor: TechBooks
Printer: Maple Press

© 2003 by **LIPPINCOTT WILLIAMS & WILKINS**
530 Walnut Street
Philadelphia, PA 19106 USA
LWW.com

Printed in the USA

Library of Congress Cataloging-in-Publication Data

Perrino, Albert C.
    A practical approach to transesophageal echocardiography / Albert C. Perrino, Scott T. Reeves.
        p. ; cm.
    Includes bibliographical references and index.
    ISBN 0-7817-3638-2
    1. Transesophageal echocardiography.   I. Reeves, Scott T.   II. Title.
    [DNLM: 1. Echocardiography, Transesophageal—methods. 2. Heart Diseases—ultrasonography.   WG 141.5.E2 P458p 2003]
    RC683.5.T83P47   2003
    616.1′207543—dc21

                                                                                   2002043396

10 9 8 7 6 5 4 3 2

To Anita, Mary, Isabella, and Juliana for sustaining another of my adventures and to Winston Churchill whose keen observation also served as a source of support.

Writing is an adventure. To begin with, it is a toy and an amusement. Then it becomes a mistress, then it becomes a master, then it becomes a tyrant. The last phase is that just as you are about to be reconciled to your servitude, you kill the monster and fling him to the public.

—Winston Churchill
ACP

To
My Savior, Jesus Christ, who gives me strength...
My wife, Cathy, who loves and puts up with me...
My children, Catherine, Carolyn, and Townsend, who give me great joy...
My patients, who inspire me to do my best daily!

STR

Contents

Contributing Authors viii

Preface xi

Part I. Essentials of Two-Dimensional Imaging

1. Principles and Technology of Two-Dimensional Echocardiography   3
   Andrew Maslow and Albert C. Perrino, Jr.

2. Two-Dimensional Examination 22
   Joseph P. Miller

3. Ventricular Systolic Performance and Pathology 37
   *J. Scott Walton, Scott T. Reeves, and
   Bruce H. Dorman, Jr.*

4. Diagnosis of Myocardial Ischemia 56
   Martin J. London

Part II. Essentials of Doppler Echocardiography

5. Doppler Technology and Technique 77
   Albert C. Perrino, Jr.

6. Quantitative Doppler and Hemodynamics 94
   Andrew Maslow and Albert C. Perrino, Jr.

7. Evaluation of Ventricular Diastolic Function 110
   Stanton K. Shernan and Michael R. Zile

Part III. Transesophageal Echocardiography in Valvular Disease and Surgery

8. Mitral Regurgitation 133
   A. Stephane Lambert

9. Mitral Valve Stenosis 145
   Colleen Gorman Koch

10. Mitral Valve Repair 159
    Kristine J. Hirsch and Gregory M. Hirsch

11. Aortic Regurgitation 177
    Ira S. Cohen

12. Aortic Stenosis 188
    Ira S. Cohen

13. Prosthetic Valves 200
    Albert T. Cheung

14. Right Ventricle, Right Atrium, Tricuspid Valve, and
    Pulmonic Valve 218
    Gautam M. Sreeram and Jonathan B. Mark

Part IV. Clinical Challenges

15. Transesophageal Echocardiography for
    Coronary Revascularization 233
    Stuart J. Weiss and John G. Augoustides

16. Transesophageal Echocardiography of the Thoracic Aorta 251
    Kim J. Payne, William M. Yarbrough,
    John S. Ikonomidis, and Scott T. Reeves

17. Transesophageal Echocardiography in the
    Intensive Care Unit 272
    Emilio B. Lobato and Felipe Urdaneta

18. Transesophageal Echocardiography for Congenital Heart Disease
    in the Adult 286
    Kathryn Rouine-Rapp and Wanda C. Miller-Hance

Part V. Man and Machine

19. Common Artifacts and Pitfalls of Clinical Echocardiography 305
    Joseph P. Miller, Albert C. Perrino, Jr., and Zak Hillel

20. Techniques and Tricks for Optimizing
    Transesophageal Images 321
    Herbert W. Dyal II, Michael D. Frith, and
    Scott T. Reeves

Appendices

Appendix 1. Transesophageal Echocardiographic Anatomy 332

Appendix 2. Summaries of Valvular Stenosis and Insufficiency 336

Answers to Questions 338

Subject Index 343

Contributing Authors

John G. Augoustides, M.D. Assistant Professor, Department of Anesthesia, University of Pennsylvania; Attending Anesthesiologist, Department of Anesthesia, University of Pennsylvania Medical Center, Philadelphia, Pennsylvania

Albert T. Cheung, M.D. Associate Professor, Department of Anesthesia, University of Pennsylvania; Staff Anesthesiologist, Department of Anesthesia, Hospital of the University of Pennsylvania, Philadelphia, Pennsylvania

Ira S. Cohen, M.D., F.A.C.C. Clinical Professor of Medicine, Department of Cardiology, Thomas Jefferson University School of Medicine, Philadelphia, Pennsylvania; and Co-Director, Heart Station, Department of Cardiology, Lankenau Hospital, Wynnewood, Pennsylvania

Bruce H. Dorman, Jr., M.D., Ph.D. Professor, Department of Anesthesia and Perioperative Medicine, Medical University of South Carolina, Charleston, South Carolina

Herbert W. Dyal II, B.H.S., R.D.C.S., R.D.M.S. Cardiovascular Clinical Applications Specialist, General Electric Company, Milwaukee, Wisconsin

Michael D. Frith, B.S., R.D.C.S., R.V.T. Account Executive, Cardiovascular Ultrasound, General Electric Company, Milwaukee, Wisconsin

Zak Hillel, Ph.D., M.D. Professor of Clinical Anesthesiology, Department of Anesthesiology, Columbia University College of Physicians and Surgeons; Director of Cardiac Anesthesia, Department of Anesthesiology, St. Lukes-Roosevelt Hospital, New York, New York

Gregory M. Hirsch, M.D., F.R.C.P.S. Associate Professor, Department of Surgery, Dalhousie University; Staff Cardiac Surgeon, Division of Cardiac Surgery, Department of Surgery, Queen Elizabeth II Health Sciences Centre, Halifax, Nova Scotia, Canada

Kristine J. Hirsch, M.D., F.R.C.P. Assistant Professor, Department of Anesthesia, Dalhousie University; Staff Anesthesiologist, Director of Perioperative Transesophageal Echocardiography, Department of Anesthesia, Queen Elizabeth II Health Sciences Centre, Halifax, Nova Scotia, Canada

John S. Ikonomidis, M.D., Ph.D. Assistant Professor, Division of Cardiothoracic Surgery, Medical University of South Carolina, Charleston, South Carolina

Colleen Gorman Koch, M.D., M.S. Department of Cardiothoracic Anesthesia, The Cleveland Clinic Foundation, Cleveland, Ohio

A. Stephane Lambert, M.D., F.R.C.P.C. Assistant Professor, Department of Anesthesia, University of Toronto; Attending Anesthesiologist, Department of Anesthesia, St. Michael's Hospital, Toronto, Ontario, Canada

Emilio B. Lobato, M.D. Associate Professor, Department of Anesthesiology, University of Florida College of Medicine; Chief, Cardiothoracic Anesthesiology, Assistant Chief of Anesthesiology, Anesthesiology Service, Malcom Randall Veterans Affairs Medical Center; and Director, Cardiac Anesthesia Shands, Gainesville, Florida

Martin J. London, M.D. Professor of Clinical Anesthesia, Department of Anesthesia and Perioperative Care, University of California, San Francisco; and Attending Anesthesiologist, San Francisco Veterans Affairs Medical Center, San Francisco, California

Jonathan B. Mark, M.D. Chief, Anesthesiology Service, Veterans Affairs Medical Center; Professor and Vice Chairman, Department of Anesthesiology, Duke University Medical Center, Durham, North Carolina

Andrew Maslow, M.D. Assistant Professor, Department of Anesthesiology, Brown Medical School; Department of Anesthesiology, Rhode Island Hospital, Providence, Rhode Island

Joseph P. Miller, M.D. Director, Cardiovascular Anesthesia, Department of Anesthesia and Operative Services, Madigan Army Medical Center, Tacoma, Washington

Wanda C. Miller-Hance, M.D. Director, Intraoperative Echocardiography for Anesthesiology and Pediatrics; Director, Research in Pediatric Cardiovascular Anesthesiology, Texas Children's Hospital; and Associate Professor, Department of Anesthesiology and Pediatrics, Baylor College of Medicine, Houston, Texas

Kim J. Payne, M.D. Assistant Professor, Department of Anesthesiology and Perioperative Medicine, Medical University of South Carolina, Charleston, South Carolina

Albert C. Perrino, Jr., M.D. Associate Professor, Department of Anesthesiology, Yale University School of Medicine; Chief, Anesthesiology Service, VA-Connecticut Healthcare System, New Haven, Connecticut

Scott T. Reeves, M.D., M.B.A., F.A.C.C. Professor, Department of Anesthesiology and Perioperative Medicine, Medical University of South Carolina, Charleston, South Carolina

Kathryn Rouine-Rapp, M.D. Associate Professor of Clinical Anesthesia, Department of Anesthesia, University of California, San Francisco, California

Stanton K. Shernan, M.D. Assistant Professor of Anesthesia, Department of Anesthesiology, Perioperative and Pain Medicine, Brigham and Women's Hospital, Harvard Medical School, Boston, Massachusetts

Gautam M. Sreeram, M.D.   Assistant Professor, Department of Anesthesiology, Duke University; Anesthesiologist, Veterans Affairs Hospital, Durham, North Carolina

Felipe Urdaneta M.D.   Assistant Professor, Department of Anesthesiology, University of Florida College of Medicine; Assistant Professor, Department of Anesthesiology, Malcom Randall Veterans Affairs Hospital, Gainesville, Florida

J. Scott Walton, M.D.   Associate Professor, Department of Anesthesia and Perioperative Medicine, Medical University of South Carolina, Charleston, South Carolina

Stuart J. Weiss M.D., Ph.D.   Associate Professor, Department of Anesthesia, University of Pennsylvania, Philadelphia, Pennsylvania

William M. Yarbrough, M.D.   Resident, Department of Surgery, Medical University of South Carolina, Charleston, South Carolina

Michael R. Zile, M.D.   Charles Ezra Daniel Professor, Cardiology Division of the Department of Medicine, Gazes Cardiac Research Institute, Medical University of South Carolina, and RHJ Department of Veterans Affairs Medical Center, Charleston, South Carolina

Preface

Transesophageal echocardiography (TEE) is the first imaging technique to enter the mainstream of intraoperative patient monitoring. The dramatic display of detailed cardiac anatomy and physiology provided in real-time by two-dimensional (2-D) and Doppler techniques quickly convinced the most skeptical among us of the remarkable clinical potential TEE offers to optimize patient management. For clinicians accustomed to invasive hemodynamic monitoring, it is something of a challenge to become an accomplished interpreter of TEE images and Doppler techniques. The multiple views and imaging planes require a readjustment of our orientation to cardiac anatomy. And the quantitative assessments of cardiovascular function, particularly those derived from blood flow velocity, also require new insights for the clinician accustomed to pressure measurements. This book provides the intraoperative clinician with a resource to readily acquire the principles and perspectives underlying the approach used in practice by accomplished intraoperative echocardiographers.

The editors have gathered contributing authors who are internationally renowned and acknowledged for their independent contributions and teaching ability. The authors were given the task of presenting a highly readable and clinically relevant survey of the current practice of perioperative echocardiography. Their enthusiasm, backed with the strong support of the publisher, has produced this book.

In contrast to the comprehensive reference texts and case atlases available on this subject, this project offers the aspiring clinician the best resource to acquire the essential skills of TEE practice. The presentation, illustrations, and content create a surprisingly portable text that is conducive to rapid appreciation of the critical elements in the use of TEE for a particular clinical challenge.

The content outline guides the reader through the physics, principles, and applications of 2-D imaging and Doppler modalities for assessing ventricular performance and the significance of coexistent valvular disease. There is particular emphasis on the use of TEE for valve repair and replacement surgery. A complete chapter is dedicated to echocardiographic artifacts and other pitfalls of interpretation that can lead to misdiagnosis. This book concludes with a section on technical issues and echocardiography machine operation. It is our intention that after an understanding of the imaging modalities has been acquired, the importance and relevance of these somewhat dry but essential concepts will be better appreciated than if they were presented as initial topics. Each chapter concludes with a series of self-assessment test questions to further emphasize important teaching points.

Certainly, the skills required to be an expert echocardiographer cannot be gained from textbooks alone. Extensive clinical training and intraoperative exposure to the application of these techniques remains paramount. In addition, we recommend the excellent educational programs on intraoperative TEE sponsored by the

American Society of Echocardiography, the Society for Cardiovascular Anesthesiology, and the American Society of Anesthesiologists. We hope this textbook will become a well-worn and valued asset to your echocardiography practice.

Albert C. Perrino, Jr., M.D.
Scott T. Reeves, M.D., M.B.A., F.A.C.C.

PART I

ESSENTIALS OF TWO-DIMENSIONAL IMAGING

Principles and Technology of Two-Dimensional Echocardiography

Andrew Maslow and Albert C. Perrino, Jr.

Two-dimensional echocardiography generates dynamic images of the heart from reflections of transmitted ultrasound. To achieve these images, the echocardiography system transmits a brief pulse of ultrasound that propagates through and is subsequently reflected from the various cardiac structures. The sound reflections travel back to the ultrasound transducer, which records the time delay for each returning reflection. Because the speed of sound in tissue is constant, the time delay allows a precise calculation of the location of the cardiac structures, and the echocardiography system can then create an image map of the heart. Not surprisingly, successful cardiac imaging requires a firm understanding of the interactions of sound and tissue. This chapter reviews the basic principles of ultrasound, its propagation through tissues, and the technologies used to create moving images of the heart.

PHYSICAL PROPERTIES OF SOUND WAVES

Vibrations

Sound is vibration of a physical medium. In clinical echocardiography, a mechanical vibrator, known as the *transducer,* is placed in contact with the esophagus (transesophageal echocardiography) or skin (transthoracic echocardiography) to create sound waves. The resulting tissue vibrations or sound waves consist of areas of **compression** (areas where molecules are tightly packed) and **rarefaction** (areas where molecules are dispersed) resembling a sine wave (Fig. 1.1).

Amplitude. The amplitude of a sound wave represents its peak pressure and is appreciated as loudness. The level of sound energy in an area of tissue is referred to as **intensity** and is an important factor regarding the potential for tissue damage with ultrasound. For example, lithotripsy uses high-intensity sound signals to fragment renal stones. In contrast, diagnostic ultrasound uses low-intensity signals to image tissue, which produces only limited bioeffects. Because levels of sound pressure vary over a large range, it is convenient to express sound wave amplitude with the decibel scale, a logarithmic scale that compares two sound wave amplitudes:

$$\text{Decibel (dB)} = 20 \log_{10} A_2 / A_1 \qquad [1]$$

where A_2 is the sound amplitude of interest and A_1 is a reference sound level.

More simply expressed, each doubling of the sound pressure equals a gain of 6 dB.

Frequency and Wavelength

Sound waves are also characterized by their **frequency** (f), or pitch, expressed in cycles per second, or Hertz (Hz), and by their **wavelength** (λ). These attributes have a significant impact on the depth of penetration of a sound wave in tissue and the image resolution of the ultrasound system.

Propagation Velocity

Sound waves travel, or propagate, through tissue from the transducer to the cardiac structures. The propagation velocity, or speed, of sound (v) can be measured or calculated. *However, it is essential to recognize that the speed of sound is determined solely by the medium through*

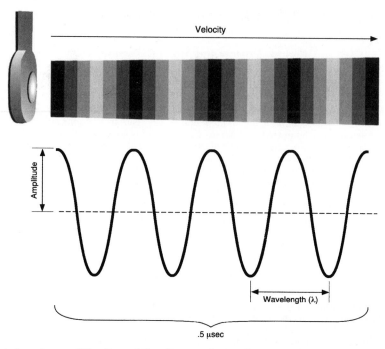

FIG. 1.1. Sound wave. Vibrations of the ultrasound transducer create cycles of compression and rarefaction in adjacent tissue. The ultrasound energy is characterized by its amplitude, wavelength, frequency, and propagation velocity. In this example, four sound waves are shown in a period of 0.5 μs. The frequency can be calculated as 4 cycles divided by 0.5 μs and equals 8 MHz.

which it passes. For example, the speed of sound in soft tissue is approximately 1,540 m/s. Alternatively, velocity can be calculated because the product of wavelength and frequency must equal the speed of sound:

$$v = \lambda \times f \qquad [2]$$

It becomes apparent that the wavelength and frequency are necessarily inversely related:

$$\lambda = v \times 1/f \qquad [3]$$

$$\lambda = (1,540 \text{ m/s})/f \qquad [4]$$

Table 1.1 lists the corresponding sound wavelengths and frequencies commonly used in clinical ultrasonography.

What's So Special about Ultrasound?

Several favorable physical properties of ultrasound explain its usefulness in clinical imaging. **Ultrasound** is sound with frequencies greater than those of the audible range for humans (20,000 Hz). In clinical echocardiography, frequencies of 2 to 10 MHz are used. The

TABLE 1.1. CORRESPONDING FREQUENCIES
AND WAVELENGTHS IN SOFT TISSUE

Frequency (MHz)	Wavelength (mm)
1.25	1.20
2.5	0.60
5.0	0.30
7.5	0.20
10.0	0.15

high-frequency, short-wavelength ultrasound beam can be more easily manipulated, focused, and directed to a specific target. Image resolution also increases when higher frequency sound waves are used (see later).

INTERACTIONS OF SOUND AND TISSUE

The propagation, or passage, of a sound wave through the body is markedly affected by its interactions with the various tissues encountered. These interactions result in reflection, refraction, scattering, and attenuation of the ultrasound signal. The exact manner in which sound is affected by the various tissues it encounters determines how they appear in the two-dimensional image (Fig. 1.2).

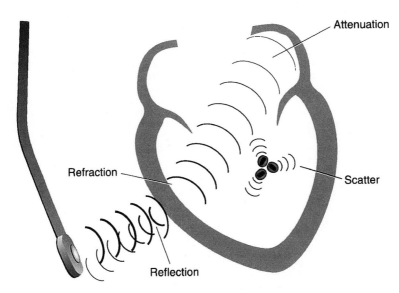

FIG. 1.2. Interactions of sound and tissue. Traveling through various tissues, sound energy is altered by four major events. Specular *reflection* creates strong echoes directed back toward the transducer. *Refraction* bends the ultrasound beam, directing it in a new path. As the ultrasound beam travels deeper in tissue, *attenuation* occurs as the beam is dispersed and the sound energy is converted to heat. *Scattering* reflections from small objects such as red cells disperse the sound energy in all directions.

TABLE 1.2. ACOUSTIC PROPERTIES OF VARIOUS TISSUES

Tissue/ medium	Speed of sound (m/s)	Acoustic impedance (kg/m^{2}s $\times$ 10^6)	Attenuation coefficient (cm^{-1} at 1 MHz)	Half-power distance (cm at 2.5 MHz)
Air	330	0.00004		0.08
Lung	600	0.26		0.05
Fat	1,460	1.35	0.04–0.09	
Water	1,480	1.52	0.0003	380.0
Blood	1,560	1.62	0.02	15.0
Muscle	1,600	1.7	0.25–0.35	0.6–1.0
Bone	4,080	7.80		0.7–0.8

Reflection

Echocardiographic imaging depends on the transmission and subsequent reflection of ultrasound energy back to the transducer. A sound wave propagates through uniform tissue until it reaches another tissue type with different acoustic properties. At the tissue interface, the ultrasound energy undergoes a dramatic alteration, after which it can be reflected back toward the transducer or transmitted into the next tissue, often in a direction that deviates from the original course. Precisely how the ultrasound beam will be affected is predicted by factoring the acoustic properties of the tissues that create the interface and the angle at which the ultrasound beam strikes this interface.

The tissue interface: acoustic impedance. An important acoustic property of a tissue is its capacity for transmitting sound, known as acoustic impedance (Z). This property is largely related to the **density** (ρ) of the material:

$$Z = \rho \times v \qquad [5]$$

As seen in Table 1.2, denser materials like bone and fluids effectively transmit ultrasound, whereas air and lung tissue have a low level of acoustic impedance and are poor transmitters of sound energy. This property explains why an amplification system is required even for a small lecture hall, yet whales can hear sound over great expanses of the ocean.

When sound reaches an interface of two tissues of similar acoustic impedance, the ultrasound beam travels across the interface largely undisturbed. When the tissues differ in impedance, a percentage of the ultrasound energy is **reflected** and the remainder is **transmitted.** *The larger the absolute difference in the levels of acoustic impedance across the interface, the greater the percentage of the ultrasound energy that is reflected.* Reflection can be calculated by using the reflection coefficient (R):

$$\text{Reflection coefficient} = \frac{(Z_2 - Z_1)^2}{(Z_1 + Z_2)^2} \qquad [6]$$

The reflective properties of an interface are key factors in the imaged appearance of a structure. *When the absolute difference between the levels of acoustic impedance of the two interfacing media is large, as when soft tissue interfaces with air or bone, more energy is reflected back to the transducer.* These interfaces are represented by echo-dense or bright signals on the echogram. When the absolute difference is small, as when soft tissue interfaces with soft tissue, the interface will not appear as bright and may even be echo-lucent or dark.

Specular and scattering reflectors. The reflection of sound also is greatly affected by the size and surface of the tissue. Two types of reflection, specular and scattered, are commonly encountered.

Specular reflection occurs when a sound wave encounters a large object with a smooth surface. Such surfaces act like an acoustic mirror, generating strong reflections that travel away from the interface at an angle equal and opposite to that at which the ultrasound beam traveled to the interface. Reflection is maximal when the angle of incidence is 90 degrees—that is, the ultrasound beam and the object are perpendicular to each another. With an angle of incidence other than 90 degrees, less energy is reflected back to the transducer. Because of the important effect of strong specular reflection on image quality, echocardiographers are constantly adjusting the position of the transesophageal echocardiographic (TEE) transducer so that the direction of its beam is perpendicular to the cardiac structure of interest.

Scattering reflection occurs when an ultrasound beam encounters small or irregularly shaped surfaces. Such small objects, such as red blood cells, scatter ultrasound energy in all directions, so that far less energy is reflected back to the transducer than in the case of a specular reflector. This type of reflection is the basis of the Doppler analysis of red blood cell movement.

Both types of reflection contribute to the two-dimensional image. Although the strongest signals and best images are obtained from interfaces that are perpendicular to the beam orientation, cardiac tissue is to a large extent irregular and nonlinear in shape. Thus, a significant component of the reflected energy comes from scattering off the smaller irregular components of tissue. An example is imaging of the lateral and septal walls of the left ventricle from esophageal windows. Although the ventricular walls are parallel to the ultrasound beam, they can be imaged as a result of both specular reflection and scattering off the irregular surfaces of the myocardium. However, the total amount of ultrasound returning to the transducer is low, which accounts for the poor quality of images, which often include dark spots called *echo dropout*. Adjusting the transducer angle or using a different echocardiographic window to orient the beam better often dramatically improves image quality.

Refraction

The portion of the ultrasound beam that is not reflected propagates through the interface, but its direction is often altered, or refracted. Refraction is most pronounced when the difference in the levels of acoustic impedance is large and the angle of incidence is acute. When the angle of incidence is 90 degrees, or when the difference in levels of acoustic impedance is minimal, refraction does not occur because the ultrasound energy either is reflected or continues to travel in the same direction.

Refraction is an important factor in the formation of artifacts. Although the ultrasound beam may proceed in an altered direction, the transducer does not recognize this change. Consequently, the refracted energy may interface with a cardiac structure outside the *intended* scanning field. The reflected energy from this interface returns to the transducer, which then incorrectly displays the structure alongside structures detected by the beam in its original course (Fig. 1.3). Altering the viewing angle so that the ultrasound energy is perpendicular to the area of interest minimizes refraction and any resultant artifact.

Attenuation

In addition to being reflected and refracted from tissue interfaces, the ultrasound signal is altered as it travels through uniform tissue. Most notable is the steady loss (i.e., attenuation) in transmitted *intensity* (watts per square meter) as a consequence of dispersion and absorption. The attenuation in ultrasound energy caused by dispersion and absorption result in less energy returning back to the transducer, and subsequently a weaker signal on the display.

Dispersion occurs as the ultrasound beam diverges in the far field. In addition, because the cellular structure of tissue is irregular, scattering further disperses the ultrasound energy. The amount of scattering varies greatly with tissue type.

Absorption occurs as frictional forces convert ultrasound energy into heat. Because friction is related to the level of tissue movement, it is not surprising that the higher the frequency of the signal and the greater the distance traveled, the greater the absorption (Fig. 1.4). The dependence of attenuation on frequency and distance is reflected in the **attenuation coefficient** (decibels per centimeter per megahertz), which allows a comparison of the degree of attenuation between tissue types. The penetration of ultrasound can also be

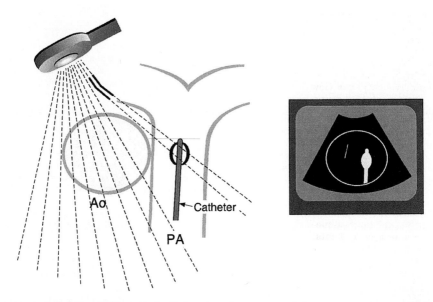

FIG. 1.3. Refraction artifact. **Left:** Refraction of a portion of the ultrasound beam in the near field (*solid line*) deflects the beam laterally where it interacts with a strong reflector, a pulmonary artery (PA) catheter. **Right:** The transducer is unable to recognize that these scan lines have been refracted and incorrectly assumes that the returning reflections have originated from the original course of the beam. Echocardiography display illustrates the resulting artifact as the reflections from the pulmonary artery catheter are mistakenly positioned within the aorta (Ao).

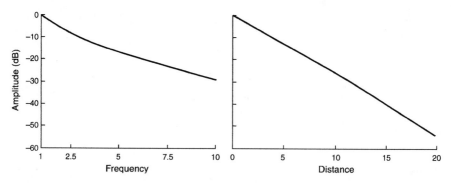

FIG. 1.4. Attenuation of ultrasound. The effects of transducer frequency and distance on signal strength are plotted in decibels. **Left:** The lower-frequency signals are less attenuated. **Right:** The amplitude of a 1-MHz signal traveling through cardiac tissue is plotted. Signals reaching the far field can be more than 60 dB less than those lying close to the transducer. These effects warrant careful selection of the transducer frequency, imaging view, and gain settings to mitigate attenuation.

expressed by the **half-power distance** specific for each tissue, which expresses the distance sound will travel until half of its original energy is lost. The acoustic properties of various tissues are summarized in Table 1.2.

As a result of these phenomena, the returning echoes from deeper structures are weakened. To decrease the negative effects of attenuation during an examination, echocardiographers may choose to use a lower-frequency signal (e.g., a 2.5- instead of a 7.5-MHz transducer frequency) and view the structure from a window closer to the structure of interest. In addition, the incoming signal can be enhanced by adjusting the gain controls to amplify the weakened returning signals. These adjustments are discussed in greater detail in Chapter 20.

TRANSDUCER DESIGN AND BEAM FORMATION

Transducer Components

The transducers used in echocardiography systems create a brief pulse of ultrasound that is transmitted into tissue (Fig. 1.5). To achieve this goal, most TEE transducer designs use the following components:

1. A *ceramic piezoelectric crystal,* which acts as an ultrasonic vibrator
2. *Electrodes,* which both conduct electric energy to stimulate the piezoelectric crystal and record the voltage from returning echoes

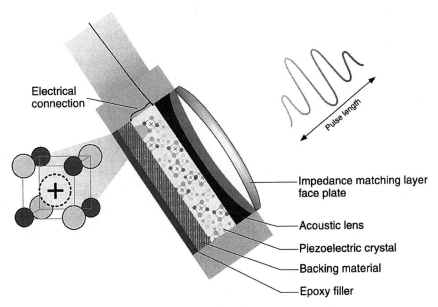

FIG. 1.5. Transducer components: creating a sound pulse. A brief transmission of alternating current from the *electric connector* causes charged particles within the matrix of the piezoelectric crystal to vibrate. The *backing material* helps to dampen the crystal vibrations quickly, keeping the pulse length short; in this example, it is 4 wavelengths. An *acoustic lens* aids in focusing the sound energy. The *faceplate* contains layers of material that match the acoustic impedance of the esophagus, to avoid unwanted reflections and ensure excellent sound transmission. *Epoxy filler* secures the working components to the probe.

3. *Backing,* which acts to dampen the vibrations of the crystal rapidly
4. *Insulation,* which prevents unwanted vibration of the transducer from standing waves or extraneous incoming waves
5. A *faceplate,* which optimizes the acoustic contact between the piezoelectric crystal and the esophagus. The faceplate may also include an acoustic lens to focus the beam.

The following sections detail the inner workings of the modern ultrasound transducer and their effects on the transmitted sound beam and the echocardiographic image.

Formation of Ultrasound Waves: The Piezoelectric Crystal

The heart of the transducer consists of a piezoelectric crystal, which contains polarized molecules trapped within a matrix. The formation of the sound wave used in echocardiography is based on the principle of **piezoelectricity.** When stimulated by an alternating electric current, the polarized particles within the crystal vibrate, generating ultrasound. Conversely, when an ultrasound wave strikes the crystal, the resulting vibrations of the polarized particles generate an alternating electric current. Thus, a piezoelectric crystal can function as both a transmitter and a receiver of ultrasound. This process is the hallmark of piezoelectricity—that is, the transformation of electric energy into mechanical energy and the reverse transformation of mechanical energy into electric energy.

For imaging purposes, the transducer emits a brief burst of ultrasound. Typically, two-dimensional transducers emit a sound pulse of two to four wavelengths. As illustrated in Figure 1.6, the shorter the length of the sound pulse, the better the axial resolution of the system. Thus, the shorter the wavelength, the shorter the resulting pulse length and the greater the axial resolution.

The Three-Dimensional Ultrasound Beam

Near and far fields. The ultrasound transducer emits a three-dimensional ultrasound beam similar to the beam of a flashlight (Fig. 1.7). The physical dimensions of this beam determine the following:

1. The specific area of the heart examined
2. The intensity distribution of ultrasound energy
3. The lateral (side-to-side) and elevational (top-to-bottom) resolution of the system.

Narrower beams are preferred because they improve resolution, increase the intensity of returning echoes, and reduce artifact. Most commonly, ultrasound beams have either a disk or rectangular shape and comprise two main zones: the **near field (Fresnel)** and **far field (Fraunhofer) zones.** Beam manipulation and image resolution are greatest within the near field. Also, ultrasound energy is more concentrated within this zone, yielding stronger echoes and better imaging.

In the near field zone, the ultrasound beam is narrow. The length of the near field zone is proportional to the radius (r) of the transducer face and inversely proportional to the wavelength:

$$L_n = r^2 / \lambda \qquad\qquad [7]$$

Distal to the near field zone, the ultrasound beam diverges, forming the far field zone. The angle of divergence (θ) is inversely related to the radius (r) of the transducer face:

$$\text{Sin } \theta = 0.61/r \qquad\qquad [8]$$

Accordingly, larger transducers with high-frequency (small λ) signals produce the most desirable beam profile: a long, narrow near field and a less divergent far field.

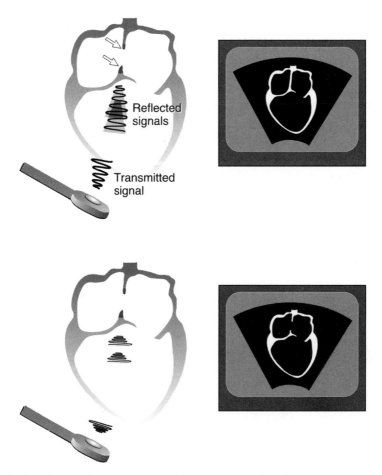

FIG. 1.6. Effect of pulse length on axial resolution. **Top:** The transducer emits a long sound pulse. Because the length of this pulse is greater than the length of the atrial septal defect (*arrows*), the reflections from the two tips of atrial septum are smeared and the defect cannot be resolved. Consequently, the resulting two-dimensional echocardiographic display (**right**) does not show the abnormality. **Bottom:** The pulse length has been shortened and is now less than the length of the atrial septal defect. The reflections from each interface are clearly identifiable, and the resulting display (**right**) shows the defect.

Focusing. Focusing can further narrow the ultrasound beam. This is accomplished in three ways:

1. By creating a concave shape in the piezoelectric crystal
2. By gluing an acoustic lens to the front of the crystal
3. Electronically with the use of annular array transducers.

The narrow beam at the focal zone enhances imaging at this location. However, the beam diverges widely distal to the focal zone, reducing the intensity of the ultrasound energy and impairing imaging of the far field. The ability of modern echocardiography systems to allow the echocardiographer to adjust the depth of the focal zone selectively provides a means to optimize image quality.

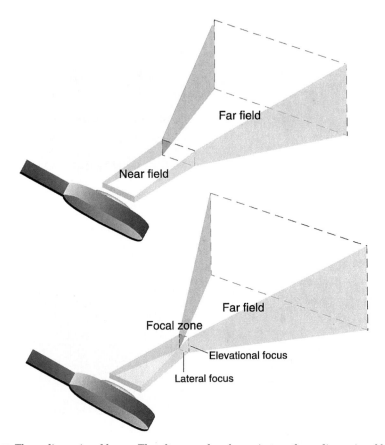

FIG. 1.7. Three-dimensional beam. The ultrasound probe projects a three-dimensional beam. The dimensions of this projection have important effects on imaging resolution and artifact. Typically, a narrow profile is preferred. **Top:** Unfocused beam. The beam is narrow in the near field and then diverges in the far field. **Bottom:** Focused beam. Focusing has resulted in a narrower beam in both the lateral and elevational planes, so that the imaging resolution of structures in the focal zone is improved. Distal to the focal zone, the beam rapidly diverges, and the images of structures in this area will be of lower quality.

Electronic beam focusing: the phased array. Modern echocardiography systems allow the echocardiographer to adjust the depth of the focal zone selectively to optimize image quality. A transducer consisting of 64 to 96 independently controlled piezoelectric crystals, known as a *phased array,* creates the beam shape. Although each individual element emits a wave front that diverges in a hemispheric pattern, the interaction of the individual sound waves emitted by each crystal creates a narrow, forwardly directed wave front (Fig. 1.8A). If the crystals at the ends of the array are electronically activated before those located at the center, the wave front becomes concave, so that it can be focused at a selected distance from the transducer face (Fig. 1.8B).

It is important to be cognizant of both the advantages and disadvantages of selecting the focus depth of the beam. As is discussed next, beam shape is of prime importance in determining the resolution of an imaging system.

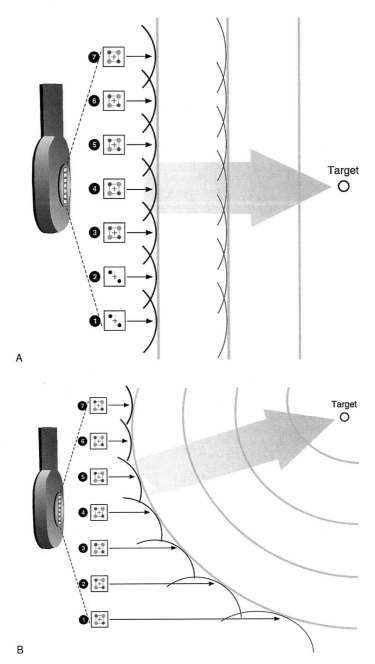

FIG. 1.8. Phased array transducers. **A:** This illustration shows seven crystal elements in an array. The interactions of the individual hemispheric wave fronts create a flat, profiled, forward-directed wave front. **B:** Phased array transducer. Here, the crystals have been activated sequentially: crystal 1 first, followed by crystal 2, and so on. This causes the beam to be steered upward toward the target. Note that crystals 7 and 8 have been activated before crystal 6, creating a concave wave front to focus the energy of the beam at the target. The ability to steer electronically and focus the beam is a major advantage of the phased array system.

Resolution

Two aspects of the resolution of an ultrasound system are usually assessed: the resolution of objects lying along the axis of the ultrasound beam (axial resolution), and the resolution of objects perpendicular to the beam orientation (lateral and elevational resolution).

Axial resolution. Axial resolution is the ability of the ultrasound system to identify two separate objects that lie along the path of the ultrasound beam axis. This is determined by the duration and wavelength of the ultrasound pulse. As seen in Figure 1.6, short pulses of high-frequency ultrasound offer the greatest axial resolution. A general rule is that the axial resolution of a system is about two times the wavelength of the system. Improved axial resolution does not come without a cost. The shorter the pulse, the lower its energy level, so that penetration and returning echoes are weaker. Similarly, high-frequency sound is quickly attenuated. Accordingly, the echocardiographer must select these parameters based on the imaging needs.

Lateral (azimuth) resolution. Lateral resolution is the ability of the ultrasound system to distinguish between objects that are side by side and perpendicular to the path of the ultrasound beam. Beam width is a primary determinant of lateral resolution. Wide beams produce a "smeared" image of two such objects, whereas narrow beams can identify each object individually.

Elevational resolution. Elevational resolution is the ability of the ultrasound system to distinguish between objects that are vertically aligned and perpendicular to the emitted ultrasound beam. Although two-dimensional images appear to display a thin slice of cardiac anatomy, in actuality the information gathered from the entire thickness of the beam is averaged and displayed. For this reason, the thinner the ultrasound beam, the better the elevational resolution of the system (Fig. 1.7).

Optimizing resolution. The interplay of the radius, frequency, and focal length of the transducer and its distance from the structure of interest determine beam width and height. The net effect is a beam that is narrowest in the near field or focal zone and divergent in the far field. Resolution is therefore better in the near field and decreases in the far field. Factors that lengthen the near field, such as a higher transducer frequency and a larger transducer radius, improve lateral and elevational resolution. Focusing further decreases the width of the ultrasound beam and improves lateral and elevational resolution at the focal point. However, focusing increases beam divergence distal to the focal zone, with an associated loss of lateral and elevational resolution. These factors explain why it is preferable to position a transducer with a relatively high frequency (smaller wavelength) and relatively large radius close to the target of interest to optimize both lateral and elevational resolution.

Extraneous Sound Beams

Side lobes. Unfortunately, in addition to the powerful main beam of sound energy produced by both single crystal and annular array transducers, additional beams of sound are emitted that travel off axis to the main beam (Fig. 1.9). These extraneous beams of sound (side lobes) significantly affect imaging quality because the transducer incorrectly processes their reflections as reflections of the main beam. Consequently, structures off axis to the imaging plane appear incorrectly located on the two-dimensional image.

Each section on the transducer face can be considered a point source of sound emission. Wherever constructive interference of the sound waves of two sections of the transducer occurs, the energy is enhanced and a side lobe is created. Because constructive interference occurs when two waves meet in phase with each other, resulting in a summation of their amplitudes, the pattern of side lobes can be predicted based on the wavelength of the emitted signal.

Grating lobes. Grating lobes are another type of eccentric beam, commonly generated by annular array transducers. In this case, the constructive interference is related to the summations of the individual sound waves emitted from each crystal. When these individual sound waves meet in phase and off axis to the main beam, a grating lobe is created. The position of a grating lobe is related to the spacing of the crystals and the wavelength of the signal.

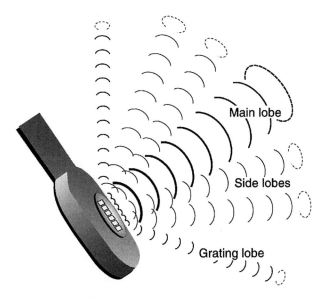

FIG. 1.9. Side lobes. The sound energy emitted from ultrasound transducers has a typical pattern. Constructive interference of the individual wave fronts concentrates most of the energy on axis, in what is called the *main lobe*. However, constructive interference of individual wave fronts also causes lobes of energy to be directed off axis; these are known as *side lobes* and *grating lobes*. Reflections from these lobes reduce image quality and are a well-described source of imaging artifact.

Side lobe artifacts. Both side and grating lobes contain less energy than the main beam and usually do not significantly affect the echocardiographic image. However, when these lobes of energy contact a highly reflective surface (catheter, prosthesis, calcium), sufficient energy can be reflected back to the transducer to create an artifact. The transducer believes these reflections have arisen from the main field and mistakenly displays them together with those from the main beam. To reduce such artifacts, the echocardiographer should minimize gain settings to decrease the likelihood of strong reflections from the weaker lobes. If they persist, to differentiate an artifact from a real structure, the field should be imaged from another window. An artifact is not likely to be reproduced in multiple planes.

SIGNAL RECEPTION AND PROCESSING

The conversion of reflected ultrasound signals into high-fidelity cardiac images is a complex process in which returning ultrasound pulses are received, electronically processed, and displayed. Understanding the basic principles of these steps is essential both to optimize image acquisition and avoid misdiagnosis caused by artifacts.

Cycling of Transducer Transmit and Receive Modes

The ultrasound transducer acts first as a transmitter and then as a receiver of sound signals. An oscillator signals the discharge of electric current to the piezoelectric crystal, thus determining the rate of sound pulse transmission. After emitting a short burst of ultrasound, the transducer switches to receive mode to listen for the returning ultrasound reflections from the tissues.

Electrical Processing

Amplification: gain controls. The echoes that return to the transducer are converted from sound energy to a radiofrequency electric signal by the piezoelectric crystal. A large portion of the sound energy is lost as the ultrasound wave travels, and the electric signal must be amplified before it can be further processed. This amplification is controlled by the **system gain** control. Furthermore, because signal attenuation is proportional to distance traveled, signals from distant structures can be 10 to 100 times weaker than those from closer structures. **Time gain compensation** allows the echocardiographer to amplify signals from structures of varying distances from the transducer individually. With this feature, signals from distant targets and weaker reflectors are boosted so that their amplitudes more closely match those from nearby structures.

Compression and display. The amplified and time gain–compensated electric signal must be processed before it can be displayed on a monitor. The radiofrequency signal has a large dynamic range of more than 100 dB, far too large for monitors to display. To reduce the dynamic range, two processes are commonly used. First, **reject** circuits filter out low-amplitude signals, which typically represent background noise or speckle. The remainder of the signal is then **compressed,** so that both low- and high-amplitude components can be displayed. **Digital scan conversion** then converts the electric signal into a standard video format for display.

Preprocessing and postprocessing. The digital scan converter requires the analog electric signal to be digitized so it can be processed and then converted to an analog video format. This process offers two important opportunities for the echocardiographer to control the display of the imaging data. By adjusting the **preprocessing settings,** which affect the analog-to-digital conversion, and the **postprocessing settings,** which affect the conversion to analog video format, the echocardiographer can modify the appearance of the displayed image. These adjustments can be used, for example, to emphasize edge detection versus tissue texture or to improve the delineation of weaker reflectors. Again, the choice of these settings is dictated by the examination and the personal preferences of the echocardiographer.

DISPLAY FORMATS

The Golden Rule: Time Is Distance

Ultrasonic imaging is based on the amplitude and time delay of the reflected signals (Fig. 1.10). Because the velocity in tissue is relatively constant, only the distance of the structure from the transducer alters the time required for the ultrasound wave to travel to and from the reflected structure:

$$\text{Distance from Transducer} = \text{Velocity} \times \text{Time}/2 \qquad [9]$$

By timing the interval between transmission and return of the reflections, the echocardiography system can precisely calculate the location of a structure.

A-Mode (Amplitude Mode)

The original display format is A-mode, in which the amplitudes of the returning signals are represented as a series of horizontal spikes along the vertical axis of the display. The horizontal spikes correspond to the distance of the reflecting tissue and the strength of the returning echoes.

B-Mode (Brightness Mode)

Current imaging is based on B-mode technology. Instead of horizontal spikes, the amplitudes of the returning echoes are represented as pixels of varying brightness along the

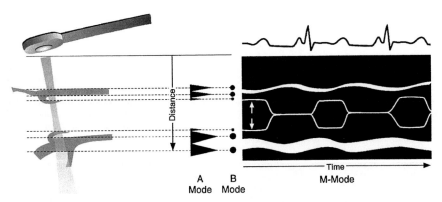

FIG. 1.10. Display formats. The ultrasound beam is directed through the aortic valve leaflets. A-mode (amplitude mode) display shows the resulting reflections as horizontal spikes. In the B-mode (brightness mode) display, the spikes are replaced with pixels of varying brightness. M-mode (motion mode) shows sequential B-mode frames to capture cardiac motion. The "boxcar" pattern depicts normal opening and closing of the aortic valve leaflets.

vertical axis of the display. The brightness correlates with the strength of the returning signal.

M-Mode (Motion Mode)

M-mode adds temporal information to B-mode by displaying a series of collected B-mode images. M-mode echocardiography provides a one-dimensional, "ice pick" view through the heart and updates the B-mode images at a very high rate, allowing dynamic real time imaging. *It is important to realize that before it emits the next pulse of energy, the transducer element must first receive the reflected energy of the previously emitted pulse.* The frequency at which the B-mode images are generated is the **frame rate.** The frame rate is very high (1000–2000 frames per second), affording a superior display of dynamic motion in comparison with other techniques. However, M-mode imaging displays only axial motion and is unable to display lateral movement. Because of its superior dynamics and axial resolution, M-mode is the best mode for examining the timing of cardiac events when displayed with the electrocardiogram.

Two-Dimensional Echocardiography

Two-dimensional echocardiography is a modification of B-mode echocardiography and the mainstay of the echocardiographic examination. Instead of repeatedly firing ultrasound pulses in a single direction, the transducer in two-dimensional echocardiography sequentially directs the ultrasound pulses across a sector of the cardiac anatomy. In this way, two-dimensional imaging can display a tomographic section of the cardiac anatomy, and unlike M-mode, it can show shape and lateral motion (Fig. 1.11).

TWO-DIMENSIONAL SCAN SYSTEMS

Both electronic and mechanical systems have been developed to sweep the beam across an area of interest. Most commonly, the transducer consists of multiple crystals (or elements) aligned next to one another in an **array.** The individual sound waves from each crystal combine to provide a unified wave front that can be better focused and directed than that of

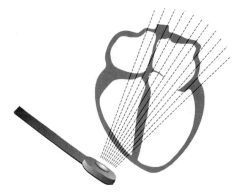

FIG. 1.11. Scan lines. Illustration of the arced sector from a phased array two-dimensional echocardiogram. Each *dotted line* represents an individual B-mode (brightness mode) scan line. Any structure that interacts with a scan line will create reflections (*dark highlight*); however, structures that lie between the scan lines are not interrogated, and the echocardiography system averages the neighboring signals to fill in this defect. Accordingly, the closer the scan lines, the better the image quality. With a phased array scan, the gap between scan lines increases with the distance from the transducer.

a single crystal. Furthermore, with alterations in the timing of the electric activation of each crystal, the beam can actually be steered without the transducer itself being moved. The advantages of an electronic system over a mechanical one, including an absence of moving parts and easy manipulation (steering, focusing, narrowing) of the ultrasound beam, have made it the dominant technology in echocardiography scanners. The two commonly used electronic scanning systems in medical ultrasound are the **linear array** and the **phased array** systems.

Linear Array

The linear array system uses a long transducer composed of several crystals. Groups of crystals are activated sequentially from one end of the transducer to the other. The firing of each group of crystals images the structures directly in front of them. With sequential firing of the groups of crystals, the anatomic features under the entire transducer are imaged. However, the disadvantage of this approach is that the transducer face must be large enough to cover a broad anatomic area effectively. The linear array is commonly used in vascular and obstetric applications.

Phased Array

The phased array system is the one most commonly used in echocardiography. This is an electronic system that by precisely timing the activation of the individual transducer elements is able to sweep the sound beam in an arc across a predetermined field. With activation of the transducer elements in different sequences, the ultrasound beam in the phased array system can be easily narrowed, steered, and focused. The ability to direct a series of beams electronically over an arced sector also makes it possible to use the smaller transducer face required for TEE and transthoracic echocardiography.

CREATING THE TWO-DIMENSIONAL IMAGE

Imaging a Sector

To construct the two-dimensional image, the echocardiographic system records the B-mode data from the first pulse, redirects the next beam, records the returning signals, and so on until the entire sector has been scanned. Typically, the scanner images a sector of 30 to 90 degrees. The orientation of each B-mode line (also called the *scan line*) is recorded so that the information can be displayed in the correct position on the display screen. The two-dimensional scanner then repeats the entire process to update the image and capture motion. Each image created by a sector scan is a **frame.** Two-dimensional imaging typically requires 100 to 200 scan lines per frame, resulting in a frame rate of 30 to 60 frames per second. Because this rate is significantly slower than that of M-mode echocardiography, two-dimensional imaging is not as precise for demonstrating dynamic motion or the timing of cardiac events.

Image Quality and Dynamic Motion

Two-dimensional imaging is characterized by several factors that are operator-controlled and have important (and often opposing) effects on image quality and dynamic motion. The proper settings vary depending on the particular examination at hand.

The **pulse repetition frequency** is the rate at which sound pulses are transmitted per second. The greater the pulse repetition frequency, the greater the number of scan lines that are emitted in a given period of time. The pulse repetition frequency is inversely related to the sector depth because a longer period of time is required for the ultrasound to travel increased distances.

The **frame rate** is the frequency at which the sector is rescanned. Each frame consists of one or two scans across the sector of interest. The information from two sweeps can be interlaced to improve image quality. A high frame rate improves the capture of movement. Typically, a frame rate greater than 30/s allows the dynamic representation of some relatively fine movements (e.g., intermediate positions of the aortic valve). The frame rate is critically dependent on the sector depth, which determines the time required for each scan line to be received, and sector width, which increases the number of scan lines to be processed. Consequently, increases in the sector size and depth come at the cost of a decreased frame rate.

The **scan line density,** calculated as the number of lines per degree of the sector, greatly affects the image quality. Line densities should be maintained at 1.5 to 2.2 lines per degree. Doubling the scan lines essentially doubles the lateral resolution. However, the cost is a decrease in the frame rate. The scan line density is calculated by dividing the number of scan lines per sweep by the angle of the sector. The greater the sector angle, the larger the area and the lower the line density. Because phased array transducers produce a fan-shaped sector, scan line density is always greater closer to the transducer and decreases in direct proportion to distance.

Image quality versus dynamic motion. It quickly becomes apparent that the echocardiographer must choose between the size of the imaging field and the frame rate. If the frame rate is too high (100 frames per second), the number of scan lines per frame is reduced, resulting in a lower line density. Although the dynamics of the image may be excellent, the image quality is decreased. We caution against the practice of assessing several structures in a single large view because it compromises both the dynamics and quality of the images. We recommend that the clinician focus each part of the examination on a given structure of interest and select the imaging plane that best delineates the structure in the near field. Motion can be then be enhanced without costs in lateral resolution by decreasing the sector angle and depth. In situations in which the maximal frame rate is desired, M-mode should be considered. This results in a very dynamic image with a high level of axial resolution. For these reasons, M-mode echocardiography remains an important adjunct to both two-dimensional and color Doppler echocardiography.

SUMMARY

Two-dimensional echocardiography is based on the interaction of ultrasound and the patient. Between the generation of the ultrasound pulse and its subsequent reflection, reception, and display, a complex series of events takes place. Echocardiographers who wantonly ignore the physical realities of the imaging process will encounter two causes of misdiagnosis: inadequate imaging and artifact. However, if they apply their understanding of the principles involved, selecting the most appropriate views and machine settings, expert echocardiographers can reliably optimize the imaging of a particular structure of interest. No patient or echocardiographic system is ideal. Rather, echocardiographers must compromise between conflicting imaging needs, such as between dynamic motion and the visual quality of an image, based on the primary diagnostic goal. We expand on the important relationship between the echocardiographer and the echocardiography machine in Chapter 20.

SUGGESTED READINGS

Geiser EA. Echocardiography: physics and instrumentation. In: Marcus ML, Skorton DJ, Schelbert AR, et al., eds. *Cardiac imaging,* 2nd ed. Philadelphia: WB Saunders, 1991.
Weyman A, ed. *Principles and practice of echocardiography,* 2nd ed. Philadelphia: Lea & Febiger, 1994:3–55.

QUESTIONS

1. All of the following statements regarding sound are true **except**
   a. Sound is a vibration in a physical medium.
   b. Wavelength and frequency are inversely related.
   c. The velocity of sound in soft tissue is relatively constant at 1,540 m/s.
   d. Higher sound frequencies result in less absorption.
2. Which of the following statements regarding reflection of ultrasound is true?
   a. Two-dimensional echocardiographic imaging consists of both specular and scattering reflections.
   b. Scattered reflections come from larger, regular surfaces.
   c. Specular reflections are greatest when the ultrasound beam and tissue interface is perpendicular to the beam.
   d. Maximal reflection occurs at a tissue interface with an acoustic mismatch of zero.
   e. **a and c.**
3. All of the following statements regarding reflection of the ultrasound beam are true **except**
   a. Reflection occurs at a tissue interface or area of acoustic mismatch.
   b. Reflection is directly related to the absolute difference between the levels of acoustic impedance of two tissues.
   c. The ultrasound beam is reflected at an angle equal and opposite to that of the incident beam.
   d. Air is highly reflective because of its high acoustic impedance.
4. All of the following statements regarding attenuation are true **except**
   a. It is caused by friction.
   b. It is caused by scattered reflection.
   c. It is caused by dispersion.
   d. Fluids rapidly absorb ultrasound energy.
5. All the following statements regarding wavelength and frequency are true **except**
   a. Resolution is improved with higher-frequency sound waves.
   b. Resolution is improved with higher wavelengths.
   c. Lower frequency sound waves are absorbed less than higher frequency sound waves.
   d. Higher frequency sound waves create longer near fields.
6. All of the following statements regarding the ultrasound beam are true **except**
   a. It is more concentrated in the near field.
   b. Width determines the axial resolution.
   c. Width determines the lateral resolution.
   d. Focusing increases far field divergence.
7. Resolution
   a. Is improved with focusing
   b. Is better with high-frequency/low-wavelength sound
   c. Is better in the near field
   d. Consists of axial, lateral, and elevational components
   e. All of the above

8. All of the following statements are true **except**
   a. Narrow ultrasound beams improve lateral resolution.
   b. Higher frequencies increase the resolution and imaging of deeper structures.
   c. Focusing improves resolution in the near field but creates a more divergent beam thereafter.
   d. Beam width is related to the frequency of the sound wave.
   e. Resolution is best in the near field.
9. All of the following statements regarding echocardiographic displays are true **except**
   a. A-mode imaging uses horizontal spikes along a vertical axis to represent tissue character and axial position.
   b. M-mode imaging is characterized by high-resolution axial imaging and superdynamic display of cardiac motion.
   c. M-mode imaging displays not only axial (vertical) motion but also lateral relations.
   d. Two-dimensional imaging displays lateral and axial relations.
   e. Two-dimensional imaging occurs at a much lower frame rate than M-mode imaging.
10. Which of the following statements is true with respect to scan systems?
    a. An array consists of a single transducer element that is mechanically moved across the field of interest.
    b. A linear array scan emits a narrow beam from a small transducer face, so that it is ideal for imaging through small apertures (echocardiographic windows).
    c. A phased array scan sweeps the ultrasound beam over a fan-shaped sector.
    d. Neither phased array nor linear array scans are subject to side or grating lobes.
    e. Electronic activation of the multiple elements of a phased array scanner allows steering of the ultrasound beam, but not focusing.

2

Two-Dimensional Examination

Joseph P. Miller

The purpose of this chapter is to demystify echocardiographic image orientation and provide a stepwise approach to image acquisition. In the eyes of the novice, learning and applying transesophageal echocardiography (TEE) may seem like an insurmountable task. With the use of this stepwise approach, TEE will quickly become an integral part of your practice and a valuable aid for intraoperative decision making (1–6).

IMAGING PLANES AND ORIENTATION

Understanding the orientation of the imaging plane is crucial for both acquisition of the desired images and correct interpretation of the displayed cardiac anatomy. Although TEE is limited to the confines of the esophagus and stomach, the ability to alter the position and orientation of the ultrasound beam allows a broad view of the cardiac anatomy.

Probe Insertion

The TEE probe is passed into the esophagus in the same manner in which an orogastric tube is placed. The easiest way to insert the probe is to perform a jaw lift by grabbing the mandible with the left hand and inserting the probe with the right. The probe is inserted with constant gentle pressure in addition to a slight turning back and forth and from left to right to find the esophageal opening. If resistance is encountered, the cause most often is excessive extension of the head and neck. Advancement of the probe is stopped after the head of the probe has passed the larynx and cricopharyngeus muscle, where a distinct loss of resistance is felt. The imaging head will lie in the upper esophagus.

Probe Manipulation

The position and orientation of the TEE probe can be altered by several types of manipulation (Fig. 2.1). By gripping the probe shaft near its entrance in the mouth, the probe can be **advanced** or **withdrawn.** The degree of insertion can be easily determined by the depth markings imprinted on the shaft. For cardiac imaging, the probe position ranges from the upper esophagus to the stomach. In the upper esophagus, the structure closest to the TEE probe is one of the great vessels. In the mid esophagus (ME), the structure closest to the TEE probe is the left atrium, and in the transgastric (TG) position, the structure closest to the TEE probe is the left ventricle. Therefore, depending on the depth of insertion, the structure at the apex of the imaging sector will be one of the great vessels (most commonly the aorta), the left atrium, or the left ventricle.

The orientation of the ultrasound beam can be further adjusted by manually **turning** the probe shaft to the left or right. The probe can be **anteflexed** or **retroflexed** by using the large knob on the probe handle. The small knob on the probe handle will **flex** the probe leftward or rightward. These maneuvers allow precise user control over the direction of the ultrasound beam to visualize the structure of interest.

The opinions or assertions contained herein are the private views of the author(s) and are not to be construed as official or as reflecting the views of the Department of Defense.

22

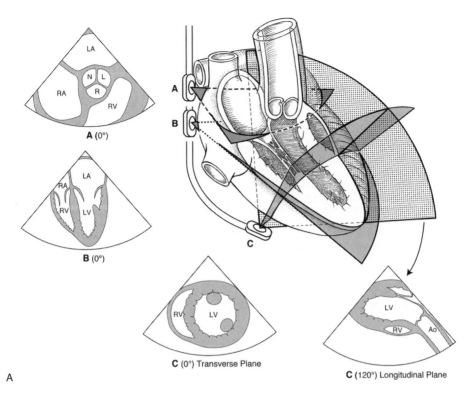

A

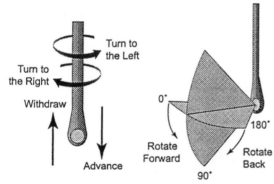

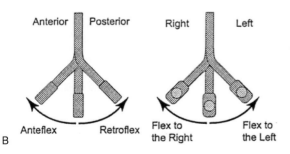

B

FIG. 2.1. A: Through simple manipulations, the TEE probe offers a multifaceted picture of the cardiac anatomy. Progressive advancement of the probe in the midesophagus provides a cross-sectional view of the aortic valve (*A*) followed by long-axis imaging of the cardiac chambers (*B*). Further advancement and anterior flexion of the probe head (*C*) allows visualization of the left ventricle in the short axis. Rotation of the imaging plane expands the imaging capacity of TEE. In this example, the left ventricle and its outflow tract have been brought into view by rotating the imaging plane to 120 degrees. **B:** Terminology used to describe manipulation of the probe and transducer during image acquisition. (From Ref. 7, with permission).

Multiplane Imaging Angle

The first clinically useful TEE probes were capable of producing a single or monoplane cross section of the heart. This imaging plane is generated perpendicular to the shaft of the probe and corresponds to the typical transverse views obtained with transthoracic echocardiography. The biplane probes of the next generation were able to produce two perpendicular views: the standard transverse cross sections and a longitudinal cross section. Today, most of the probes in use in adult TEE are multiplane probes. Through an electronic switch on the probe handle, the operator selectively rotates the orientation of the imaging plane from 0 degree (transverse plane) through 180 degrees in 1-degree increments. This capability offers many advantages with respect to image acquisition but can also generate tremendous confusion for novice echocardiographers.

Experts rely on two key points to determine image orientation quickly. First, independent of the imaging plane, the ultrasound beam always originates from the esophagus or stomach and projects anteriorly. Consequently, on the monitor the apex of the sector displays structures that are closest to the TEE probe. As a general rule of thumb, structures seen near the apex of the image sector (i.e., closest to the TEE probe) will be posterior structures, and those close to the arc of the sector (i.e., more distant from the TEE probe) will be anterior structures.

Second, left and right orientation depends on the degree of rotation of the scan head. A simple way to orient yourself is to place your right hand on your chest with your palm facing upward and your fingers pointing to your left. This is the orientation of the imaging scan at 0. Your fingers point toward the structures that will be displayed on the right side on the monitor (Fig. 2.2).

Increases in the imaging plane angle proceed in a counterclockwise manner. For example, when the imaging plane is rotated to 60 degrees, the imaging orientation is mirrored by taking your hand and rotating it counterclockwise 60 degrees (Fig. 2.3).

At 90 degrees, the hand is further rotated counterclockwise to point at your head, 12 o'clock (Fig. 2.4).

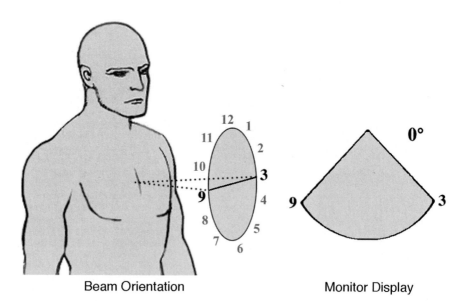

Beam Orientation   Monitor Display

FIG. 2.2. With a beam orientation of 0 degree (transverse plane), in a clock face analogy, the right side of the display will contain structures on the patient's left (3 o'clock). The left side of the display will contain structures on the patient's right (9 o'clock).

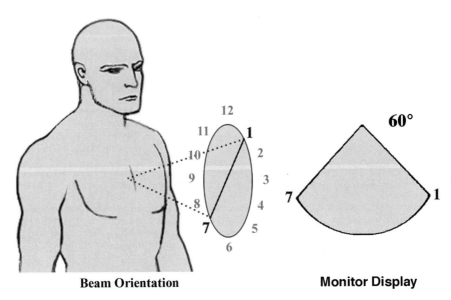

Beam Orientation   **Monitor Display**

FIG. 2.3. In a clock face analogy, the right side of the monitor display will contain structures on the patient's left and cephalad (1 o'clock). The left side of the monitor display will contain structures on the patient's right and caudad (7 o'clock).

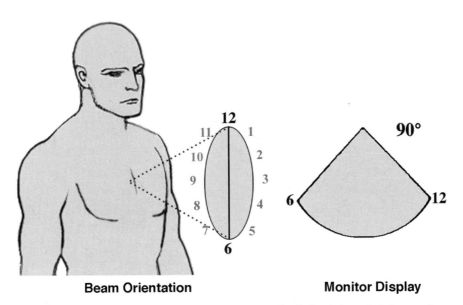

Beam Orientation   **Monitor Display**

FIG. 2.4. With a beam orientation of 90 degrees (longitudinal plane), in a clock face analogy, the right side of the display will contain structures toward the patient's head (12 o'clock). The left side of the display will contain structures toward the patient's feet (6 o'clock).

1. ME AV SAX

~40°-60°

2. ME RV I-O

~60°-80°

3. ME RV I-O w/ CFD of PV

~60°-80°

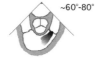

4. ME AV LAX

~110°-140°

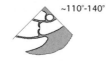

5. ME AV LAX w/ CFD of AV

~110°-140°

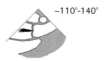

6. ME Bicaval

~110°

7. ME 4C

~0°-10°

8. ME 4C w/ CFD of MV

~0°-10°

9. ME 4C w/ CFD of TV

~0°-10°

10. ME 2C

~90°

11. TG Mid SAX

~0°

12. TG 2C

~90°

13. Desc Aorta SAX

~0°

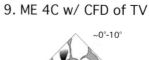

14. UE Aortic Arch SAX

~90°

15. Desc Aorta LAX

~90°

GOALS OF THE EXAMINATION

TEE examinations, whether comprehensive or abbreviated, should display all pertinent structures in the heart. Each cardiac chamber and valve should be visualized in two orthogonal planes. All segments of the myocardium should also be visualized. This approach helps ensure the diagnosis of any significant abnormalities and minimizes the incorrect identification of artifacts.

Echocardiographers differ in their approach to a diagnostic TEE examination. Many prefer to start with those views that examine known pathology. Others believe the examination should first systematically examine for unknown pathology before the area of concern is evaluated. A common approach starts with TG views of the left ventricle because of the frequent abnormalities detected with these views. Each of these approaches has its pluses and minuses, and there is no one correct way. However, the goal of any approach must be a complete examination of all structures of the heart. A joint task force including members of the American Society of Echocardiography and the Society of Cardiovascular Anesthesiologists has published guidelines for performing a comprehensive intraoperative multiplane TEE examination (7) (see Appendix 1). However, no consensus has been reached regarding whether all 20 cross sections described in the guidelines should be acquired in every patient.

THE STEPWISE EXAMINATION

A recommended examination sequence follows (8) (Fig. 2.5). It can be completed in 3 to 5 minutes and focuses on pathologic conditions that require immediate therapy. This examination functions well as a preliminary screening tool in the evaluation of a patient before cardiopulmonary bypass and is just as applicable in the evaluation of refractory hypotension after the induction of anesthesia.

The cardiac examination is performed at three locations. The first location is the ME at the aortic valve level, the second is a few centimeters distal in the ME at the level of the mitral valve, and the final location is in the stomach at the level of the left ventricle. After completion of the cardiac examination, the aorta is then evaluated throughout its thoracic course. The major advantages of this systematic approach are twofold. First, it minimizes manipulation of the TEE probe, thereby shortening the examination time. Second, the progressive advancement of the probe maintains an anatomic orientation.

Aortic Valve Level

Midesophageal aortic valve short-axis view. After probe insertion, the probe is advanced until the leaflets of the aortic valve are seen. The imaging plane is then rotated to approximately 45 degrees to obtain the ME aortic valve short-axis view. The primary structure visualized is the aortic valve in short axis. The size of the aortic valve in comparison with the atrial chambers in addition to the mobility of the aortic leaflets and any leaflet calcification are carefully noted.

The primary diagnostic goals of this view are to define the general morphology of the aortic valve (e.g., bicuspid vs. tricuspid) and to determine if aortic stenosis is present. The relative sizes of the aorta and the atria should be noted. The intraatrial septum can be observed for openings consistent with an atrial septal defect or patent foramen ovale. In addition, look for continuous deviation to one side or the other away from an atrium with elevated pressures.

FIG. 2.5. The author's recommended basic transesophageal echocardiography cardiac examination. ME, midesophageal; AV, aortic valve; CFD, color Doppler flow; TV, tricuspid valve; RV, right ventricular; I-O, inflow-outflow; PV, pulmonary valve; TG, transgastric; SAX, short-axis; LAX, long-axis; Desc, descending; 2C, two-chamber; 4C, four-chamber. (Modified from Miller JP, Lambert SA, Shapiro WA, et al. The adequacy of basic intraoperative transesophageal echocardiography performed by experienced anesthesiologists. *Anesth Analg* 2001;92:1103–1110, with permission.)

Midesophageal Aortic Valve Short-Axis View
Imaging Settings

- Angle ~40 to 60 degrees
- Sector depth ~8 cm

Probe Adjustment

- Neutral

Primary Diagnostic Uses

- Aortic stenosis
- Valvular morphology

Required Structures

- Three leaflets
- Commissures
- Coaptation point

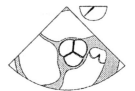

Midesophageal right ventricular inflow-outflow. After completion of the ME short-axis view of the aortic valve, the next three views are obtained at the level of the aortic valve in the longitudinal plane. The first view is the ME right ventricular inflow-outflow view. Start at the ME aortic valve short axis and, without moving the probe, change the rotation of the imaging angle to approximately 60 to 90 degrees. The desired imaging plane will visualize the tricuspid valve, right ventricular outflow tract, and proximal pulmonary artery. Note that the right atrium will be at 10 o'clock, the tricuspid valve at 9 o'clock, the right ventricular cavity at 6 o'clock, and the pulmonary valve and pulmonary artery at 3 o'clock.

The primary diagnostic goals of this view are to gauge the right ventricular chamber and pulmonary artery size and to evaluate the pulmonic valve. This view is often superior to the ME four-chamber view for Doppler interrogation of the tricuspid valve. In adults with prior congenital heart surgery, evaluation of the right ventricular outflow tract and pulmonary valve may provide important diagnostic information.

Midesophageal Right Ventricular Inflow-Outflow
Imaging Settings

- Angle ~60 to 80 degrees
- Sector depth ~10 cm

Probe Adjustment

- Neutral

Primary Diagnostic Uses

- Pulmonic valve disease
- Pulmonary artery pathology
- Right ventricular outflow tract pathology

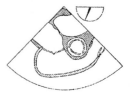

(Continued on next page)

Required Structures

- Pulmonic valve
- Tricuspid valve
- Main pulmonary artery (at least 1 cm distal to the pulmonic valve)
- Right ventricular outflow tract (at least 1 cm proximal to the pulmonic valve)

Midesophageal aortic valve long-axis view. The ME aortic valve long-axis view is obtained by further rotating the imaging angle to approximately 110 to 130 degrees. A slight turn of the probe toward the patient's right may be necessary to optimize this image. The view is complete when the left ventricular outflow tract, aortic valve, and proximal ascending aorta are displayed together. Additional structures to observe are the outflow tract itself, the sinus of Valsalva, and the sinotubular junction.

The primary diagnostic goal of this view is to evaluate aortic valve function. The proximal ascending aorta should be inspected for calcification, enlargement, and protruding atheroma. An important limitation of this view is that the aortic cannulation site in the distal ascending aorta cannot be visualized. After completion of a two-dimensional examination, aortic valve function is evaluated further with color flow Doppler.

Midesophageal Aortic Valve Long-Axis View

Imaging Settings

- Angle ~110 to 140 degrees
- Sector depth ~8 cm

Probe Adjustment

- Neutral

Primary Diagnostic Uses

- Aortic valve pathology
- Aortic pathology (ascending aorta and root)
- Left ventricular outflow tract pathology

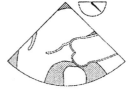

Required Structures

- Left ventricular outflow tract (at least 1 cm proximal to the aortic valve)
- Aortic valve (visualized cusps approximately equal in size)
- Ascending aorta (at least 1 cm distal to the sinotubular junction)

Midesophageal bicaval view. The ME bicaval view is then obtained by turning the probe further to the patient's right. This image is often best with 5 to 15 degrees less rotation than in the ME aortic valve long-axis view. The key structures in this view are the left atrium, right atrium, superior vena cava, intraatrial septum, and right atrial appendage.

The primary diagnostic goals of this view are to examine for atrial chamber enlargements and the presence of a patent foramen ovale or an atrial septal defect, and to detect intraatrial air. If the integrity of the intraatrial septum is questioned, color flow Doppler or bubble contrast should be performed.

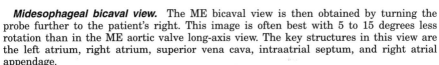

Midesophageal Bicaval View

Imaging Settings

- Angle ~110 degrees
- Depth ~10 cm

Probe Adjustment

- Neutral with rightward turn

Primary Diagnostic Uses

- Atrial septal defect
- Tumor

Required Structures

- Right atrial free wall (or appendage)
- Superior vena cava (at least its entry into the right atrium)
- Interatrial septum

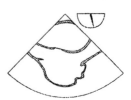

Mitral Valve Level

Midesophageal four-chamber view. After completion of the ME bicaval view, the imaging angle is returned to 0 degree and the TEE probe is advanced to the mitral valve level. In the transverse plane, the ME four-chamber view is obtained. This view allows visualization of all the chambers of the heart. The image rotation is approximately 0 to 10 degrees with some posterior flexion of the probe. The key structures to observe are the left atrium, left ventricle, right atrium, right ventricle, the mitral and tricuspid valves, and the septal and lateral walls of the myocardium. If a portion of the left ventricular outflow tract and aortic valve is displayed (the so-called five-chamber view), retroflexion of the probe and slight advancement or rotation of the imaging plane to 5 to 10 degrees should produce the ME four-chamber view. Remember that the aortic valve and left ventricular outflow tract are anterior structures, and these maneuvers will produce a true cross section of the more posteriorly located ME four-chamber view.

The ME four-chamber view is one the most diagnostically valuable views in TEE. The diagnostic goals of this view include evaluation of chamber size and function, valvular function (both mitral and tricuspid), and regional motion of the septal and lateral walls of the left ventricle. An additional important use of this view is to look for intraventricular air following cardiopulmonary bypass. After two-dimensional interrogation of this view, color flow Doppler should be placed on the mitral and tricuspid valves to detect valvular insufficiency and stenosis.

Midesophageal Four-Chamber View

Imaging Settings

- Angle ~0 to 20 degrees
- Sector depth ~14 cm

Probe Adjustment

- Neutral to retroflexed

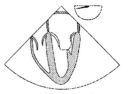

(Continued on next page)

Primary Diagnostic Uses

- Atrial septal defect
- Chamber enlargement/dysfunction
- Mitral disease
- Tricuspid disease
- Detection of intracardiac air

Required Structures

- Left atrium
- Left ventricle
- Mitral valve
- Tricuspid valve (maximal diameter)

Midesophageal two-chamber view. From the ME four-chamber view, rotate the imaging angle to approximately 60 to 90 degrees to obtain the ME two-chamber view. This view is identified by the presence of the left atrial appendage and the absence of right-sided heart structures, and it allows visualization of the anterior and inferior walls of the left ventricle. Occasionally, turning the probe shaft to the right will improve chamber alignment and visualization of the true left ventricular apex, so that the long axis of the ventricle can be seen in its entirety. Care must be taken to ensure that the apex is seen. The apex is mechanically silent and therefore will not contract. The anterior and inferior walls should contract inward, like the narrowing of a V. If the apex rises with contraction, you are viewing the muscular wall of the heart and not seeing the true apex, and the probe position should be adjusted. Ventricular thrombus or hypokinesis at the apex is often best appreciated in this view.

The primary goals of this view are to evaluate left ventricular function (especially the apex) and anterior and inferior regional wall motion. It can also be used to look for thrombus of the left ventricular apex and left atrial appendage. Another frequent use is to verify the correct position of a retrograde cardioplegia catheter in the coronary sinus.

Midesophageal Two-Chamber View

Imaging Settings

- Angle ~90 degrees
- Sector depth ~14 cm

Probe Adjustment

- Neutral

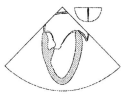

Primary Diagnostic Uses

- Left atrial appendage mass/thrombus
- Left ventricular apex pathology
- Left ventricular systolic dysfunction (apical segments)

Required Structures

- Left atrial appendage
- Mitral valve
- Left ventricular apex (i.e., maximal left ventricular length)

Left Ventricular Level

Transgastric midpapillary short-axis view. After completion of the interrogation of the heart at the aortic and mitral levels, the imaging plane is returned to 0 degree and the probe is advanced into the stomach to obtain the TG views. The first is the TG mid short-axis view. The probe is then anteflexed and withdrawn until contact is made with the wall of the stomach. The key structures to visualize are the left ventricular walls and cavity in addition to the posteromedial and anterolateral papillary muscles. A true short-axis cross section of the left ventricle is confirmed when the two papillary muscles are approximately of equal size. Fine-tuning this image may be difficult, but it is done in two phases. In the first phase, the depth of the probe is altered, and in the second phase, the degree of flexion is altered. The proper depth of the probe is obtained by focusing on the posteromedial papillary muscle, which is the papillary muscle closest to the apex of the scan. If chordae tendineae are visible, the probe is too high and should be advanced. If no papillary muscle is visible, most often the probe is too low and should be withdrawn. Once the depth of the probe is appropriate, the flexion is adjusted to bring the anterolateral papillary muscle into the correct position. If any of the anterolateral chordae tendineae are visible, the probe is excessively anteflexed, and relaxation of the large wheel on the probe handle should bring the papillary muscle into the correct position.

The primary diagnostic goals of this view are assessment of left ventricular systolic function, left ventricular volume, and regional wall motion.

Transgastric Mid Short-Axis View

Imaging Settings

- Angle ~0 degree
- Sector depth ~12 cm

Probe Adjustment

- Neutral

Primary Diagnostic Uses

- Hemodynamic instability
- Left ventricular enlargement
- Left ventricular hypertrophy
- Left ventricular systolic dysfunction (global and regional)

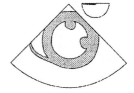

Required Structures

- Left ventricular cavity
- Left ventricular walls (≥50% of circumference with visible endocardium)
- Papillary muscles (approximately equal in size and distinct from ventricular wall)

Transgastric two-chamber view. After completion of the TG mid short-axis view, the imaging angle is rotated to approximately 90 degrees and the TG two-chamber view is obtained; this provides a long-axis view of the left ventricle, with the apex to the left of the display and the mitral valve to the right. The primary diagnostic goal of this view is analysis of regional wall motion and evaluation of the support structures of the mitral valve. If desired, further rotation of the imaging plane to 120 to 140 degrees will visualize the anterior structures of the left ventricular outflow tract and aortic valve (the TG long-axis view).

Transgastric Two-Chamber View

Imaging Settings

- Angle ~90 degrees
- Sector depth ~12 cm

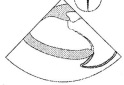

Probe Adjustment

- Neutral

Primary Diagnostic Uses

- Left ventricular systolic dysfunction (basal segments)

Required Structures

- Mitral leaflets
- Mitral subvalvular apparatus
- Left ventricle (basal and mid segments)

Aortic Examination

Descending aorta short-axis view. After completion of the preliminary evaluation of the heart, the aorta is examined. From the TG two-chamber view, the imaging angle is rotated to 0 degree and the probe shaft is turned to the patient's left and slightly withdrawn until a transverse view of the descending aorta is obtained (the descending aorta short-axis view). Key factors in imaging the aorta are its small size and its proximity to the TEE probe head in the esophagus. Consequently, the following maneuvers are necessary to optimize aortic imaging. First, the image depth in reduced to enlarge the displayed aortic image. Second, the time gain compensation in the near field may have to be increased because it is often set at low levels during the cardiac examination. Finally, the frequency of the transducer can be increased to enhance resolution. In the author's experience, these changes in the settings have allowed the visualization of aortic atheromas that were not evident before the adjustments were made. The aorta is then visualized along its course as the probe is slowly withdrawn. When the aorta begins to appear elongated, you have reached the level of the aortic arch.

Descending Aorta Short-Axis View

Imaging Settings

- Angle ~0 degree
- Sector depth ~6 cm

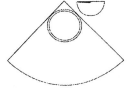

Probe Adjustment

- Neutral

Primary Diagnostic Uses

- Aortic atherosclerosis
- Aortic dissection

Required Structures

- Aorta in cross section in transverse plane (0 degree)

Upper esophageal aortic arch short-axis view. From the level of the aortic arch, the imaging angle is then turned to 90 degrees to obtain the upper esophageal aortic arch short-axis view. Small left and right turns of the probe shaft will allow you to interrogate the arch for calcification, enlargement, and foreign bodies. You may see the origins of the great vessels at approximately 3 o'clock in the short axis of the aortic arch. The origin of the left subclavian artery is visualized in this view.

Upper Esophageal Aortic Arch Short-Axis View
Imaging Settings

- Angle ~90 degrees
- Sector depth ~8 cm

Probe Adjustment

- Neutral

Primary Diagnostic Uses

- Aortic atherosclerosis
- Aortic dissection

Required Structures

- Aortic arch in cross section in longitudinal plane (90 degrees)

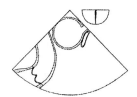

Descending aorta long-axis view. From the upper esophageal aortic arch short-axis view with the imaging plane maintained at 90 degrees, the probe is advanced to obtain the longitudinal view of the descending aorta (the descending aorta long-axis view). Again, as the probe is advanced, small left and right turns of the probe permit better interrogation of the aortic walls.

Descending Aorta Long-Axis View
Imaging Settings

- Angle ~90 degrees
- Sector depth ~6 cm

Probe Adjustment

- Neutral

Primary Diagnostic Uses

- Aortic atherosclerosis
- Aortic dissection

Required Structures

- Aorta in long axis in longitudinal plane (90 degrees)

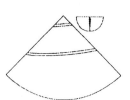

LOST AND FOUND

Mastering the two-dimensional echocardiographic examination requires an understanding of the imaging planes and practical experience. No two patients' anatomy is identical, and the images obtained in clinical practice vary from the textbook examples. Some TEE views cannot be obtained in certain patients. A common setback is disorientation with the displayed images. To recover your anatomic orientation, it is often best to return the imaging plane to 0 degree because many structures are more easily identified from the transverse plane. Next, identify the structure at the apex of the scan. This structure will be one of the great vessels (most often the aorta), the left atrium, or the left ventricle. Next, advance or withdraw the probe until you can identify a major structure in the view (e.g., aortic valve). Finally, with the known structures in view, rotate the imaging plane. In this way, an unknown structure can be identified by its association with the neighboring anatomy.

SUMMARY

The stepwise approach detailed earlier ensures an efficient yet systematic examination of the pertinent anatomy. By following such an approach, the examiner avoids the all too common error of not assessing clinically important and unrecognized abnormalities. With experience, you can easily incorporate this examination into your clinical practice.

REFERENCES

1. Sheikh KH, De Bruijn NP, Rankin JS, et al. The utility of transesophageal echocardiography and Doppler color flow imaging in patients undergoing cardiac valve surgery. *J Am Coll Cardiol* 1990;15:363–372.
2. Sheikh KH, Bengtson JR, Rankin JS, et al. Intraoperative transesophageal Doppler color flow imaging used to guide patient selection and operative treatment of ischemic mitral regurgitation. *Circulation* 1991;84:594–604.
3. Stevenson JG. Adherence to physician training guidelines for pediatric transesophageal echocardiography affects the outcome of patients undergoing repair of congenital cardiac defects. *J Am Soc Echocardiogr* 1999;12:165–172.
4. Ungerleider RM, Kisslo JA, Greeley WJ, et al. Intraoperative echocardiography during congenital heart operations: experience from 1,000 cases. *Ann Thorac Surg* 1995:S539–S542.
5. Savage RM, Lytle BW, Aronson S, et al. Intraoperative echocardiography is indicated in high-risk coronary artery bypass grafting. *Ann Thorac Surg* 1997;64:368–374.
6. Practice guidelines for perioperative transesophageal echocardiography. A report by the American Society of Anesthesiologists and the Society of Cardiovascular Anesthesiologists Task Force on Transesophageal Echocardiography. *Anesthesiology* 1996;84:986–1006.
7. Shanewise JS, Cheung AT, Aronson S, et al. ASE/SCA guidelines for performing a comprehensive intraoperative multiplane transesophageal echocardiographic examination: recommendations of the American Society of Echocardiography Council for Intraoperative Echocardiography and the Society of Cardiovascular Anesthesiologists Task Force for Certification in Perioperative Transesophageal Echocardiography. *Anesth Analg* 1999;89:870–884.
8. Miller JP, Lambert SA, Shapiro WA, et al. The adequacy of basic intraoperative transesophageal echocardiography performed by experienced anesthesiologists. *Anesth Analg* 2001;92:1103–1110.

QUESTIONS

1. The large knob on the TEE hand piece controls
   a. Anteflexion/retroflexion
   b. Left/right flexion
   c. Image rotation
   d. Image depth

2. The small knob on the TEE hand piece controls
   a. Anteflexion/retroflexion
   b. Left/right flexion
   c. Image rotation
   d. Image depth
3. When a standard orientation is used, at 0 degree, the image seen on the right side of the display is
   a. On the patient's left
   b. On the patient's right
   c. Cephalad
   d. Caudad
4. When a standard orientation is used, at 90 degrees, the image seen on the right side of the display is
   a. On the patient's left
   b. On the patient's right
   c. Cephalad
   d. Caudad
5. The primary diagnostic purpose of the ME aortic valve short-axis view is to
   a. Identify aortic valve stenosis
   b. Identify aortic valve insufficiency
   c. Measure the sinotubular junction
   d. **a** and **b**
6. The view that best visualizes the left ventricular apex is the
   a. ME two-chamber view
   b. TG two-chamber view
   c. TG mid short-axis view
   d. ME four-chamber view
7. The view that is not commonly useful in assessing LV systolic function is the
   a. ME four-chamber view
   b. ME two-chamber view
   c. TG mid short-axis view
   d. ME bicaval view
8. Increasing the near field time gain compensation is especially important in an interrogation of the
   a. Left atrium
   b. Right atrium
   c. Left ventricle
   d. Aorta
9. The origins of the great vessels (e.g., carotid, subclavian) can be seen in the
   a. ME four-chamber view
   b. Descending aorta short-axis view
   c. Descending aorta long-axis view
   d. Upper esophageal aortic arch short-axis view
10. The left atrial appendage is best seen in the
    a. ME bicaval view
    b. ME two-chamber view
    c. TG mid short-axis view
    d. TG two-chamber view

Ventricular Systolic Performance and Pathology

J. Scott Walton, Scott T. Reeves, and Bruce H. Dorman, Jr.

The blood flow provided by the left ventricle (LV) is essential in maintaining a steady supply of oxygen to the tissues and removing the waste products of cellular metabolism. Because of the vital importance of the LV and the myriad of factors that can impair its functioning during surgery, assessment of the LV is among the most important indications for intraoperative transesophageal echocardiography (TEE). Intraoperative TEE is often undertaken to determine the reason(s) for hemodynamic instability when conventional diagnostic measures yield inconclusive results or are not available. With two-dimensional imaging of the LV, the two most crucial questions regarding hemodynamic stability can be rapidly answered. First, is the heart adequately filled, and second, is LV contractility adequate? This chapter focuses on the use of TEE in the evaluation of global LV systolic function and conditions such as LV hypertrophy and the cardiomyopathies. The role of TEE in assessing LV diastolic performance and regional function is discussed in subsequent chapters.

VENTRICULAR SYSTOLIC PERFORMANCE

Preferred Imaging Views for the Assessment of Left Ventricular Function

Assessment of the LV is usually the first or among the first priorities in an intraoperative TEE examination. After a complete diagnostic TEE examination has been performed, most anesthesiologists monitor ventricular function continuously with two-dimensional TEE. To be clinically relevant, intraoperative assessment of the LV must produce meaningful information quickly and in real time. Extensive manipulation and analysis of images are impractical in the dynamic intraoperative setting. *By far the most commonly used view for the evaluation of systolic function is the transgastric (TG) midpapillary short-axis view.* Because the heart contracts primarily along its short axis (as opposed to the limited motion of the apex toward the base), the TG midpapillary short-axis view is the preferred view for the rapid evaluation of ventricular volume status and global ventricular function. This view also allows for a quick assessment of regional wall motion abnormalities because the perfusion beds supplied by each of the three major coronary arteries (left anterior descending, circumflex, and right coronary arteries) are visualized. This is discussed further in Chapter 4.

Additional views, such as the midesophageal (ME) two-chamber and four-chamber views, are necessary when the TG midpapillary short-axis view is suboptimal or the position of the heart is distorted, such as during off-pump coronary artery bypass surgery. Others, such as the TG long-axis and deep TG views, are preferred for Doppler assessments of ventricular ejection and cardiac output.

Fractional Shortening

Fractional shortening is among the simplest methods for quantifying LV systolic function. Fractional shortening is the percentage of change in LV cavity dimension with systolic contraction and is expressed by Formula 3.1:

$$\frac{LVED - LVES}{LVED} \times 100 \qquad [1]$$

where LVED is the LV end-diastolic dimension and LVES is the LV end-systolic dimension.

LV measurements are performed with M-mode (motion mode) or two-dimensional echocardiography just beyond the mitral valve at the chordal level and perpendicular to the long

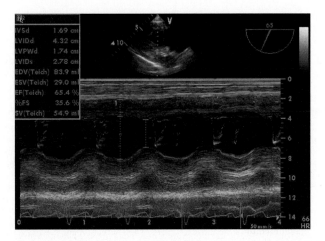

FIG. 3.1. Transgastric long-axis view demonstrating the measurements needed to calculate fractional shortening of the left ventricle. LVIDd, left ventricular diastolic internal dimension; LVIDs, left ventricular systolic internal dimension.

axis of the ventricle. The measurements are made from inner edge to inner edge of the endocardium (1). Figure 3.1 demonstrates the calculation of LV fractional shortening. The normal range for fractional shortening is 25% to 45%.

Fractional shortening is conceptually a one-dimensional measure of ejection fraction. The advantage of fractional shortening over calculated ejection fraction is that the measurements are simply and quickly obtained. In addition, the values are not cubed, so any errors in measurement are not magnified. Its major limitation is the use of a single image view with resultant single cavitary dimensions in diastole and systole that may not accurately reflect global LV function. This typically is problematic in dilated cardiomyopathy when the dilated internal dimensions measured may not be reflective of the whole LV (2).

Ejection Fraction and Left Ventricular Volumes

In contrast to fractional shortening, which depends on a single cavitary dimension in systole and diastole, the ejection fraction examines the entirety of myocardial contraction by expressing stroke volume as a percentage of end-diastolic LV volume (Formula 3.2):

$$LVEF = \frac{LVEDV - LVESV}{LVEDV} \times 100 \qquad [2]$$

where LVEF is the LV ejection fraction, LVEDV is the LV end-diastolic volume, and LVESV is the LV end-systolic volume.

The LVEF represents a composite of cardiac performance in that it is dependent on preload, contractility, and afterload. It is widely regarded as a predictor of outcome and survival. The following sections review the approaches used to calculate LV volumes and hence ejection fraction by both quantitative and qualitative methods.

Quantitative Measurements of Left Ventricular Dimensions

Quantitative measurement of the LVEF starts by obtaining two-dimensional views of the LV of adequate quality to perform tomographic measurements of length and area. Images with clear endocardial definition and borders must be obtained at both end-systole and end-diastole. These measurements are then applied to geometric models to estimate the three-dimensional intracavitary volume.

The use of two-dimensional measurements to calculate three-dimensional values entails several limitations. The first is that assumptions must be made regarding the geometry of the heart. Even normal hearts may vary considerably in individual geometry. The second limitation is that some formulas require that the measured values be cubed, which greatly magnifies any errors. Finally, the more images and measurements that must be obtained, the more time-consuming and therefore the less valuable the method in a dynamic setting.

Calculation of left ventricular volume. A number of geometric formulas are used for LV volume calculation, which vary greatly in their complexity and assumptions. The most common methods are discussed, with the simplest presented first.

Cubed formula: $V = D^3$ (Formula 3.3). The simplest approach to the quantitative measurement of LV volume is the cubed formula that allows volume in either systole or diastole to be estimated from a single linear dimension (3). The major assumption of the model is that the long-axis dimension is twice the short-axis dimension; hence, $V = D^3$. Figure 3.2 is a simplistic prolate ellipsoid model of the LV, where $V = D^3$.

All the measurements are taken from the inner margins of the endocardial echoes. Although the cubed formula is the simplest of the geometric models, it is also the least accurate. In particular, the cubed formula may profoundly overestimate the volume of larger ventricles. This happens because the LV typically dilates primarily along the short axis and becomes more spherical in shape.

Single-plane ellipsoid model: $V = 8A^2/3\pi L$ (Formula 3.4). Because of the irregular outline of the LV, the location and direction of the minor-axis measurements may be difficult to assess accurately. This limitation can be overcome by using the ventricular area (A) (Fig. 3.3). *The single plane used must include the true ventricular long axis to be valid; thus, for TEE applications, the ME four-chamber or two-chamber view is used, with the assumption that the complete LV is visualized.*

The area is obtained by using the internal software package of the echocardiography machine and tracing the inner border of the LV created by the endocardium. The long-axis length is obtained in the same view by using the calipers of the machine.

The single-plane ellipsoid formula assumes that the LV can be modeled as a prolate ellipse and that the echocardiographic long-axis view is representative of the true LV long axis and is actually visualized. It fails to account for the volume displaced by the papillary muscles, trabeculae, and mitral valve apparatus.

Simpson's rule of discs, method of discs: The use of a series of discs ($\geq$20) from the apex to base of the LV to calculate LV volume is known as *Simpson's rule* and is represented below (Formula 3.5):

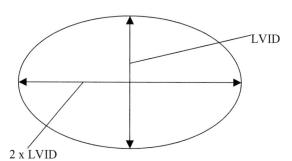

2 x LVID

FIG. 3.2. LVID = left ventricular internal dimension = D. Cubed formula model: $V = D^3$. Classically, the left ventricular internal dimension has been measured in M-mode (motion mode) from the parasternal long-axis transthoracic view just below the mitral valve. For transesophageal echocardiography, the midesophageal four-chamber view can be used. Note that volume measurements must be individually obtained in both systole and diastole. (Modified from Weyman AE, ed. *Cross-sectional echocardiography.* Philadelphia: Lea & Febiger, 1982:284.)

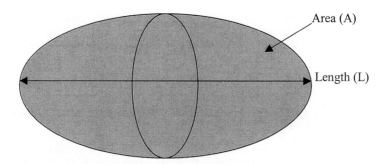

FIG. 3.3. Single-plane ellipsoid model: $V = 8A^2/3\pi L$. The single-plane ellipsoid model overcomes the difficulties of measuring the minor axis encountered with the cubed formula model by using measurements of area. (Modified from Weyman AE, ed. *Cross-sectional echocardiography*. Philadelphia: Lea & Febiger, 1982:284.)

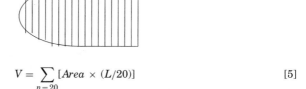

$$V = \sum_{n=20} [Area \times (L/20)] \qquad [5]$$

The mathematical formula is complex but is frequently found on modern echocardiographic systems. The formula recommended by the American Society of Echocardiography is the modified Simpson's rule (1), expressed by Formula 3.6:

$$V = (A_1 + A_2)h + \left(\frac{A_3 h}{2}\right) + \left(\frac{\pi h^3}{6}\right) \qquad [6]$$

where A_1 indicates the short-axis cross-sectional area at the level of the mitral valve, A_2 is the short-axis cross-sectional area at the level of the papillary muscles, A_3 is the short-axis cross-sectional area at the level of the apex, and h equals one-third the LV length.

Figure 3.4 shows TEE images obtained for measurement of the dimensions to be used in calculating the LVEF with the modified Simpson's rule. Modern echocardiographic machines use internal software to assist in calculating the ejection fraction with the multiple disc method (Simpson's rule). Because multiple measurements are used ($n \geq 20$), this technique is one of the most accurate available and is relatively easy to perform on modern echocardiography machines.

Fractional area change and acoustic quantification. The complexity of the echocardiographic determination of the LV volumes needed to calculate the ejection fraction has led to the widespread use of a surrogate index, fractional area change (FAC). FAC is a two-dimensional measurement that is easily obtained from the TG mid short-axis view. FAC is derived from Formula 3.7:

$$FAC = \frac{EDA - ESA}{EDA} \times 100 \qquad [7]$$

where EDA is the end-diastolic area and ESA is the end-systolic area.

With the use of freeze-frame images, planimetry of the endocardial borders in both systole and diastole is performed so that these measurements are easily obtained. Normal values for FAC are between 50% and 75%.

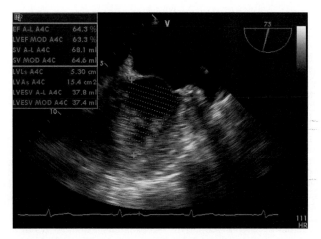

FIG. 3.4. Midesophageal two-chamber view demonstrating application of the method of discs (Simpson's rule) to calculate a left ventricular ejection fraction of 64%.

An automated method of obtaining FAC in real time is possible with an acoustic quantification technique available on some machines. Acoustic quantification enables automated border detection of the endocardial borders and calculation of the LV cavity dimensions, including ESA and EDA. Analysis of the images is performed in real time by the machine, and the FAC is reported for each cardiac cycle. Acoustic quantification is very sensitive to image quality for machine identification of the endocardial borders (Fig. 3.5). The endocardial borders of the septal and lateral walls often can be difficult to image throughout the cardiac cycle. In one study, adequate images could be obtained in only 73% of patients (4).

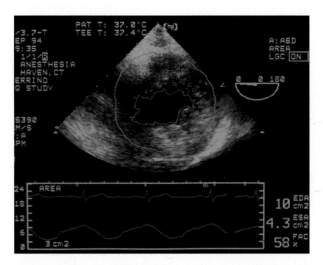

FIG. 3.5. Transgastric mid short-axis view with an acoustic quantification–derived fractional area change (*FAC*) of 58%.

TABLE 3.1. FACTORS THAT AFFECT THE ACCURACY OF QUALITATIVE DETERMINATIONS OF LEFT VENTRICULAR EJECTION FRACTION

Experience and expertise of the examiner
Quality of the image (especially endocardial border definition)
Number of views obtained for examination
Asynchronous contraction patterns (conduction abnormalities, pacing)
Regional wall motion abnormalities

Qualitative Assessment of the Ejection Fraction

Intraoperatively, the LVEF is most commonly determined by a qualitative visual estimation. It is the authors' experience that quantitative methods are most useful for research purposes and to assure "beginners" that their estimates of the LVEF are realistic.

Visual estimates of the ejection fraction produce results in real time. No time is spent manipulating images, tracing borders, or performing algebraic calculations. To determine the ejection fraction by visual estimation, the examiner examines a full-motion video of the TG midpapillary short-axis view. When time allows, additional views of the LV can be obtained to describe global ventricular function more completely.

When learning TEE, one should evaluate as many views as is practical given the intraoperative situation and then report the ejection fraction in a way that conveys the imprecise nature of the measurement: normal, mildly reduced, moderately reduced, or severely reduced. Alternatively, when performed by an experienced echocardiographer, intraoperative visual estimation of the ejection fraction provides accurate data and is comparable with quantitative analysis. It is typically reported as a range (e.g., 40–50%), or the value may be reported as an approximate value (e.g., ~45%).

Multiple factors can affect the accuracy and reproducibility of qualitative estimates of the LVEF and are outlined in Table 3.1. Caution must be exercised when the LVEF is determined on-line in the operating room versus off-line in the echocardiography laboratory. The former is more difficult, and the misinterpretation rate tends to be higher. Errors in LVEF estimates can be diminished by increased experience of the echocardiographer, the use of cine loop technology, and frequent, continuous training for quality improvement (5).

Stroke Volume and Cardiac Output

TEE allows the clinician to calculate cardiac output. Cardiac output, the product of stroke volume and heart rate, is widely used to track cardiovascular performance and response to therapy. TEE assesses the stroke volume by measuring the transit of blood volume through a confined area, such as the LV outflow tract (LVOT), aorta, or pulmonary artery. This calculation requires the assumptions that flow is laminar (i.e., not turbulent) and that the conduit being measured is an unchanging circular orifice such that it has the area of πr^2. Figure 3.6 demonstrates the calculation of cardiac output within the LVOT. Integration of the Doppler time-velocity integral (TVI) will give the cumulative distance that blood travels during a single cardiac cycle. The volume of blood moved during that single cardiac cycle is the product of the TVI and the cross-sectional area of the conduit through which the blood is moving. Therefore, cardiac output is derived as demonstrated in Figure 3.6. *The accuracy of the cardiac output calculation depends on parallel alignment of the ultrasound beam to the blood flow and an accurate determination of the vessel diameter.* Properly performed, TEE estimates of cardiac output are within thermodilution estimates by 0.5 to 1 L/min (6).

Isovolemic Rate of Pressure Rise

As discussed above, most measurements, including stroke volume and ejection fraction, are composite indices. Their values depend not only on myocardial contractility but also on

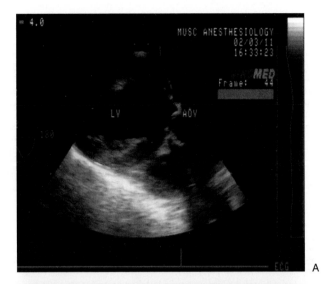

A

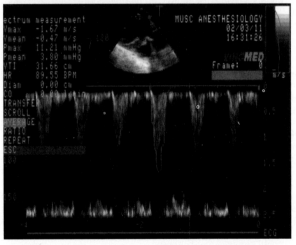

B

FIG. 3.6. A: Transgastric long-axis view demonstrating the left ventricular outflow tract (LVOT) and aorta (AO). **B:** The continuous wave Doppler is aligned parallel to the blood flow to obtain the velocity profile and resulting time-velocity integral (TVI) of the LVOT, which has a diameter of 2 cm. The patient's heart rate is 90 beats/min. $SV = CSA_{LVOT} \times TVI_{LVOT}$; $SV = \pi r_{LVOT}^2 \times TVI_{LVOT} = 3.14(1)^2 \times 31.66 = 99.41$; $CO = SV \times HR = 99.41 \times 90 = 8.9$ L/min. CO, cardiac output; CSA, cross-sectional area; HR, heart rate; SV, stroke volume.

several other factors, most notably loading conditions. Because loading conditions can fluctuate widely in the perioperative period, an accurate interpretation of most LV systolic indices is difficult. Thus, the search for a load-independent parameter that reflects the contractile state of the myocardium has been the Holy Grail of physiologists and clinicians.

Several indicators have been proposed as a load-independent measure of myocardial contractility. Currently, pressure-volume relations are the most widely used in laboratory studies, and with the advent of acoustic quantification, clinical echocardiographers have been able use this approach in the operating room. However, the complexity of obtaining a series of pressure-volume relations limits their role to investigative studies.

The maximal rate of pressure rise during isovolemic contraction ($\Delta P/\Delta t$) is a widely regarded systolic parameter and is used primarily in invasive catheterization laboratories (Fig. 3.7). This technique is not affected by alterations in loading conditions and is of proven value is assessing the myocardial function of patients undergoing mitral valve replacement.

A noninvasive determination of $\Delta P/\Delta t$ is possible with Doppler echocardiography. By applying the Bernoulli equation to the velocities measured from a mitral regurgitant jet, the generation of LV pressures can be tracked:

$$P_{LV} = P_{LA} + 4v_{MR}^2$$

where

P_{LV} indicates LV pressure, P_{LA} is left atrial pressure, and v_{MR} is the velocity of the mitral regurgitation jet.

As seen in Figures 3.7 and 3.8, by using the hemodynamic data, $\Delta P/\Delta t$ is calculated as the slope of the LV pressure rise from 4 to 36 mm Hg above the baseline LA pressure:

$$\Delta P/\Delta t_{max} = \frac{36 - 4\,mmHG}{\Delta t\,msec} = \frac{32\,mmHG}{\Delta t\,msec}$$

The echocardiographic approach to calculate $\Delta P/\Delta t$ is equally simple:

1. Optimize visualization of the MR jet with color flow Doppler by adjusting the imaging plane from the ME four-chamber view.
2. Place the continuous wave cursor to obtain a spectral waveform of the MR velocities. Capture a freeze frame of the waveform.
3. From the Bernoulli equation, a gradient of 4 mm Hg correlates with an MR jet velocity of 1 m/s, and 36 mm Hg converts to a velocity of 3 m/s. Simply place the ultrasound cursor at the 1-m/s and 3-m/s velocities, and the ultrasound system will calculate Δt in milliseconds. Use this Δt in the above formula to calculate the maximal rate of pressure rise (Fig. 3.8).

The superiority of $\Delta P/\Delta t$ in comparison with FAC and cardiac output as a monitor of LV systolic function during alterations of loading conditions in the perioperative period has been confirmed (7). The technique is limited in patients in whom an MR jet is not present or is poorly defined by continuous wave Doppler.

Optimizing Ventricular Performance

Frank–Starling relationship. Optimizing ventricular performance is one of the most important roles of intraoperative TEE. This is not a simple task because systolic ventricular function is predicated on a complex combination of factors, including the underlying metabolic condition of the heart, heart rate, contractility, preload, and afterload. Of these determinants, only the heart rate is easily measured. Consequently, most clinicians rely on an intuitive approach to optimizing the intraoperative cardiac status based on the Frank–Starling relationship.

Frank–Starling quantified the effect of ventricular preload on systolic performance (8). Figure 3.9 demonstrates the classic Frank–Starling curvilinear relationship, in which increases in LVEDV result in a greater stroke volume. An increase in contractility, as occurs with the addition of an inotrope, shifts the curve upward, resulting in an increased stroke

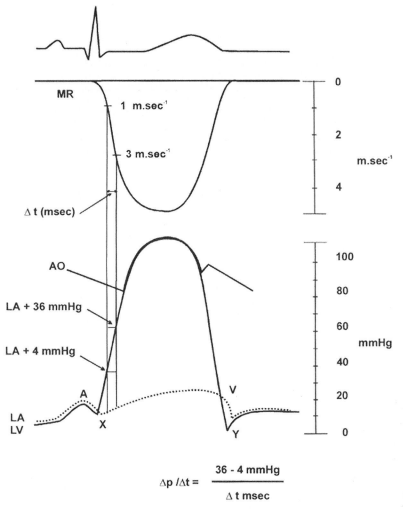

FIG. 3.7. Determination of rate of left ventricular (*LV*) pressure rise ($\Delta P/\Delta t$) with Doppler echocardiography. ΔP is the magnitude of the rise in LV pressure during the increase in mitral regurgitant velocity from 1 to 3 m/s (32 mm Hg because left atrial pressure does not significantly rise during this period). Δt is the time taken for mitral flow velocity to rise from 1 to 3 m/s. AO, aorta; LA, left atrium; MR, mitral regurgitation. (Modified from Pai RG, et al. Doppler-derived rate of left ventricular pressure rise: its correlation with postoperative left ventricular function in mitral regurgitation. *Circulation* 1990;82:514–520, with permission.)

volume for any given LVEDV. Increases in afterload, on the other hand, are inversely related to stroke volume (Fig. 3.9).

Echocardiographic determination of the Frank–Starling relationship and the optimal fluid status. The necessary parameters for deriving the Frank–Starling relationship, preload and cardiac output, can be monitored intraoperatively with TEE. TEE is a superb means of quantitatively assessing the preload and monitoring its adequacy throughout

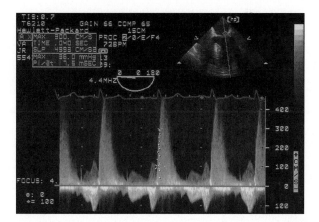

FIG. 3.8. Midesophageal four-chamber view demonstrating ease of $\Delta P/\Delta t$ measurements. Note that velocities at 1 and 3 seconds correspond to Bernoulli-derived pressure gradients of 4 and 36 mm Hg, respectively. $\Delta P = 36 - 4 = 32$ mm Hg; $\Delta t = 0.04$ s; $\Delta P/\Delta t = 32/0.04 = 800$ mm Hg/ms.

surgery. Typically, LV preload is assessed by determining the LVEDA in the TG midpapillary short-axis view. However, preexisting cardiac disease, acute alterations in ventricular compliance, and increased metabolic demands disturb this relationship, and the optimal intraoperative LVEDA often exceeds the normal value. For these reasons, we advise against using a single parameter, in this case the LVEDA, as the basis for clinical fluid management. Rather, we recommend using LVEDA measures of preload combined with matched Doppler measurements of stroke volume. This approach allows the clinician to approximate an intraoperative Starling curve for the patient and effectively titrate fluid and vasoactive therapy to optimize the cardiovascular status. Typically, boluses of intravenous fluids are administered until a satisfactory endpoint is achieved while distention of the LV is avoided. Great care must be used when volume challenging a depressed ventricle. Also, it must be

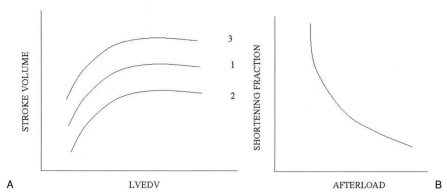

FIG. 3.9. Frank-Starling relationship. **A:** The effect of increasing left ventricular end-diastolic volume (LVEDV), or preload, on the resulting stroke volume in the normal heart (*1*), failing heart (*2*), and heart exposed to an inotrope (*3*). **B:** The inverse relationship occurs with increasing afterload, as evidenced by a decreasing shortening velocity.

remembered that the right ventricle may become distended before the desired endpoint is achieved without LV distension (9). This technique is particularly valuable in patients with hemorrhagic or septic shock.

VENTRICULAR PATHOLOGY

Left Ventricular Hypertrophy

LV hypertrophy is a compensatory adaptation of the ventricle to stress. *Concentric hypertrophy* is a thickening of the ventricular wall as a consequence of parallel replication of sarcomeres without significant chamber enlargement; it occurs secondary to chronic pressure overload of the ventricle, as in systemic hypertension and aortic stenosis. *Eccentric hypertrophy* is an enlargement or dilation of the LV chamber as a consequence of serial replication of sarcomeres and occurs secondary to chronic volume overload of the ventricle; aortic regurgitation is the classic example.

Concentric hypertrophy. Increased impedance to ejection causes marked rises in ventricular wall stress. Concentric hypertrophy is a compensatory response that reduces wall stress and enables the ventricle to develop the exaggerated intracavitary pressures necessary to contract effectively against the increased afterload. This results in an increased systolic wall stress that is somewhat mitigated by the increased LV wall thickness. Other physiologic alterations of the ventricle that occur in concentric hypertrophy include a prolongation of isovolumetric relaxation, a reduction in compliance that leads to diastolic dysfunction, and eventual worsening of cardiac function as compensatory limits are reached. Echocardiographic analysis of concentric hypertrophy involves a determination of LV thickness or LV mass (10,11).

Determination of left ventricular mass. Although the details are beyond the scope of this chapter, LV mass can be calculated from two-dimensional echocardiography by an area-length method or a truncated ellipsoid formula:

$$\text{LV mass (grams)} = 1.04\,[(\text{LVID} + \text{PWT} + \text{IVST})^3 - \text{LVID}^3] \times 0.8 + 0.6$$

where LVID indicates LV internal dimension, PWT is the posterior wall thickness, IVST is the interventricular septal thickness at end-diastole, 1.04 is the specific gravity of the myocardium, and 0.8 is a correction factor.

An easier approach involves the calculation of total LV myocardial volume by tracing the epicardial borders and then subtracting the volume of the cavity, estimated by tracing the endocardial borders. The resulting difference is then multiplied by the specific density of the myocardium to derive the LV mass. Hence, LV mass = (total LV volume − LV chamber volume) × 1.04 (12). This approach is problematic when the epicardial border definition is not satisfactory; hence, wall thickness is most frequently used.

Determination of left ventricular wall thickness. LV wall thickness historically has been measured by transthoracic echocardiography at end-diastole in M-mode from the parasternal long-axis view. The beam is placed at the mitral chordal level just beyond the mitral leaflet tips, perpendicular to the long axis of the ventricle. With TEE and anatomic M-mode, the ME four-chamber view can be used (Fig. 3.10), or the TG midpapillary view is used if anatomic M-mode is not a machine option. An LV wall thickness greater than 1.1 cm is considered hypertrophic (Table 3.2).

Left Ventricular True Aneurysm

Most LV aneurysms are located at the apex and are predominantly a consequence of anterior myocardial infarctions. Within 90 days after an anterior myocardial infarction, LV aneurysms develop in 22% of patients (13). No new true aneurysms develop more than 3 months after myocardial infarction. Early aneurysm formation, within the first 5 days after myocardial infarction, is associated with increased mortality.

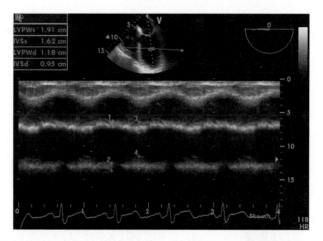

FIG. 3.10. Midesophageal four-chamber view demonstrating anatomic M-mode (motion mode) measurement of left ventricular wall thickness.

Two-dimensional characteristics. A ventricular aneurysm is characterized as a dilated dyskinetic area with myocardial thinning. A narrow band of myocardium lines a "true" aneurysm and distinguishes it from a pseudoaneurysm (discussed later). As demonstrated in Figure 3.11, a smooth, gradual transition is seen between the aneurysm and normal myocardium, with a gradual, obtuse tapering of myocardium into a dilated, thinned area that has a wide neck or opening. The ratio of the size of the aneurysmal opening from the ventricle to the maximal aneurysmal diameter ranges between 0.9 and 1.0 (14).

Associated findings. Intraoperative TEE is useful to detect thrombus formation within the aneurysm. Thrombus appears as an area of increased echogenicity that can be clearly delineated from the endocardium and is a frequent finding as a consequence of stasis of blood within the dilated aneurysm.

Left Ventricular Pseudoaneurysm

The ability to distinguish a true aneurysm from a pseudoaneurysm is critical because pseudoaneurysms have a high incidence of spontaneous rupture and thus require surgical

TABLE 3.2. NORMAL TRANSESOPHAGEAL ECHOCARDIOGRAPHIC MEASUREMENTS IN ADULTS

	Mean ± SD	Range	View-axis	Technique
Aortic root	28 ± 3	21–34	AV-short	2-D
LV diameter (diastole) anterior-posterior	43 ± 7	33–55	LV-short	2-D
LV diameter (diastole) medial-lateral	42 ± 7	23–54	LV-short	2-D
LV diameter (systole) anterior-posterior	28 ± 6	18–40	LV-short	2-D
LV diameter (systole) medial-lateral	27 ± 6	18–42	LV-short	2-D
LV wall thickness		≤11	LV-short	M-mode
Proximal descending thoracic aorta diameter	21 ± 4	18–40	Ao-short	2-D
Distal descending thoracic aorta diameter	20 ± 4	18–42	Ao-short	2-D

All measurements are in millimeters.

SD, standard deviation; AV, aortic valve; 2-D, two-dimensional; LV, left ventricle; Ao, aorta; M-mode, motion mode.

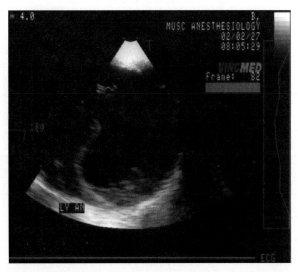

FIG. 3.11. Partial midesophageal four-chamber view demonstrating an apical left ventricular aneurysm. Note the wide neck of the aneurysm.

correction (14). A pseudoaneurysm represents a chronic ventricular rupture contained by pericardium. Thus, a pseudoaneurysm is a saccular structure that communicates directly with the pericardial space.

Two-dimensional characteristics. A pseudoaneurysm is characterized by a narrow orifice (neck) arising from the ventricular chamber; the ratio of the size of the orifice to the maximal aneurysmal diameter is less than 0.5 (Fig. 3.12). The size of the small neck rarely exceeds half the maximal parallel internal diameter of the aneurysmal sac (15). The LV cavity size decreases in systole while the false aneurysm gradually expands.

Quantitative Doppler characteristics. Doppler echocardiography has proved useful in diagnostically difficult cases and demonstrates bidirectional flow of blood between the pseudoaneurysm and the LV. Color Doppler echocardiography usually demonstrates mosaic jets exiting the LV in systole and entering the pseudoaneurysm cavity. In diastole, this mosaic pattern occurs within the LV, confirming the turbulent ebb and flow of blood to and from the pseudoaneurysm. One may also see a profound variation in maximal Doppler flow velocity throughout the respiratory cycle, with inspiration causing a significant increase in the maximal flow velocity (15).

Associated findings. Spontaneous echo contrast and thrombus within the pseudoaneurysm cavity are frequent findings.

Dilated Cardiomyopathy

Dilated cardiomyopathy accounts for more than 90% of all cases of cardiomyopathy. Potential causes are numerous and include parasitic and viral infections, toxic exposure, autoimmune diseases, metabolic abnormalities, hemochromatosis, and sarcoidosis; the condition may also be idiopathic or occur postpartum (16). Although echocardiography is not particularly useful in establishing the cause of a dilated cardiomyopathy, it is of paramount importance in providing a diagnosis, contributing prognostic data, and evaluating the efficacy of treatment regimens. Both the left and right ventricular ejection fraction should be estimated. Multivariate analysis has determined that only the ejection fraction is a significant predictor of outcome as defined by death or the need for heart transplantation (17).

Two-dimensional characteristics. The two-dimensional hallmarks of dilated cardiomyopathy are severe contractile dysfunction of the LV with a reduced ejection fraction and

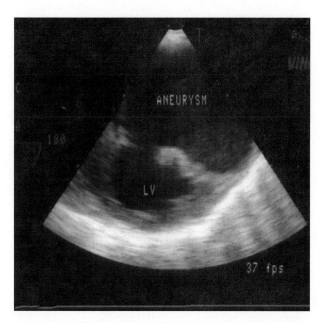

FIG. 3.12. Transgastric view demonstrating an inferior pseudoaneurysm (aneurysm) with a narrow entrance neck. Note the spontaneous echo contrast within the pseudoaneurysm.

dilation of all four cardiac chambers (16). Enlargement of the cardiac chambers is not associated with an appropriate increase in ventricular septal or free wall thickness (Fig. 3.13). Therefore, the two-dimensional echocardiographic evaluation of a patient with dilated cardiomyopathy includes imaging of all four cardiac chambers for a determination of size and a qualitative assessment of LV function.

The LV chamber dimensions and volumes should be documented at end-systole and end-diastole in both short- and long-axis views. The prognosis of patients with a more spherical LV appears to be poorer, irrespective of systolic cavity dimension, fractional shortening, or wall thickness, than that of patients with a smaller LV end-diastolic short-axis dimension (18).

Associated findings. The tricuspid and mitral valve leaflets are structurally normal, but significant regurgitation can occur secondary to abnormal displacement of the papillary muscles, or secondary to ventricular and annular dilation with incomplete coaptation of the valve leaflets. Additional evidence for a low cardiac output includes decreased excursion of the mitral leaflets. Other secondary features that should be evaluated by two-dimensional echocardiography in dilated cardiomyopathy include apical thrombus and enlarged atrial cavities.

Hypertrophic Cardiomyopathy

Introduction and classification. Hypertrophic cardiomyopathy is an inherited autosomal dominant disorder of the myocardium. The essential features of this disease include asymmetric LV hypertrophy, normal LV systolic function, and compromised diastolic function (19,20). In all forms, the basal posterior LV wall is normal. Hypertrophy isolated to the anterior portion of the ventricular septum is classified as type I. Hypertrophy confined to the anterior and posterior aspects of the septum is type II. Type III involves the entire myocardium with the exception of the basal posterior wall. Type IV is a rare form in which only the apical segment of the LV is hypertrophic.

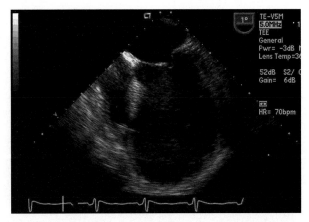

FIG. 3.13. Dilated cardiomyopathy: midesophageal four-chamber view.

Two-dimensional characteristics. *Hypertrophy of the interventricular septum that is disproportionate to hypertrophy of the free wall of the LV is the classic finding in hypertrophic cardiomyopathy.* Multiple TEE imaging views are necessary to delineate the hypertrophic segments completely and to determine the type, as previously described. The ME two-chamber view allows an assessment of the posterior basal wall contained between the mitral valve and papillary muscle. This region is not thickened in patients with asymmetric hypertrophic cardiomyopathy, which differentiates this disorder from concentric hypertrophy. The ME four-chamber and TG long-axis views allow documentation of the effect of septal hypertrophy on the patency of the outflow tract and of the degree of systolic anterior motion of the mitral valve with associated MR. An apical view of the LV should always be obtained in patients with suspected hypertrophic cardiomyopathy so that the diagnosis of isolated apical hypertrophy (type IV) is not missed. LV function is preserved in hypertrophic cardiomyopathy.

Associated findings

1. Asymmetric septal hypertrophy may result in a dynamic systolic subaortic obstruction (21). During systole, bulging of the thickened septum narrows the LVOT and causes outflow obstruction (Fig. 3.14).
2. Systolic anterior motion of the mitral valve is present.

Exaggerated anterior motion of the mitral valve may accompany the septal encroachment during systole and can accentuate the outflow obstruction, typically late in systole. The cause of systolic anterior motion of the mitral valve is controversial. Vigorous contraction of the septum may generate a "Venturi" effect, in which the rapid acceleration of blood through a narrowed LVOT causes the anterior mitral leaflet and valve apparatus to be drawn toward the septum. Systolic anterior motion of the mitral valve may also be related to the contraction of papillary muscles with an altered orientation secondary to the hypertrophic process or to inadequate mobility or coaptation of the posterior leaflet (22). Notably, the mitral valve is abnormal in most patients with hypertrophic cardiomyopathy; increased leaflet length and area and anomalous papillary muscle insertion directly into the anterior leaflet may predispose to obstruction secondary to flow drag, the pushing force of flow (21). Anterior motion of the mitral valve into the outflow tract during systole results in MR with a posteriorly directed jet. The aortic valve opens normally in early systole, but fluttering of the leaflets and premature closure are a consequence of the mid-to-late systolic outflow obstruction.

Intraoperative considerations. Echocardiography is necessary to define the extent and location of septal hypertrophy before surgery. The surgeon uses this information to establish the extent of muscle that should be resected. This preparation is especially important because the limited intraoperative view across the aortic valve does not allow a complete picture of the

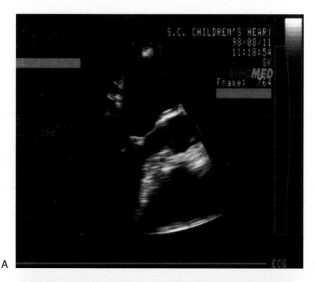

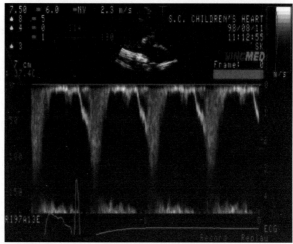

FIG. 3.14. A: Midesophageal long-axis view demonstrating profound asymmetric septal hypertrophy (ASH) involving the left ventricular outflow tract (LVOT). Note the acute narrowing of the LVOT at the proximal border of the area of septal hypertrophy. **B:** High pulse repetition frequency Doppler demonstrating the classic "dagger" flow velocity pattern of dynamic outflow obstruction.

degree of septal thickening or of the orientation of the septum to the outflow tract. Finally, intraoperative echocardiography also documents the adequacy of repair and the presence of any residual obstruction (23–25).

SUMMARY

The ability of the intraoperative echocardiographer to assess LV function and volume status rapidly is paramount in the surgical environment. This chapter has emphasized the echocardiographic indices of systolic performance and the ways in which echocardiography can be used to optimize LV performance. Also discussed are other commonly encountered alterations of systolic function, including LV hypertrophy and dilated cardiomyopathy.

REFERENCES

1. American Society of Echocardiography Committee on Standards, Subcommittee on Quantitation of Two-Dimensional Echocardiogram. Recommendations for quantitation of the left ventricle by two-dimensional echocardiography. *J Am Soc Echocardiogr* 1989;2:361–367.
2. Otto CM, ed. *Textbook of clinical echocardiography,* 2nd ed. Philadelphia: WB Saunders, 2000;103–104.
3. Feigenbaum H, Popp RL, Wolfe SB. Ultrasound measurements of the left ventricle: a correlative study with angiocardiography. *Arch Intern Med* 1972;129:461–467.
4. Perrino AC, Luther MA, O'Connor TZ, et al. Automated echocardiographic analysis: examination of serial intraoperative measurements. *Anesthesiology* 1995;83:285–292.
5. Mathew JP, Fontes ML, Garwood S, et al. Transesophageal echocardiography interpretation: a comparative analysis between cardiac anesthesiologists and primary echocardiographers. *Anesth Analg* 2002;94:302–309
6. Perrino AC, Harris SN, Luther MA. Intraoperative determination of cardiac output using multiplane transesophageal echocardiography. *Anesthesiology* 1998;89:350–357.
7. Broka SM, Dubois PE, Jamart J, et al. Effects of acute decrease in systemic afterload on accuracy of Doppler-derived left ventricular rate of pressure rise measurement in anesthetized patients. *J Am Soc Echocardiogr* 2001;14:1161–1165.
8. Guyton AC, Hall JE, eds. *Textbook of medical physiology,* 9th ed. Philadelphia: WB Saunders, 1996;115–116.
9. Swenson JD, Harkin C, Pace NL, et al. Transesophageal echocardiography: an objective tool in defining maximum ventricular response to intravenous fluid therapy. *Anesth Analg* 1996;83:1149–1153.
10. Hanrath P, Mathey DG, Siegert R, et al. Left ventricular relaxation and filling pattern in different forms of left ventricular hypertrophy: an echocardiographic study. *Am J Cardiol* 1980;45:15–23.
11. Devereux RB, Alonso DR, Lutas EM, et al. Echocardiographic assessment of left ventricular hypertrophy: comparison to necropsy findings. *Am J Cardiol* 1986;57:450–458.
12. Devereux RB, Reichek N. Echocardiographic determination of left ventricular mass in man. *Circulation* 1977:55;613–618
13. Visser CA, Kan G, Meltzer RS, et al. Incidence, timing and prognostic value of left ventricular aneurysm formation after myocardial infarction: a prospective, serial echocardiographic study of 158 patients. *Am J Cardiol* 1986;57:729–732.
14. Brown SL, Gropler RJ, Harris KM. Distinguishing left ventricular aneurysm from pseudoaneurysm. A review of the literature. *Chest* 1997;111:1403–1409.
15. Roelandt JRTC, Sutherland GR, Yoshida K, et al. Improved diagnosis and characterization of left ventricular pseudoaneurysm by Doppler color flow imaging. *J Am Coll Cardiol* 1988;12:807–811.
16. Koga Y, Toshima H, Tanaka M, et al. Therapeutic management of dilated cardiomyopathy. *Cardiovasc Drugs Ther* 1994;8:83–88.
17. Julliere Y, Barbier G, Feldmann L, et al. Additional predictive value of both left and right ventricular ejection fractions on long-term survival in idiopathic dilated cardiomyopathy. *Eur Heart J* 1997;18:276–280.
18. Douglas PS, Morrow R, Toli A, et al. Left ventricular shape, afterload and survival in idiopathic dilated cardiomyopathy. *J Am Coll Cardiol* 1989;13:311–315.
19. Wigle ED, Rakowski H, Kimball BP, et al. Hypertrophic cardiomyopathy: clinical spectrum and treatment. *Circulation* 1995;92:1680–1692.
20. Spirito P, Maron BJ, Chiarella F, et al. Diastolic abnormalities in patients with hypertrophic cardiomyopathy: relation to magnitude of left ventricular hypertrophy. *Circulation* 1985;72:310–316.

21. Sherrid MV, Chu CK, Delia E, et al. An echocardiographic study of the fluid mechanics of obstruction in hypertrophic cardiomyopathy. *J Am Coll Cardiol* 1993;22:816–825.
22. Schwammenthal E, Nakatani S, He S, et al. Mechanism of mitral regurgitation in hypertrophic cardiomyopathy. Mismatch of posterior to anterior leaflet length and mobility. *Circulation* 1998;98:856–865.
23. Louie EK, Edwards LC. Hypertrophic cardiomyopathy. *Prog Cardiovasc Dis* 1994;36:275–308.
24. Grigg LE, Wigle ED, Williams WG, et al. Transesophageal Doppler echocardiography in obstructive hypertrophic cardiomyopathy: clarification of pathophysiology and importance in intraoperative decision making. *J Am Coll Cardiol* 1992;20:42–52.
25. Marwick TH, Stewart WJ, Lever HM, et al. Benefits of intraoperative echocardiography in the surgical management of hypertrophic cardiomyopathy. *J Am Coll Cardiol* 1992;20:1066–1072.

QUESTIONS

1. The following vital signs were obtained from a patient undergoing mitral valve repair:

   Heart rate, 100
   Body surface area, 1.8 m^2
   LVOT diameter, 1.9 cm
   LVOT TVI, 14.47 cm

   Calculate the following:
   a. Stroke volume
   b. Cardiac output
   c. Cardiac index.
2. A patient has the following LV measurements:

   LVID in diastole, 5.2 cm
   LVID in systole, 3.1 cm

   A. Calculate the fractional shortening.
   B. Is the LV function normal based on this measurement?
3. Which parameters measured by TEE correlate with systolic ventricular performance?
   a. Cardiac output
   b. Ejection fraction
   c. Fractional shortening
   d. FAC
   e. All of the above
4. Explain the difference between adequate and optimal ventricular preload. Does an "empty ventricle" require treatment with intravenous fluids?
5. Explain why quantitative methods of determining the cardiac output or ejection fraction are not frequently used for the intraoperative measurement of systolic ventricular performance.
6. All of the following are echocardiographic manifestations of an LV pseudoaneurysm **except**
   a. A wide neck opening
   b. A decreasing LV cavity size in systole while the pseudoaneurysm expands
   c. Spontaneous echo contrast within the pseudoaneurysm cavity
   d. Demonstration by color Doppler of bidirectional flow into the pseudoaneurysm
7. All of the following statements regarding dilated cardiomyopathy are true **except**
   a. The ventricular end-diastolic pressure is increased.
   b. Severe contractile dysfunction is present.
   c. Only the LA and LV are enlarged.
   d. The RVEF and LVEF are predictors of death.

8. In dilated cardiomyopathy
   a. The mitral leaflets are typically normal
   b. Abnormal displacement of the papillary muscles can cause significant MR
   c. Annular dilation can cause incomplete coaptation of the mitral valve leaflets
   d. The mitral leaflet excursion may be decreased
   e. All of the above
9. All of the following statements about asymmetric septal hypertrophy are true **except**
   a. It is an autosomal dominant disorder.
   b. Outflow obstruction occurs during systole.
   c. Narrowing of the LV outflow tract initiates the obstruction.
   d. The basal posterior LV wall is also extremely thickened.
10. Which of the following statements has been proposed as an explanation of mitral valve pathology in asymmetric septal hypertrophy?
    a. Anterior motion of the mitral valve may exaggerate the LVOT obstruction.
    b. A "Venturi" effect may occur through the narrowed LVOT, thereby drawing the anterior leaflet toward the septum.
    c. An altered orientation of the papillary muscles leads to systolic anterior motion of the mitral valve.
    d. The anterior leaflet is usually enlarged in asymmetric septal hypertrophy.
    e. All of the above.

4

Diagnosis of Myocardial Ischemia

Martin J. London

Perioperative transesophageal echocardiography (TEE) is a valuable monitor for detecting myocardial ischemia, capable of rapidly and decisively guiding antiischemic therapy. Currently, the qualitative recognition of regional wall motion abnormalities (RWMAs) is the basis of the clinical use of TEE for ischemia detection. Although newer technologies may allow easier, more precise, and quantitative analysis, the basic physiologic principles underlying RWMAs are not likely to change in the near future.

CLINICAL RELEVANCE OF TRANSESOPHAGEAL ECHOCARDIOGRAPHY IN DIAGNOSING MYOCARDIAL ISCHEMIA

TEE may improve the outcome in certain high-risk subsets of patients (1). However, the magnitude of this effect, relative to the greater expense and training required for TEE than for other commonly used methods of perioperative monitoring (e.g., electrocardiography [ECG], pulmonary artery catheterization [PAC]), remains controversial. Early clinical studies of TEE, particularly during vascular surgery, were somewhat overly optimistic about its value because it was mistakenly thought that new intraoperative RWMAs identified *all patients sustaining perioperative myocardial ischemia*. However, cardiology research subsequently documented more complex manifestations of myocardial ischemia, particularly myocardial stunning and hibernation, that complicate the *immediate assessment* of myocardial viability (2,3) (Table 4.1). More recent studies report a much lower predictive value for new intraoperative RWMAs as they relate to postoperative myocardial ischemia, and enthusiasm for "routine" TEE monitoring in noncardiac surgery *for the sole purpose of detecting ischemia* has waned (4,5).

In contrast, the use of TEE for ischemia detection and other applications during coronary artery bypass graft (CABG) surgery continues to increase (6). Given that epidemiologic studies convincingly demonstrate long-term survival advantages of CABG relative to medical therapy or percutaneous coronary interventions (i.e., percutaneous transluminal coronary angioplasty), particularly in patients with a depressed ejection fraction, it is likely that clinical interest in monitoring patients at high risk for ischemia with TEE will continue to grow (7). Also, the use of off-pump CABG (OPCAB) has increased dramatically. In OPCAB, TEE is useful in evaluating the early efficacy of revascularization and, perhaps of greater importance, assessing the impact of surgical complications (e.g., inadequate anastomosis, inability to tolerate temporary occlusion of a distal vessel, hemodynamic consequences of cardiac displacement by stabilizers) (8,9).

The intraoperative echocardiographer must have a firm grounding in the physiologic, technical, and clinical aspects of ultrasound imaging as it relates to acute and chronic myocardial ischemia and infarction. Although ischemia and infarction lie at the ends of a continuous physiologic spectrum, obvious physiologic differences and morphologic changes specific to myocardial infarction (e.g., chronic wall thinning, calcification, septal rupture) may substantially affect clinical decision making with TEE. These changes tend to reduce the sensitivity and specificity of TEE, although recognition of the chronic irreversible consequences of infarction can have important implications for hemodynamic management. Also, the detection of thrombus in an infarcted segment or aneurysm can prevent devastating cerebrovascular consequences.

The American Society of Anesthesiologists/Society of Cardiovascular Anesthesiologists practice guidelines for the use of perioperative TEE accorded TEE only a category II indication (i.e., supported by weaker evidence than category I, possibly useful in improving clinical outcomes but appropriate indications less certain) for use in patients at increased risk for ischemia and infarction (10). It was given an even lower rating (category III: little

TABLE 4.1. CHARACTERISTICS OF CURRENTLY POSTULATED FORMS OF MYOCARDIAL ISCHEMIA

	Conventional ischemia	Stunned myocardium	Hibernating myocardium	Preconditioned myocardium
Regional function	Reduced, usually in proportion to reduction in CBF	Reduced	Reduced	Possibly reduced during preconditioning stimulus, protected with repeated stimulus
Coronary blood flow	Severe reduction for akinesia, dyskinesia	Partial to full restoration after relief of ischemia	Moderate reduction to normal at rest, reduced with stress	Dependent on clinical situation, reduced during OPCAB
Energy metabolism	Reduced during low CBF	Normal to moderate reduction	Reduced in relation to contractile decrease	Reduced during preconditioning stimulus
Duration	Minutes to hours	Hours to weeks	Days to months	Minutes to hours after stimulus
Outcome	Infarction if severe enough	Full to partial recovery	Full recovery with revascularization	Decreased postischemic infarct or ischemic damage
Perioperative implications	Most "treatable" form	Common following CPB	May show immediate improvement after CPB	Sometime used during OPCAB, volatile anesthesia preconditioning effects

CBF, cerebral blood flow; OPCAB, off-pump coronary artery bypass; CPB, cardiopulmonary bypass.
Modified from Opie LH. The multifarious spectrum of ischemic left ventricular dysfunction: relevance of new ischemic syndromes. *J Mol Cell Cardiol* 1996;28:2403–2414, with permission.

current scientific or expert support) for evaluating myocardial perfusion, coronary artery anatomy, or graft patency. Given the logistic difficulties of performing clinical research on the impact of monitoring technology on patient outcomes, it is unlikely that the indications will be upgraded in subsequent revisions of these somewhat dated guidelines. However, significant clinical research based on newer technology continues to show promise for a wider application of TEE in ischemia monitoring.

PHYSIOLOGIC BASIS FOR THE DETECTION OF ISCHEMIA

Experimental animal and human clinical studies document the extraordinary sensitivity of ultrasound technology in detecting the rapid reduction in regional myocardial function associated with an acute reduction in myocardial blood flow in the perfusion territory of an affected coronary artery. These changes usually occur within a significantly shorter time than either ST-segment changes on the ECG or increased filling pressures noted by PAC, allowing earlier diagnosis. Although the ECG is also sensitive for ischemia detection, a number of physiologic factors lower its specificity (e.g., bundle branch block, pacing, Q waves or nonspecific ST-segment changes), so that *at least during the intraoperative period,* TEE is useful in a wider range of patients (11).

The most sensitive change associated with ischemia is a reduction or cessation of systolic wall thickening, which normally increases by 50% of the end-diastolic value (12) (Fig. 4.1). With a complete cessation of coronary flow, systolic *wall thinning* may occur, leading to outward bulging of the affected wall (Fig. 4.2). However, because the function of the heart is to eject blood *via a reduction in chamber size* by inward motion of the endocardial surface during systole, a reduction in *endocardial excursion* is a more obvious sign, especially when referenced to movement of the normal walls. It is also well established that in unaffected, nonischemic regions, exaggerated inward movement (termed *compensatory hyperkinesis*) develops, off-setting the adverse effects of regional dysfunction on cardiac stroke volume. This is the principal reason why changes in systemic hemodynamics with ischemia are a late (and particularly ominous) sign and usually occur only with very severe regional (particularly dyskinetic) or global ischemia.

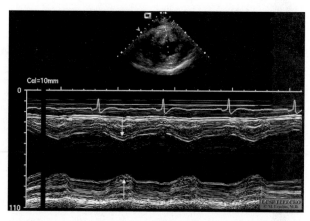

FIG. 4.1. Normal wall motion M-mode (motion mode). Normal inward endocardial excursion and wall thickening are illustrated on an M-mode image through the inferior (**top**) and anterior (**bottom**) walls in the transgastric short-axis view (**top inset**). Systole starts at the onset of the QRS complex and ends near the end of the T wave (*arrows*). M-mode imaging through transesophageal echocardiography can on occasion provide helpful information regarding the timing of wall motion, particularly when coupled with the electrocardiogram. (Courtesy of M. London, M.D., http://www.ucsf.edu/teeecho)

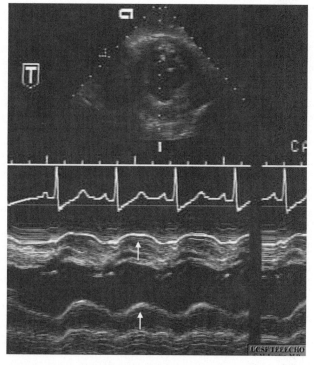

FIG. 4.2. M-mode (motion mode) dyskinesis. Dyskinetic outward motion of the inferior wall (*upper arrow*) in a patient with a chronic inferior wall infarction (note the increased density of the myocardium on both the M-mode and two-dimensional images). Orientations are identical to those in Figure 4.1. (Courtesy of M. London, M.D., http://www.ucsf.edu/teeecho)

TABLE 4.2. ENDOCARDIAL EXCURSION VERSUS WALL THICKENING

Endocardial excursion	Wall thickening
Advantages	
Relies on a more readily defined interface (endocardium)	Independent of a center of reference
More readily measured around the entire circumference of the ventricle	Unaffected by translation or rotation
Disadvantages	Unaffected by shape changes
Centroid (center of mass)–dependent	Difficult to measure around the entire circumference of the ventricle because of poor epicardial definition
Affected by translation and rotation of the left ventricle in the chest	Tends to be "all or none" phenomenon
	More difficult to correlate with other imaging modalities (i.e., radionuclide or contrast ventriculograms)

From Mann DL, Gillam LD, Weyman AE. Cross-sectional echocardiographic assessment of regional left ventricular performance and myocardial perfusion. *Prog Cardiovasc Dis* 1986;29:1, with permission.

When wall motion is scored, it should be appreciated that our eyes (and brain) can integrate several factors, particularly the translation and rotation movements of the heart in the chest, in "real time" to arrive at the "semiquantitative" classification of wall motion agreed on by echocardiographers (13) (Tables 4.2 and 4.3; Fig. 4.3). These same factors greatly complicate computer analysis. Currently, despite the promotion of automated boundary detection techniques and their refinements (i.e., color kinesis), which are based on the detection of very low-level echo signals ("tissue backscatter"), the visual analysis of wall motion is the only viable option for use in clinical practice (14).

It is important to appreciate that in most experimental studies, changes in endocardial excursion substantially overestimate the area of hypoperfused ischemic myocardium, whereas wall thickening more closely approximates it (15). The leading explanation for this overestimation is "tethering" of the abnormal myocardium to adjacent muscle segments, with complex mechanical effects (16). The clinician should always remember that endocardial excursion substantially overestimates the degree of ischemia. It is also critical to appreciate that other physiologic and morphologic conditions can "mimic" ischemia by causing abnormal endocardial excursion (discussed later). However, in these situations, *systolic wall thickening should be normal*. Finally, it is important to recognize that the magnitude of endocardial excursion and wall thickening can vary between different regions of the heart and between different "normal" individuals (17). Thus, using the patient's baseline status as a control is necessary.

Precise numeric relations between coronary blood flow and regional function are controversial. The subendocardium, with its higher metabolic requirements and greater susceptibility to the adverse effects of elevated intracavitary filling pressures, is more sensitive to flow reduction and shows earlier change in thickening (12). In the nonsurgical setting, myocardial infarction is usually related to coronary obstruction at the epicardial level and, depending on the site of obstruction and the status of the collateral circulation, results in transmural or

TABLE 4.3. SCORING OF SEGMENTAL WALL MOTION ABNORMALITIES

Grade	Endocardial excursion (%)	Wall thickening (%)
Normal	>30	30–50
Hypokinesis		
Mild	10–30	30–50
Severe	<10	<30
Akinesis	0	<10
Dyskinesis	Outward bulging	Absent or systolic thinning
Hyperkinesis	>"Normal"	>"Normal"

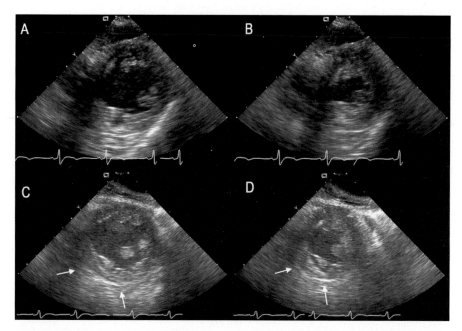

FIG. 4.3. Anteroseptal akinesis following cardiopulmonary bypass. The upper frames show normal endocardial excursion and wall thickening from end-diastole (**A**) to end-systole (**B**) in the transgastric short-axis view in a patient undergoing coronary artery bypass grafting. The lower frames show akinesis of the mid anterior and anteroseptal segments (*arrows*) on weaning from coronary bypass. **C:** End-diastole. **D:** End-systole. (Courtesy of M. London, M.D., http://www.ucsf.edu/teeecho)

subendocardial ischemia. An often quoted cardiology study suggests that regional function may cease with only a 20% reduction in transmural flow (18). This observation forms the basis for the considerable interest of cardiologists in assessing myocardial viability because an RWMA in the resting state indicates little regarding potential improvement (i.e., return to normal wall motion) after medical or surgical intervention. Myocardial viability is most commonly assessed with measures of metabolism (positron emission tomography), intact microvascular circulation (thallium imaging, perfusion contrast echocardiography), and, of particular interest to the cardiac anesthesiologist, mechanical contractile reserve (dobutamine stress testing). Each of these methods yields slightly different (and complementary) information (19).

Increasing emphasis is being placed on dobutamine stress testing for risk stratification before noncardiac surgery and for assessing the early postoperative wall motion response to CABG. With low doses of dobutamine, normal myocardium becomes hyperkinetic and coronary blood flow increases (20). The development of hypokinesis or akinesis in a previously normal segment with dobutamine indicates myocardial ischemia. A chronic transmural infarction will not increase wall thickening in response to either low or high doses of dobutamine. Improvement of function in an akinetic segment with low-dose dobutamine indicates the presence of *viable myocardium with contractile reserve,* called *stunned myocardium.* A *biphasic response,* in which improvement occurs at a low dose followed by deterioration at a higher dose, is characteristic of *hibernating myocardium.* One study suggests a potential role for intraoperative dobutamine stress testing before revascularization during CABG (21). However, in most centers, dobutamine stress echo or other tests of viability are routinely performed during the preoperative workup for CABG. The development of short-term myocardial stunning during cardiopulmonary bypass (CPB) can complicate the early interpretation of viability. *Although early studies suggested that the development of new RWMAs on termination of CPB was an indication for graft revision, a more widespread appreciation of the complexities of myocardial stunning suggests that only when the surgeon suspects technical problems (e.g., intramyocardial vessel, difficulty in locating proper vessel, need for endarterectomy of the vessel, intimal flaps,) should a new RWMA prompt a potentially morbid return to CPB.*

Despite these complexities, the anesthesiologist will most commonly encounter ischemia related to more dynamic changes in coronary blood flow during surgical manipulation (i.e., with retraction of the heart during OPCAB) or to hemodynamic abnormalities caused by surgery (e.g., profound hypotension, tachycardia, marked increase in afterload). In these situations, new RWMAs are more likely to be coupled to acute changes in coronary blood flow caused by the altered hemodynamics and thus are usually more amenable to immediate treatment.

ECHOCARDIOGRAPHIC DETECTION OF ISCHEMIA

Anatomic Localization of Ischemia: The 16-Segment System

The precise anatomic localization of left ventricular (LV) RWMAs is essential to guide clinical decision making, particularly in localizing the likely diseased coronary artery, and to gauge the impact of therapy. It is also important for accurate documentation in the medical record and for communication with surgeons and cardiologists. The 16-segment model adopted by the American Society of Echocardiography in 1989 forms the basis of the Society of Cardiovascular Anesthesiologists comprehensive intraoperative protocol and is universally accepted in this country (13,22) (Figs. 4.4–4.7; see Color Plates 1–4 following page 212). This system is based on division of the LV into apical, mid, and basal zones. The basal and mid zones each contain six segments, whereas the apical zone with its smaller area has only four. To assess all 16 segments completely requires interrogation of five imaging planes: the midesophageal (ME) four-chamber, two-chamber, and long-axis views, and the transgastric (TG) mid and basal views.

In the author's experience, the basal TG view can be problematic to obtain, and interpreting wall motion in this region so close to the fibrous atrioventricular (AV) skeleton of the heart can be challenging. Thus, some clinicians omit this view, substituting the three longitudinal

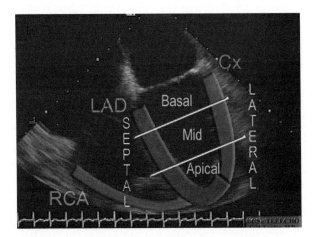

FIG. 4.4. Midesophageal four-chamber anatomic segments and perfusion. Segmental anatomy of the left ventricle in the midesophageal four-chamber view according to the American Society of Echocardiography classification system. Also depicted are the approximate perfusion zones of the left anterior descending (*LAD*), circumflex (*CX*), and right coronary (*RCA*) arteries. (Courtesy of M. London, M.D., http://www.ucsf.edu/teeecho) (See Color Plate 1 following page 212.)

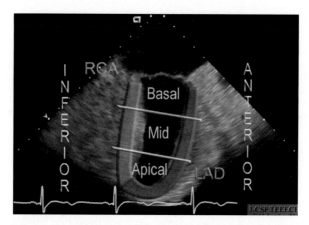

FIG. 4.5. Midesophageal two-chamber anatomic segments and perfusion. Segmental anatomy of the left ventricle in the midesophageal two-chamber view according to the American Society of Echocardiography classification system. Also depicted are the approximate perfusion zones of the left anterior descending (*LAD*) and right coronary (*RCA*) arteries. (Courtesy of M. London, M.D., http://www.ucsf.edu/teeecho) (See Color Plate 2 following page 212.)

ME views to assess the basal segments. Although this method allows visualization of at least a portion of each of the six basal segments, it is technically *incomplete* because the entire radius of each segment is not visualized. However, if these segments appear normal in the longitudinal orientation, it is likely that the remaining portion will be. It is important to remember that to obtain a "true" ME four-chamber view, one must rotate the multiplane transducer approximately 10 degrees to "remove" the anteriorly located LV outflow tract, which allows visualization of the basal septal segment.

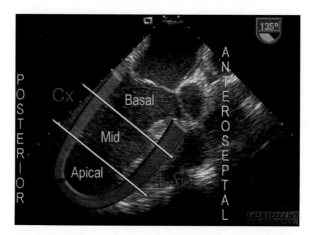

FIG. 4.6. Midesophageal long-axis anatomic segments and perfusion. Segmental anatomy of the left ventricle in the midesophageal long-axis view according to the American Society of Echocardiography classification system. Also depicted are the approximate perfusion zones of the major left anterior descending (*LAD*) and circumflex (*CX*) arteries. (Courtesy of M. London, M.D., http://www.ucsf.edu/teeecho) (See Color Plate 3 following page 212.)

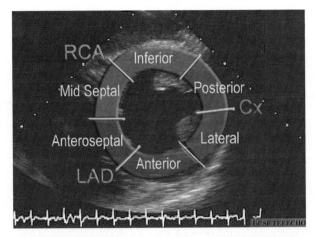

FIG. 4.7. Transgastric short-axis anatomic segments and perfusion. Segmental anatomy of the left ventricle in the transgastric short-axis view according to the American Society Echocardiography classification system. Also depicted are the approximate perfusion zones of the major left anterior descending (*LAD*), circumflex (*CX*), and right coronary (*RCA*) arteries. (Courtesy of M. London, M.D., http://www.ucsf.edu/teeecho) (See Color Plate 4 following page 212.)

Although assessing all 16 segments can be laborious for the busy clinician, it is important for the effective communication of findings.

Clinical caveat: imaging the apical segments. Recognition by the clinician that new apical RWMAs are commonly encountered in patients undergoing CABG and that complications of infarction, particularly aneurysm and thrombus formation, are commonly encountered in this region mandates careful attention to the apex during the baseline echocardiographic examination.

It is difficult to obtain a transverse apical image, although it is facilitated by retroflexion at the level of the TG short-axis view (Fig. 4.8). Thus, assessment of the apex is nearly exclusively performed with the ME longitudinal orientations. However, TEE has documented limitations for assessing the "true apex," and it is well known that TEE long-axis images can be "foreshortened," with the echo beam exiting the ventricle somewhere above the true apex (23). The ability of transthoracic echocardiography (TTE) to image the apex more reliably given the ability of the echocardiographer to move the transducer freely on the chest wall is one of the few advantages of TTE over TEE. Despite these limitations, TEE imaging of the apex can be accomplished in nearly all patients with focused effort by an experienced echocardiographer. Given that the apex is in the "far field" of the image, it is important to optimize gain/time gain compensation settings in this region. To optimize visualization of the apex, place the focal zone over the apex, select as low a frequency as is consistent with optimal resolution (usually no higher than 6 MHz), and if the ultrasound system allows, use the "zoom" feature. The TG long-axis view can be of particular value in further assessing anterior and inferior wall motion in a complementary fashion to the TG short-axis view, particularly when imaging from the ME planes is poor. However, apical imaging is not possible from this view.

Coronary artery perfusion zones. The 16-segment system was adopted by the American Society of Echocardiography in part because the coronary artery perfusion territories are relatively constant in the various segments (Figs. 4.4–4.7; see Color Plates 1–4 following page 212). One of the reasons for the popularity of the TG short-axis view (besides that it is the easiest one in which to assess intracavitary area/volume continuously) is that it is the only view in which *a portion of the territories of all three main coronary arteries perfusing the LV can be visualized.* (In the four-chamber view, right coronary perfusion of the right ventricular [RV] free wall, but not of the LV, can be assessed.) Thus, with a significant

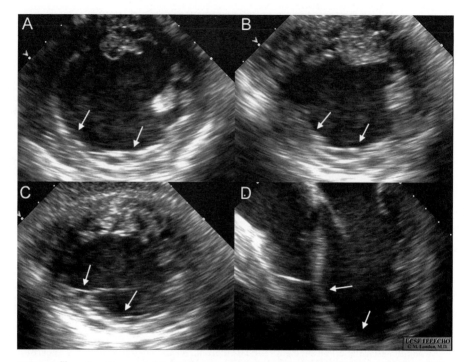

FIG. 4.8. Chronic anteroseptal infarction in multiple views. A large area of infarction in the anteroseptal region is characterized by chronic wall thinning (approximately outlined by *arrows*), and akinesis is visualized in multiple imaging planes. **A:** Basal transgastric short-axis view. **B:** Midtransgastric short-axis view. **C:** Apical transgastric short-axis view. **D:** Midesophageal four-chamber view. A "hinge point" characteristic of the junction between normal and infarcted myocardium is evident at the *top arrow* in the frame. Calcification of the anteromedial papillary muscle is also evident. (Courtesy of M. London, M.D., http://www.ucsf.edu/teeecho)

reduction in flow in one of the three main coronary arteries, one will *usually* see a new RWMA. However, if ischemia is caused by stenosis in a vessel distal to this region (i.e., perfusing the apical segments), wall motion will remain normal in the TG short-axis view, and the clinician must remain "vigilant" and use other views.

Variation in the normal coronary anatomy further complicates simple mapping of the coronary artery distributions by anatomic segments. The most important factor is the origin of the posterior descending artery from the right coronary artery in a *right-dominant system* versus its origin from the circumflex coronary artery in the less common left-dominant system. The size of the perfusion zone can vary by individual, and overlap between territories is usual, most commonly in the posterior segments and the inferoapical and lateral apical segments. The left anterior descending coronary artery usually perfuses these apical segments, although the posterior descending (inferoapical segment) or circumflex (lateral apical segment) coronary artery may also be present.

Wall motion score index. Once wall motion has been scored in each of the 16 LV segments, a global wall motion score can easily be calculated by assigning an integer score to each category of wall motion (increasing the number with increasing severity of wall motion) (13). The sum for all the segments is divided by the total number of segments visualized (with the realization that all segments may not be adequately imaged) to obtain a wall motion score index. This approach has been validated by cardiology studies comparing echo wall motion analysis with other imaging modalities, particularly thallium perfusion methods. However, given that akinesis can occur with flow reductions affecting only 25% of wall thickness, the correlation of a wall motion index with myocardial viability, particularly in acute myocardial infarction, can be variable. It is rarely if ever used by anesthesiologists, and there is no literature basis for its value in the perioperative period.

Ischemic Mitral Regurgitation

Mitral regurgitation (MR) is commonly associated with acute, severe ischemia and provides valuable information regarding its severity and, more importantly, the efficacy of therapy as it resolves. In a previously normal mitral valve, the regurgitation is central in origin and is associated with marked elevation of the pulmonary artery pressures. A variety of theories about etiologic factors have been proposed, including acute ventricular dilation leading to incomplete leaflet coaptation, ischemic dysfunction of one or both papillary muscles, and hypokinesia of the ventricular segment underlying an otherwise normally functioning papillary muscle (24). Newer studies based on three-dimensional modeling have noted acute annular enlargement with displacement of the papillary muscle tips, resulting in what is termed *loitering* (i.e., a slow response of the mitral valve leaflets to coapt properly in early systole) (25). It may occur with severe global subendocardial ischemia. *In the author's experience, MR occurs almost universally in sudden, severe intraoperative ischemia.* Thus, rapid color flow interrogation of the mitral valve should be a "second nature" maneuver for the clinician who suspects that ischemia may be present.

With myocardial infarction, additional factors contributing to MR include LV cavity and annular dilation, aneurysmal or pseudoaneurysmal changes, particularly of the basal segments, and in the most severe and life-threatening situation, papillary muscle rupture. Rupture most commonly involves the posteromedial muscle in the setting of either a right or circumflex infarction because the posteromedial papillary muscle is perfused by a single coronary artery, whereas the anteromedial papillary muscle has a dual arterial supply.

Recognizing the Complications of Myocardial Infarction

It is important to recognize the chronic manifestations and complications of myocardial infarction for the following reasons:

1. Often, the myocardial infarction will preclude monitoring for ischemia in the affected segments.
2. Certain complications, if unrecognized, can have serious or fatal consequences (e.g., mural thrombus causing a cerebrovascular accident, ruptured pseudoaneurysm causing pericardial tamponade) (Table 4.4 and Fig. 4.9).

An end-diastolic wall thickness of 0.6 cm or less has been shown to exclude the potential for recovery of function with myocardial revascularization (26). Recognition of a chronically infarcted, fibrotic, or, in the later phases, calcified segment is important to distinguish these findings from acute ischemia. However, the dyskinesis seen in these longstanding conditions does not have the ominous potential that results from acute dyskinesis (with wall thinning) in a previously normal segment, although it is obvious that the latter situation is more likely to be amenable to therapy.

Mural thrombi may pose a particular challenge because they are often difficult to appreciate on routine echocardiographic examination. The sessile, laminated thrombus that commonly occurs with a large anterior infarction may blend in with the wall. Apical thrombi are more likely to be recognized because they may present as unique shapes in the apex, occasionally as pedunculated masses. Recognition of thrombi is important because the use of an LV vent during CABG or valve surgery can dislodge thrombus, with potentially fatal consequences.

Clinical Caveats: Detection of Ischemia

Digital capture of cine loops. To monitor for RWMAs, the clinician must accurately distinguish between systole and diastole. Although this seems trivial, in fact it can be quite challenging, particularly if the patient has abnormal resting function or morphology

TABLE 4.4. COMPLICATIONS OF ACUTE MYOCARDIAL INFARCTION

Acute phase
  LV systolic dysfunction
  Rupture
    Free wall rupture
    Ventricular septal defect
    Papillary muscle rupture
    Subepicardial aneurysm
  Mitral regurgitation
    LV diltation
    Papillary muscle dysfunction
    Papillary muscle rupture
  LV thrombus
  Pericardial effusion/tamponade
  RV infarct
  LV outflow tract obstruction
Chronic phase
  Infarct expansion
  Ventricular aneurysm
    True aneurysm
    Pseudoaneurysm
  LV thrombus

LV, left ventricular; RV, right ventricular.
Adapted from Oh JK, Seward JB, Tajik AJ. *The echo manual,* 2nd ed. Philadelphia: Lippincott Williams & Wilkins, 1999:77.

(particularly LV hypertrophy) or if the ventricle is paced (as often occurs after separation from bypass) and loading conditions are markedly abnormal. Application of a three-lead ECG cable from the ultrasound machine to the patient is standard operating procedure in the echocardiography laboratory and should also be used routinely in the operating room, particularly if images are acquired digitally and displayed as "cine loops." When the capture button is pushed, digital image capture is triggered as the R wave signals the onset of systole. In the absence of an ECG R-wave trigger, a capture of 1 second or

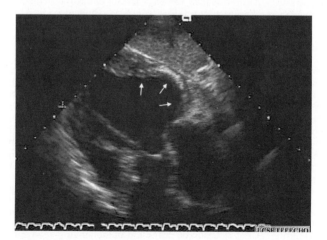

FIG. 4.9. Inferobasal aneurysm. Aneurysm (boundaries noted by *arrows*) of the inferobasal segment imaged in the transgastric long-axis view. Note the increased density of the myocardium, consistent with fibrosis. (Courtesy of M. London, M.D., http://www.ucsf.edu/teeecho)

more is acquired. Although this is more than adequate to capture several complete cardiac cycles, a lack of precise timing (i.e., onset of systole) at the start of image capture makes it difficult to play clips acquired at different time periods in a quad or split screen format *in a synchronized manner*. This makes careful comparison of loops considerably more difficult.

Imaging pitfalls. A variety of technical and patient-specific factors may complicate the detection of ischemia. The most common technical factor is endocardial "dropout," common in segments parallel to the ultrasound beam. In this situation, use of an echo "contrast agent" will in most instances precisely delineate the endocardial border. However, given the expense of these agents and storage issues, their use in the operative setting is uncommon. Foreshortening of the apex is also commonly encountered and can prevent accurate imaging of the apex. In the author's experience, with careful probe manipulation, the apex can be adequately imaged. An oblique orientation of the probe in the TG short-axis view can lead to misinterpretation of septal motion as a consequence of incorporation of a portion of the LV outflow tract into the image. This is usually easily recognized because the ventricle chamber will not be circular but oblique in shape.

Abnormal loading conditions. Common patient-specific factors include abnormal loading conditions, which at either end of the volume or pressure spectrum complicate the interpretation of RWMAs (27). With hypervolemia or an elevated afterload secondary to severe hypertension, wall motion can appear severely hypokinetic. This is usually easily recognized, especially in that all walls are affected equally and wall motion promptly returns to normal with a reduction in pressure or volume. Hypovolemia is more problematic because it accentuates any regional disparity in endocardial excursion and can cause "pseudo" dyskinetic motion in an already akinetic segment. Usually, this occurs only with gross hypovolemia. However, in a long case with major fluid shifts, clinicians may "lose" their frame of reference as to what constitutes normovolemia. Thus, a baseline image acquired shortly after the induction of anesthesia (with care taken to note any obvious loading changes during induction) is helpful when displayed alongside the later images.

Other causes of abnormal wall motion. Patients with severe LV hypertrophy are more difficult to image, and appreciating changes in wall motion is challenging. The intracavitary area may be reduced, so that the appreciation of changes in endocardial excursion becomes more difficult. In the worst-case scenario, hypertrophic cardiomyopathy, the ground glass appearance of the myocardium, greatly complicates the assessment of wall motion. Pacing of the ventricle, particularly ventricular pacing with endocardial wires during open chest cardiac procedures, can be problematic. Earlier studies suggested that septal wall motion abnormalities were particularly common in the post-CPB setting, either caused by the release of pericardial restraint or accentuated by pacing. However, in the author's clinical practice, major septal abnormalities resulting from these factors sufficiently significant to be confused with ischemia are rare.

Right Ventricular Ischemia and Infarction

The RV is a complex and important part of the heart that is often overlooked by the busy intraoperative echocardiographer. Although major abnormalities of RV function and ischemia are infrequently encountered in routine adult surgical practice, when they occur, they can be very difficult to treat. Given the anterior location of the RV in the chest and its thin walls, it is more susceptible than the LV to incomplete myocardial preservation, particularly with radiant warming during CPB. When severe RV failure occurs, as evidenced by the absence of a response to inotropic and vasodilator support, a very invasive pulmonary artery balloon pump or RV assist device may be required.

The right coronary artery perfuses most of the RV, although the conus branch of the left anterior descending artery may supply a small portion of the RV free wall (28). Patients with severe chronic obstructive pulmonary disease and coronary artery disease are particularly susceptible to RV ischemia/failure during CABG. Tricuspid regurgitation commonly accompanies RV ischemia and is severe during RV failure. The preferred imaging plane for the detection of RV ischemia is usually the ME four-chamber view, although portions of the RV can be imaged in other views, including TG planes. Gross RV dilation is common and in the absence of a major elevation of pulmonary artery pressure is usually diagnostic of RV ischemia.

CLINICAL APPLICATIONS

Use of Preoperative Data to Guide Monitoring

The clinician can tailor TEE monitoring to the particular patient by a careful consideration of the results of preoperative diagnostic testing. Obviously, careful assessment of a preoperative echocardiographic study will allow the most direct comparison of any change in the patient's state, particularly new or worsened RWMAs, worsened ventricular function, and MR. Results of a preoperative dobutamine stress test can be particularly helpful in identifying which segments are at greatest jeopardy for becoming ischemic and warrant the closest monitoring (29).

Recommendations for Monitoring

Several intraoperative factors will influence the monitoring plan for a specific patient. Patient-, clinician-, and procedure-specific variables must be considered. The availability of imaging planes based on the location of surgery, the particular patient's body habitus, and other mechanical factors clearly affect the ability to assess wall motion in all 16 segments. The level of difficulty of the surgery and the time available (or lack thereof) for the clinician to focus on the TEE images are also major factors. Given the variable impact of TEE on patient outcome during different types of surgery, the most basic recommendation is to attempt to perform as complete an examination of all segments, valvular function, and contractility as is possible under the clinical circumstances immediately after induction of anesthesia. Cardiac surgical procedures in which CPB is used usually involve additional examinations just before CPB is applied and immediately after weaning. The clinician's choice of a monitoring plane that is continuously displayed between comprehensive examinations is variable; many clinicians prefer the TG mid short-axis view, which allows a rapid estimation of cavitary area and wall motion, whereas others prefer the ME long-axis view, particularly the four- or five-chamber view, which allows continuous assessment of mitral valve structure and apical wall motion.

Primary Coronary Artery Bypass Grafting (with Cardiopulmonary Bypass)

As noted earlier, a careful assessment of wall motion is advised at several points during the procedure, although the speed at which many private surgeons operate may on occasion mandate an abbreviated examination that should focus on the individual patient's "high-risk" anatomy. Transient ischemia during CABG has numerous causes, the detection of which is greatly facilitated by the use of TEE (Table 4.5).

TABLE 4.5. CAUSES OF ACUTE ISCHEMIA DURING CORONARY ARTERY BYPASS GRAFTING

Pre-CPB ischemia
 Hemodynamic abnormalities (tachycardia, hypotension most common)
 Sudden ventricular fibrillation
 Ischemia during cannulation (hypotension most common)
 Dislodgement of atheromatous debris from previous graft (redo CABG)
Post-CPB ischemia
 Low cardiac output states
 Graft problems (intimal flap, total occlusion from thrombus, inadvertent graft into vein, graft too short or kinked during closure of chest)
 Air embolus from pooled air in cardiac apex or from pulmonary veins (most commonly right coronary distribution)
 Sudden ventricular fibrillation

CPB, cardiopulmonary bypass.

Redo Coronary Artery Bypass Grafting

Patients undergoing redo CABG are at high risk for the development of ischemia in the pre-bypass period, particularly during the manipulation of existing grafts, which can be easily damaged during dissection and are likely to contain atheromatous debris that can readily form emboli, resulting in catastrophic ischemia. Hemodynamic perturbations, particularly hypotension and tachycardia, may precipitate ischemia in the setting of multiple occluded grafts.

Off-Pump Coronary Artery Bypass

The use of OPCAB is increasing rapidly, adding new challenges to anesthetic management. TEE imaging is compromised when surgical packing is placed posteriorly and the heart is lifted to facilitate surgical exposure of the arteries (9). The best images are usually obtained during the left anterior descending artery anastomosis because only minor displacement is required. However, during circumflex and right coronary artery dissection, imaging is poor and TG planes are usually not possible. Monitoring with ME four- or two-chamber views often reveals very distorted LV anatomy but is usually the only option during this period. Fortunately, newer stabilization devices allow the elimination of posteriorly placed surgical packing and improve TEE visualization.

Because the stabilizer apparatus "tethers" the adjacent myocardium during the procedure, wall motion is usually grossly abnormal, so that analysis of regional wall motion is not reliable for detecting ischemia. Preconditioning for each of the vessels is controversial, and not all surgeons use it. For those who do use preconditioning, assessing the wall motion response (in the absence of the stabilizer) can be helpful. It is not uncommon to see new wall motion abnormalities that last for a short period of time after completion of the anastomosis, presumably caused by myocardial stunning (8). However, these should resolve relatively quickly, and if they do not, either reinspecting the anastomosis or using on-graft Doppler imaging to verify graft patency should be considered.

Transmyocardial Laser Revascularization

In this new (and controversial) procedure, a laser is used to burn approximately 1-mm trans-mural channels (approximately one channel per square centimeter) through myocardium not amenable to routine revascularization (30). The mechanism of angina relief is controversial, although some form of angioneogenesis is the leading explanation. These patients are at high risk for the development of ischemia and may have impaired ventricular function as a result of previous infarction. A complete examination of the LV segments is mandatory to monitor for ischemia. In this procedure, the echocardiographer has the important and unique responsibility of notifying the surgeon when the laser has penetrated the full thickness of the myocardium. This is easily recognized by the sudden appearance of numerous bubbles within the LV cavity (Fig. 4.10). The task is important because a burn that is too deep or too long can damage the mitral valve chordae or other valvular components. Thus, careful examination of the mitral and aortic valves by two-dimensional and color Doppler imaging before and after a series of laser treatments is mandatory.

Valve Surgery

Ischemia can develop during valve surgery secondary to either concurrent coronary artery disease or embolism. The latter is most commonly caused by air that often originates from the pulmonary veins or cardiac apex (31). Because the anteriorly located ostia of the right coronary artery is at a 90-degree angle to the aortic root, air exiting the ventricle in large quantities can cause clinically significant ischemia in this distribution. Prompt recognition of coronary air embolism is important because it can be easily treated by "blowing the air through" and using high doses of phenylephrine or returning to CPB. Ischemia can also be

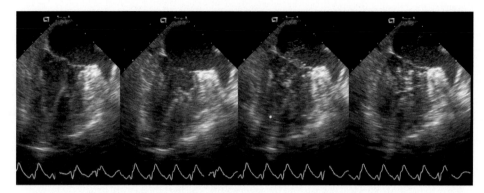

FIG. 4.10. Sequential image frames from a transmyocardial laser revascularization procedure illustrating penetration of the laser beam into the left ventricle, evidenced by microbubbles at the point of entrance in the basal portion of the anterior wall (midesophageal two-chamber view). Note the temporary current of injury on the electrocardiogram. (Courtesy of M. London, M.D., http://www.ucsf.edu/teeecho)

caused by subendocardial hypoperfusion during low cardiac output states following a technically difficult valve repair/replacement requiring a very long pump run or a failed repair.

SUMMARY

The detection of myocardial ischemia is an important priority for the practicing clinician, especially as our population ages and the incidence of coronary artery disease increases. A clinically based framework for the anatomic, physiologic, technical, and procedure-specific factors involved in ischemia has been presented here. These are only the basics, and with the increasing sophistication of echocardiographic technology (particularly applications of integrated backscatter technology and tissue Doppler imaging), the methods will undergo further refinement. It is likely that newer technology will facilitate capture of the earliest presentations of ischemia, a scenario that ultimately should enhance patient outcome.

REFERENCES

1. Savage RM, Lytle BW, Aronson S, et al. Intraoperative echocardiography is indicated in high-risk coronary artery bypass grafting. *Ann Thorac Surg* 1997;64:368–373; discussion 373–374.
2. Kloner RA, Jennings RB. Consequences of brief ischemia: stunning, preconditioning, and their clinical implications: part 1. *Circulation* 2001;104:2981–2989.
3. Kloner RA, Jennings RB. Consequences of brief ischemia: stunning, preconditioning, and their clinical implications: part 2. *Circulation* 2001;104:3158–3167.
4. London MJ, Tubau JF, Wong MG, et al. The natural history of segmental wall motion abnormalities in patients undergoing noncardiac surgery. S.P.I. Research Group. *Anesthesiology* 1990;73:644–655.
5. Dodds TM, Burns AK, DeRoo DB, et al. Effects of anesthetic technique on myocardial wall motion abnormalities during abdominal aortic surgery. *J Cardiothorac Vasc Anesth* 1997;11:129–136.
6. Morewood GH, Gallagher ME, Gaughan JP, et al. Current practice patterns for adult perioperative transesophageal echocardiography in the United States. *Anesthesiology* 2001;95:1507–1512.

7. Eagle KA, Guyton RA, Davidoff R, et al. ACC/AHA guidelines for coronary artery bypass graft surgery: executive summary and recommendations: a report of the American College of Cardiology/American Heart Association Task Force on Practice Guidelines (committee to revise the 1991 guidelines for coronary artery bypass graft surgery). *Circulation* 1999;100:1464–1480.

8. Malkowski MJ, Kramer CM, Parvizi ST, et al. Transient ischemia does not limit subsequent ischemic regional dysfunction in humans: a transesophageal echocardiographic study during minimally invasive coronary artery bypass surgery. *J Am Coll Cardiol* 1998;31:1035–1039.

9. Mathison M, Edgerton JR, Horswell JL, et al. Analysis of hemodynamic changes during beating heart surgical procedures. *Ann Thorac Surg* 2000;70:1355–1360.

10. Anonymous. Practice guidelines for perioperative transesophageal echocardiography. A report by the American Society of Anesthesiologists and the Society of Cardiovascular Anesthesiologists Task Force on Transesophageal Echocardiography. *Anesthesiology* 1996;84:986–1006.

11. London MJ, Kaplan JA. Advances in electrocardiographic monitoring. In: Kaplan JA, Reich DL, Konstadt SN, eds. *Cardiac anesthesia,* 4th ed. Philadelphia: WB Saunders, 1999:359–400.

12. Gallagher KP, Kumada T, Koziol JA, et al. Significance of regional wall thickening abnormalities relative to transmural myocardial perfusion in anesthetized dogs. *Circulation* 1980;62:1266–1274.

13. Schiller NB, Shah PM, Crawford M, et al. Recommendations for quantitation of the left ventricle by two-dimensional echocardiography. American Society of Echocardiography Committee on Standards, Subcommittee on Quantitation of Two-Dimensional Echocardiograms. *J Am Soc Echocardiogr* 1989;2:358–367.

14. Koch R, Lang RM, Garcia MJ, et al. Objective evaluation of regional left ventricular wall motion during dobutamine stress echocardiographic studies using segmental analysis of color kinesis images. *J Am Coll Cardiol* 1999;34:409–419.

15. Buda AJ, Zotz RJ, Pace DP, et al. Comparison of two-dimensional echocardiographic wall motion and wall thickening abnormalities in relation to the myocardium at risk. *Am Heart J* 1986;111:587–592.

16. Homans DC, Asinger R, Elsperger KJ, et al. Regional function and perfusion at the lateral border of ischemic myocardium. *Circulation* 1985;71:1038–1047.

17. Pandian NG, Skorton DJ, Collins SM, et al. Heterogeneity of left ventricular segmental wall thickening and excursion in two-dimensional echocardiograms of normal human subjects. *Am J Cardiol* 1983;51:1667–1673.

18. Lieberman AN, Weiss JL, Jugdutt BI, et al. Two-dimensional echocardiography and infarct size: relationship of regional wall motion and thickening to the extent of myocardial infarction in the dog. *Circulation* 1981;63:739–746.

19. Oh JK, Seward JB, Tajik AJ. Stress echocardiography. In: *The echo manual,* 2nd ed. Philadelphia: Lippincott Williams & Wilkins, 1999:91–101.

20. Lualdi JC, Douglas PS. Echocardiography for the assessment of myocardial viability. *J Am Soc Echocardiogr* 1997;10:772–780.

21. Aronson S, Dupont F, Savage R, et al. Changes in regional myocardial function after coronary artery bypass graft surgery are predicted by intraoperative low-dose dobutamine echocardiography. *Anesthesiology* 2000;93:685–692.

22. Shanewise JS, Cheung AT, Aronson S, et al. ASE/SCA guidelines for performing a comprehensive intraoperative multiplane transesophageal echocardiography examination: recommendations of the American Society of Echocardiography Council for Intraoperative Echocardiography and the Society of Cardiovascular Anesthesiologists Task Force for Certification in Perioperative Transesophageal Echocardiography. *Anesth Analg* 1999;89:870–884.

23. Smith MD, MacPhail B, Harrison MR, et al. Value and limitations of transesophageal echocardiography in determination of left ventricular volumes and ejection fraction. *J Am Coll Cardiol* 1992;19:1213–1222.

24. Kono T, Sabbah HN, Rosman H, et al. Mechanism of functional mitral regurgitation during acute myocardial ischemia. *J Am Coll Cardiol* 1992;19:1101–1105.

25. Glasson JR, Komeda M, Daughters GT, et al. Early systolic mitral leaflet "loitering"

during acute ischemic mitral regurgitation. *J Thorac Cardiovasc Surg* 1998;116:193–205.

26. Cwajg JM, Cwajg E, Nagueh SF, et al. End-diastolic wall thickness as a predictor of recovery of function in myocardial hibernation: relation to rest-redistribution Tl-201 tomography and dobutamine stress echocardiography. *J Am Coll Cardiol* 2000;35:1152–1161.

27. Seeberger MD, Cahalan MK, Rouine-Rapp K, et al. Acute hypovolemia may cause segmental wall motion abnormalities in the absence of myocardial ischemia. *Anesth Analg* 1997;85:1252–1257.

28. Bowers TR, O'Neill WW, Grines C, et al. Effect of reperfusion on biventricular function and survival after right ventricular infarction. *N Engl J Med* 1998;338:933–940.

29. Boersma E, Poldermans D, Bax JJ, et al. Predictors of cardiac events after major vascular surgery: role of clinical characteristics, dobutamine echocardiography, and beta-blocker therapy. *JAMA* 2001;285:1865–1873.

30. Lee LY, O'Hara MF, Finnin EB, et al. Transmyocardial laser revascularization with excimer laser: clinical results at 1 year. *Ann Thorac Surg* 2000;70:498–503.

31. Orihashi K, Matsuura Y, Sueda T, et al. Pooled air in open heart operations examined by transesophageal echocardiography. *Ann Thorac Surg* 1996;61:1377–1180.

QUESTIONS

1. TEE is useful in OPCAB for
   a. Evaluating the adequacy of the coronary anastomosis
   b. Evaluating the ability of the patient to tolerate vessel occlusion
   c. Evaluating the hemodynamic consequences of cardiac displacement
   d. All of the above
2. The most sensitive TEE indicator of myocardial ischemia is
   a. A reduction of systolic wall thickening
   b. The presence of systolic wall thinning
   c. A reduction in endocardial excursion
   d. The presence of compensatory hyperkinesis
3. Which of the following statements is false regarding dobutamine stress echo testing?
   a. Low doses will cause normal myocardium to become hyperkinetic.
   b. New-onset hypokinesis indicates myocardial ischemia.
   c. A biphasic response with improvement at low doses and deterioration at higher doses of dobutamine is termed *stunned myocardium*.
   d. A chronic transmural infarction will show no response to low-dose dobutamine.
4. All of the following statements are true regarding digital cine loops **except**
   a. ECG monitoring from the echocardiographic machine should be standard practice.
   b. The cine loop captures off the P wave.
   c. In the absence of an ECG tracing, a capture of 1 second or more is acquired.
   d. Ventricular systole is more difficult to determine with paced rhythms.
5. The 16-segment model for assessing wall motion adopted by the American Society of Echocardiography/Society of Cardiovascular Anesthesiologists requires evaluation of all the following views **except**
   a. ME four-chamber
   b. ME two-chamber
   c. ME long-axis
   d. TG basal short-axis
   e. TG mid short-axis
6. All of the following "tricks" are helpful in attempting to visualize the LV apex **except**
   a. Retroflexion at the level of the TG short-axis view
   b. Optimizing far field gain and time gain compensation settings
   c. Moving the focal zone over the apex
   d. Maximally increasing the frequency of the transducer in the midesophageal four-chamber view

7. The TG mid short-axis view is commonly used for monitoring during CABG surgery because
   a. Changes in intracavitary volume are easily determined
   b. Territories of all three main coronary arteries perfusing the LV are visualized
   c. The papillary muscles serve as a useful reference point to ensure that the same territory is being evaluated
   d. All of the above
8. All of the following are common imaging pitfalls in attempting to diagnose myocardial ischemia with TEE **except**
   a. Endocardial dropout
   b. Images of poor quality
   c. Oblique orientation of the TG mid short-axis view
   d. Foreshortening of the apex
9. The following may be associated with wall motion abnormalities:
   a. Hypervolemia
   b. Hypovolemia
   c. Hypertrophic cardiomyopathy
   d. Ventricular pacing
   e. All of the above
10. Chronic ischemic MR is postulated to occur through all the following mechanisms **except**
    a. Ventricular dilation with incomplete leaflet coaptation
    b. Papillary muscle rupture
    c. Ischemic dysfunction of one or both papillary muscles
    d. Hypokinesis of the ventricular segment underlying a normal papillary muscle

PART II

ESSENTIALS OF DOPPLER ECHOCARDIOGRAPHY

Doppler Technology and Technique

Albert C. Perrino, Jr.

The high-resolution display of cardiac structures in motion obtained with two-dimensional echocardiography is remarkable. Yet despite the ability to reveal the most intricate anatomic detail, two-dimensional imaging is unable to visualize blood flow. Blood flow in cardiac chambers and the great vessels is simply presented in black on the two-dimensional display. Because the movement of blood is the *raison d'être* of the cardiovascular system, this limitation presents a serious challenge to the diagnostic capability of echocardiography. Doppler ultrasound overcomes this limitation in the assessment of blood flow. Its color flow display affords the echocardiographer dramatic views of blood flow. Additionally, spectral Doppler provides the tools to quantify the magnitude and direction of flow. Because Doppler evaluation is quantitative, it provides a means of grading the severity of disease in many cases in which two-dimensional echocardiography merely demonstrates the presence of an abnormality. As such, mastery of Doppler examinations is a critical element in the training of a perioperative echocardiographer.

DOPPLER FREQUENCY SHIFT

Doppler examinations are based on principles fundamentally different from those underlying two-dimensional imaging. As is addressed in the sections that follow, these differences necessitate altered approaches and techniques when Doppler examinations are performed. Many times, the required view and imaging frequencies are contrary to those selected for two-dimensional imaging of the same anatomic region. To obtain an optimal assessment of both the form and function of the desired cardiac structure, it is essential to remain cognizant of the underlying physical principles of the two approaches and how they differ.

The Doppler Effect

As explained in Chapter 1, two-dimensional imaging is based on the intensity and time delay of reflected ultrasound. *To determine the velocity of blood flow, Doppler systems examine the change in frequency of the ultrasound reflected from red blood cells.* Our ability to use the movement of red blood cells to gauge blood flow velocity dates back to the experiments of the Austrian physicist Christian Doppler. So that the effects of motion on sound frequency could be examined, trumpeters on a high-speed locomotive played a tone at a specific pitch. A second group of musicians stationed on a loading dock played the same tone as the train passed by. As Doppler had predicted, the two tones were audibly different. The change in pitch, known as the *Doppler effect,* occurs because the motion of an object causes the sound wave to be compressed in the direction of the motion and expanded in the direction opposite to the motion.

Signal Frequency and Blood Flow

Red blood cells reflect ultrasound as they travel through the blood stream. By directing an ultrasound signal at flowing blood and listening for the change in frequency produced by the red cell reflections, Doppler echocardiography can assess the direction and speed of blood flow.

Figure 5.1 illustrates the principle of the Doppler effect for cardiac applications. When ultrasound is transmitted to blood, it is scattered by the multitude of red blood cells, and a small portion of this scattering is reflected back toward the transducer. The strength of the echoes returning to the transducer is related to the number of particles reflecting the

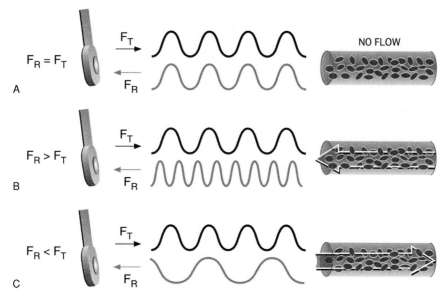

FIG. 5.1. Detecting blood flow: effects of red cell motion on ultrasound frequency. The motion of an object alters the frequency of a reflected ultrasound signal. **A:** The reflected echoes from a stationary target are of the same frequency as the transmitted signal. **B:** Objects such as red blood cells moving toward the transducer compress the sound signal, and the reflected frequency is increased. **C:** When red cells travel away for the transducer, the frequency of the reflected echoes is decreased. These modulations in the frequency of the reflected ultrasound are used to detect blood flow.

ultrasound. If the hematocrit is increased, more interfaces are available for reflection and the ultrasound signal is stronger. However, this effect is self-limited because at a hematocrit exceeding 30%, the reflected signal strength is weakened by destructive interference. Modern echocardiography systems are designed to detect Doppler signals over a wide range of hematocrit values.

If the red cells are stationary, the signal is reflected at the same frequency as the transmitted signal. Because no Doppler frequency shift occurs, the situation is similar to that of two-dimensional echocardiography. When blood flows toward the ultrasound transducer, the reflected signal is compressed by the motion of the red cells, and its frequency is higher than that of the transmitted signal. Conversely, when blood flows away from the ultrasound transducer, the frequency of the reflected signal received by the transducer is lower than that of the transmitted signal. The technical term for the alterations in the frequency of the ultrasound signals caused by the Doppler effect is *modulation*. Through analysis of the modulated signal, both the direction and speed of the red blood cells can be determined.

DOPPLER ANALYSIS

The Doppler Equation: Linking the Frequency Shift to Velocity

The *Doppler equation* describes the relationship between the alteration in ultrasound frequency and blood flow velocity (Fig. 5.2):

$$\Delta f = v \times \cos\theta \times 2f_t/c$$

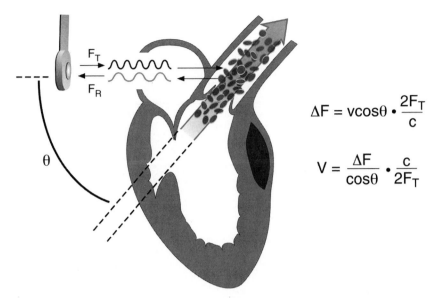

$$\Delta F = v\cos\theta \cdot \frac{2F_T}{c}$$

$$V = \frac{\Delta F}{\cos\theta} \cdot \frac{c}{2F_T}$$

FIG. 5.2. Calculating blood flow velocity: the Doppler equation. The Doppler equation calculates blood flow velocity based on two variables: the Doppler frequency shift (ΔF) and the cosine of the angle of incidence between the ultrasound beam and the blood flow. The Doppler frequency shift is measured by the echocardiographic system, but $\cos\theta$ is unknown, and manual entry by the echocardiographer is required for its estimation. V, blood flow velocity; F_T, transmitted signal frequency; F_R, reflected signal frequency; ΔF, difference between F_R and F_T; c, speed of sound in tissue; θ, angle of incidence between the orientation of the ultrasound beam and that of the blood flow.

where Δf is the difference between transmitted frequency (f_t) and received frequency, v is blood velocity, c is the speed of sound in blood (1,540 m/s), and θ is the angle of incidence between the ultrasound beam and blood flow.

Conceptually, the equation can be simplified based on the observation that the change in ultrasound frequency is directly related to just two variables: blood velocity and $\cos\theta$. The remaining factors in the equation, the speed of sound in blood (c) and the transmitted frequency (f_t), are constants. The Doppler signal is shifted only by the component of the blood velocity that is in the direction of the beam path (i.e., $v\cos\theta$). For example, when the direction of the ultrasound beam is parallel to the blood flow, the observed Δf fully reflects total blood velocity ($\cos\theta = 1$). With nonparallel orientation of the ultrasound beam to blood flow, Δf is reduced by the factor $\cos\theta$. As illustrated in Figure 5.3, when the beam angle divergence is small, the effects on Δf are limited. However, *with angles greater than 30 degrees, the value of $\cos\theta$ decreases rapidly*. When the direction of the beam is perpendicular to the blood flow (90 degrees, $\cos 90 = 0$), the movement of blood is no longer appreciated by the Doppler system ($\Delta f = 0$).

Implications of Beam Orientation

The effect of the beam angle on Doppler measurements has important clinical implications. In clinical practice, the ultrasound system measures the frequency shift to calculate velocity. By rearranging the Doppler equation, the calculated blood velocity is derived as follows:

$$v = \Delta f / \cos\theta \times c/2f_t$$

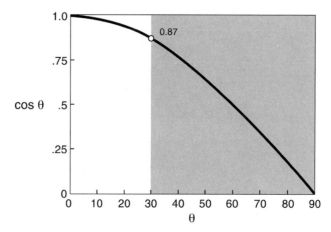

FIG. 5.3. Cosine relationship. Most devices default to a simplified Doppler equation in which cos θ is ignored, with the assumption that the Doppler beam is nearly parallel to the blood flow so that the cos θ factor is negligible. However, at angles between beam and blood flow greater than 30 degrees, a precipitous drop in the cosine curve results in a substantial underestimation of blood flow velocity.

The angle of incidence between the beam and the blood flow is not easily determined. Although a two-dimensional image of the blood vessel allows the echocardiographer to estimate the angle in the x- and y-planes, the orientation in the z-plane remains indeterminate. Assessment of the interrogation angle is further complicated by eccentrically directed blood flow, as in mitral regurgitation. Most Doppler systems default to a value of cos θ of 1, with the assumption that the echocardiographer has directed the ultrasound beam to be nearly parallel with the blood flow of interest. This approach has the advantages of stronger Doppler signals and a lower rate of errors as a consequence of the plateau shape of the cosine curve at angles of low incidence. Thus, in clinical practice, the transducer should be positioned such that the beam and blood flow are nearly parallel for accurate velocity calculations. Figure 5.3 illustrates the basis for the clinical practice of requiring the beam angle to be within 30 degrees of the direction of blood flow, so that the rate of angle-related errors remains less than 15%. The assumption that the orientation of the ultrasound beam is parallel to the blood flow leads to a common error in Doppler velocity calculations. *Because of the shape of the cosine curve, when the incident angle between the beam and the blood flow is greater than 30 degrees, the blood flow is markedly underestimated* (Fig. 5.4). However, even the 30-degree standard may not be acceptable in certain conditions. For example, when very high velocities are interrogated, as in aortic stenosis, even a 15% underestimation will correspond to a large difference in velocity and may result in an underestimation of the severity of aortic stenosis.

Clinical Caveats in Transesophageal Echocardiographic Doppler Examinations

1. Positioning the transesophageal echocardiography (TEE) probe so that the orientation of the Doppler beam is parallel to the blood flow is often a significant challenge. Unlike the position of a transthoracic probe, which can be moved freely about the chest wall to achieve proper orientation, the position of the TEE probe is limited to the confines of the esophagus and stomach.

2. The standard views used for two-dimensional imaging are often inadequate for Doppler assessments. Optimal two-dimensional images are obtained by directing the beam perpendicular to the structure of interest to obtain strong, mirrorlike reflections. Paradoxically, Doppler measurements are best obtained when the beam is parallel to the blood flow to avoid

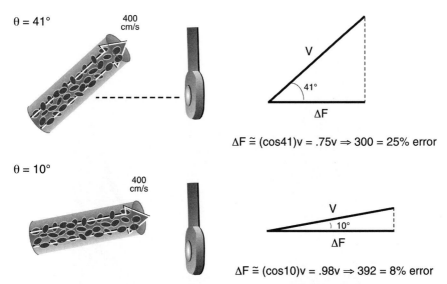

$\Delta F \cong (\cos 41)v = .75v \Rightarrow 300 = 25\%$ error

$\Delta F \cong (\cos 10)v = .98v \Rightarrow 392 = 8\%$ error

FIG. 5.4. Underestimation of blood flow velocity with nonparallel beam orientation. **Top:** With an angle of 41 degrees, the vector component of blood flow velocity in the direction of the ultrasound beam is only 75% of the total. Thus, a velocity estimation based on ΔF alone will lead to a clinically unacceptable underestimation of the true blood flow velocity of 25%. **Bottom:** With an angle of 10 degrees, the vector component of blood flow velocity in the direction of the ultrasound beam is 92%, and the practice of ignoring the $\cos \theta$ leads to a clinically acceptable 8% underestimation of velocity.

underestimates of blood flow velocity. The view that provides the best two-dimensional image of a structure typically provides only limited flow information and can result in a failure to detect abnormal flow. Figure 5.5 illustrates the application of this principle in examining the aortic valve.

Isolating the Doppler Frequency Shift

For the Doppler system to determine the frequency shift caused by red blood cells, it must first distinguish red cell–modulated echoes from all the other non–frequency-shifted echoes created by reflections from tissue (Fig. 5.6). This *demodulation process* is often accomplished by comparing the returning echoes with internal reference signals that are in phase and 90 degrees out of phase with the transmitted signal, a process known as *quadrature demodulation*. Once the Doppler signal has been isolated, its frequency content can then be determined by means of the *fast Fourier transform* technique. This approach transforms the demodulated Doppler signal into its individual frequency components. The process is analogous to identifying the individual harmonics that comprise a musical chord. At each time point, the analysis provides the range of frequencies (i.e., velocities) detected and their magnitude (i.e., the number of red cells moving at this speed).

PRESENTATION OF DOPPLER DATA

Audible Broadcast

Blood flow in the heart and great vessels creates a Doppler frequency shift in the kiloHertz range, with a high-velocity aortic stenotic jet generating a Doppler frequency shift in the

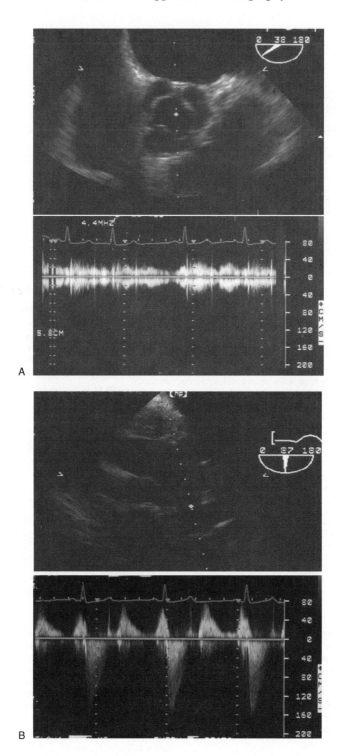

order of 20 kHz. Because these frequencies are within the audible range, most echocardiography machines provide a sound system that amplifies and broadcasts the signal to the operator. *By listening to the loudness and pitch of the broadcast Doppler frequencies, the echocardiographer can precisely position the Doppler beam to interrogate the desired flow signal.* Typically, the ideal location is identified when the signal reaches its highest frequency and greatest loudness. Soft, low-decibel signals indicate that the Doppler beam is misdirected and is only glancing a small part of the blood flow. In addition, the texture and pitch of the Doppler signal are useful in diagnosis. For example, when transvalvular flow across the aortic valve is examined, a coarse, high-pitched signal is diagnostic of a high-velocity, turbulent jet caused by aortic stenosis and contrasts markedly with the smooth-sounding, low-pitched signals generated by the laminar flow in a normal aortic valve. The ability to use the audible Doppler signal to guide beam positioning is a favored technique of experienced echocardiographers, and development of this skill remains a goal for all trainees.

Spectral Display

Presenting Doppler data as a time-velocity plot is known as a *spectral display* (Fig. 5.7). At each point in time, the spectrum of velocities detected by the Fourier transformation are displayed. Frequencies with greater amplitude (loudness) are marked with brighter pixels. The excellent temporal resolution of the spectral display allows beat-to-beat assessment of blood flow and is the basis for the quantitative calculations of cardiovascular hemodynamics. Measurement of peak velocity, acceleration ($\Delta v/\Delta t$), and the time-velocity integral (represented by the area under the velocity-time plot from a single cardiac cycle) are examples of the many important measurements that are easily obtained from the spectral display (see Chapter 6 for a detailed examination of the use of these measurements in clinical echocardiography.)

Despite the ease with which velocity measurements are made from the spectral display, vigilance is required on the part of the echocardiographer. The measurements will be accurate only when the underlying principles of good Doppler technique have been followed. First, the Doppler beam must be properly positioned to interrogate the targeted blood flow. For example, small alterations in beam position determine whether the displayed spectral velocities represent a targeted high-frequency jet of mitral stenosis or the lower blood flow velocities found along its perimeter. Second, the direction of the Doppler beam must be parallel to the path of the targeted blood flow. Errors in diagnosis are often related to failure to meet these essential requirements.

Poor ultrasound technique can often be detected by an examination of the spectral display. High-quality signals result in a pattern commonly referred to as a *clean envelope,* denoted by a sharply demarcated border, bright pixels, and clear peaks. When these features are lacking, the echocardiographer should be reluctant to accept the data from the spectral display and improve the Doppler signal through alterations in probe position or imaging view (Fig. 5.8). Inexplicably, seemingly minor alterations can resolve difficulties in obtaining a flow signal. In this regard, there is no substitute for perseverance and experience.

FIG. 5.5. Comparison of views selected for two-dimensional imaging versus Doppler flow measurement. **A:** Two-dimensional echocardiography from the midesophageal aortic valve short-axis view (**top**) provides high-fidelity images of the valve leaflets and their excursion. Because the direction of blood flow is orthogonal to the ultrasound beam in this view, the continuous wave Doppler measurement of blood flow velocity (**bottom**) will substantially underestimate blood flow velocity. **B:** After repositioning of the probe to obtain the transgastric long-axis view (**top**), the direction of the ultrasound beam is parallel to the left ventricular outflow tract and ascending aorta, providing excellent continuous wave measurements of blood flow velocity (**bottom**).

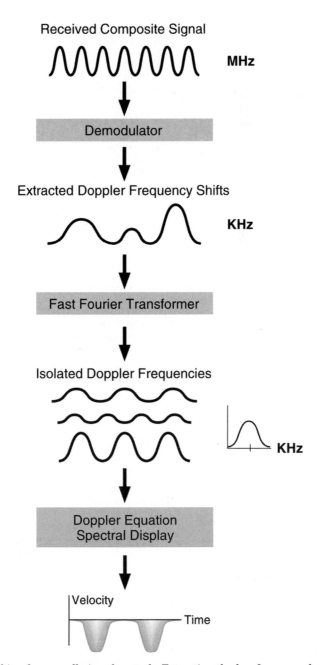

FIG. 5.6. Looking for a needle in a haystack. Extracting the low-frequency, low-amplitude Doppler signal for the received composite signal is a technical challenge requiring several procedures, including demodulation and fast Fourier transform. Once isolated, the Doppler frequencies can be analyzed and displayed.

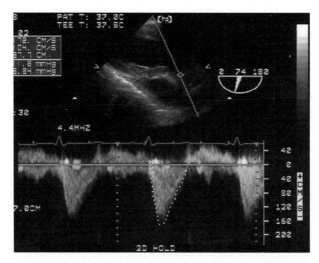

FIG. 5.7. Doppler spectral display. Blood flow through the left ventricular outflow tract and aorta is captured by using continuous wave Doppler directed from the transgastric long-axis view. This time-velocity display shows the Doppler-calculated velocities on the x-axis, with flow toward the transducer as positive deflections and flow away from the transducer as negative deflections. Planimetry of the velocity waveform has been performed by the operator, and the machine's analysis package calculates the velocity-time integral and the mean and peak flow velocities.

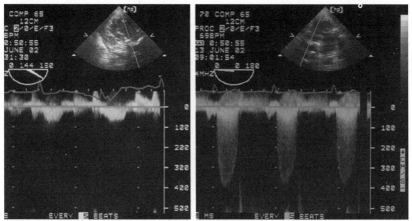

FIG. 5.8. Hunting for the jet core. **A:** Despite high-quality two-dimensional imaging of the transgastric long-axis view, Doppler interrogation of the transvalvular flow fails to detect the high-velocity flow of aortic stenosis. The wispy signal waveform provides no clear definition of peak velocities. **B:** After adjustment of the probe position to obtain the deep transgastric long-axis view, the resulting Doppler interrogation detects a 400-cm/s high-velocity jet, revealing aortic stenosis. Note the potential for misdiagnosis if the echocardiographer bases the diagnosis on the initial signal obtained in **A.**

DOPPLER TECHNIQUES

Two Doppler techniques, *pulsed wave* and *continuous wave,* are commonly used to evaluate blood flow. A thorough understanding of the advantages and disadvantages of each technique is critical in selecting the one most appropriate for the clinical setting at hand.

In clinical practice, pulsed wave and continuous wave Doppler are frequently used in conjunction with two-dimensional imaging. The two-dimensional image is used to identify the area of interest and guide the echocardiographer in precisely localizing the sampling volume in a pulsed wave study or in directing the beam in a continuous wave study.

Pulsed Wave Doppler

The pulsed wave transducer uses a single crystal as both the emitter and the receiver of ultrasound waves. Like the pulsed echo system described for two-dimensional imaging, the pulsed wave Doppler system transmits a short burst of ultrasound toward the target and then switches to receive mode to interpret the returning echoes. Because the speed of sound (c) in tissue is constant, the time delay for a signal to reach its target and return to the transducer depends solely on the distance (d) to the target:

$$\text{Time delay} = 2d/c$$

Consequently, reflected signals from locations more distant from the transducer return after a greater time interval. The electronic circuitry of the pulsed wave transducer interprets returning echoes only after a predetermined time period has elapsed since the transmission of an ultrasound pulse. In this way, only those signals associated with a specific depth or location are selected for evaluation, a process known as *time gating.* It is important to remember that the transducer transmits a three-dimensional beam. Thus, the small portion of reflected sound accepted by the time-gating process corresponds to a volume of blood at a specific location, called the *sample volume.* The pulse length, which equals the product of the wavelength and the number of cycles contained in each sound pulse, determines the length of the sample volume. The width and height of the sample volume are related to the transducer size, signal frequency, and beam focus.

Clinical caveats for pulsed wave Doppler. Because red cells scatter the ultrasound signal, the reflected Doppler signal returning to the transducer represents only a fraction of the transmitted signal. Thus, the returning signal is much weaker than the strong specular reflections from tissue interfaces. Accordingly, the clinician faces a tradeoff between good range resolution (i.e., a small sample length) and an accurate determination of velocity. *In contrast to the preferred settings in two-dimensional echocardiography, in which axial resolution is a priority and the pulse length is kept very short, large Doppler sample volumes (length >10 mm) are preferred by most echocardiographers to improve the accuracy of the velocity measurement because they provide more wavelength for demodulation.* A more powerful Doppler signal is produced because the signal-to-noise ratio is increased.

In summary, pulsed wave Doppler allows the echocardiographer to select both the location and dimensions of the sample volume to determine blood flow velocity at a discrete location. The ability to select a sample volume from which to record blood velocities was a major advancement in the diagnostic capability of echocardiography.

Pulsed wave Doppler system processing. The pulsed Doppler system uses a repeating pattern of ultrasound transmission and reception. After producing a short burst of ultrasound, it waits for a period of time, proportional to the selected distance, to receive the signal from the sample volume. The transducer then sends another burst of ultrasound, waits and receives, and so on. The rate at which the device repeatedly generates sound bursts is known as the *pulse repetition frequency.* The longer the pulsed wave system waits for the returning echoes, the lower the pulse repetition frequency. Because the speed of sound through tissue is a constant, the pulse repetition frequency is directly related to the depth of the sample volume. The pulse repetition frequency is analogous to the frame rate of a movie camera. Like the multiple frames on a roll of movie film, each ultrasound pulse interacts with the blood flow for a brief period of time, and just as a series of movie frames display motion, a series of pulsed cycles are consecutively analyzed to determine the blood flow. The demodulation process examines the returning echoes from a series of pulses to determine the Doppler frequency shift and calculate blood flow velocity.

Limitations of pulsed wave Doppler. Because the Doppler data are collected intermittently, the maximal frequency and blood flow velocity that can be accurately measured by pulsed wave Doppler are limited. The maximal frequency, which equals one-half the pulse repetition frequency, is known as the *Nyquist limit.* Figure 5.9 illustrates the principle of the Nyquist limit with the example of an orbiting comet. A similar effect is seen in movie animation, in which a rapidly spinning wheel appears to spin backward because of the slow frame rate. At Doppler shifts above the Nyquist limit, analysis of the returning signal becomes ambiguous, so that the velocity is indeterminate. This ambiguous signal for frequencies above the Nyquist limit, known as *aliasing,* appears on the spectral display as a signal on the other side of the baseline, often referred to as *wraparound* (Fig. 5.10). The intermittent sampling of the pulsed system can resolve only frequencies that are less than half the pulse repetition rate.

Maximizing pulsed wave velocity measurements. The echocardiographer has several techniques available to maximize the velocity performance of a pulsed wave system:

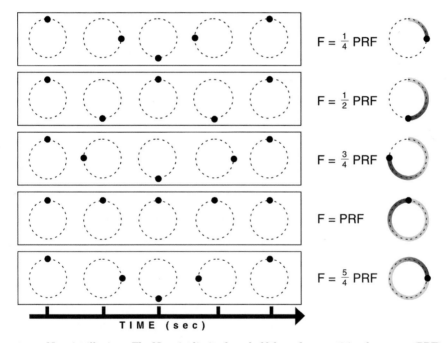

FIG. 5.9. Nyquist illusions. The Nyquist limit of one-half the pulse repetition frequency (PRF) applies to any system based on intermittent observation. In this illustration, the position of the orbiting comet at each observation point is displayed. The orbiting velocity of the comet is progressively increased from the top to the bottom rows. At the low orbiting velocity of one-fourth the pulse repetition frequency, the serial observations properly portray the comet as moving in a clockwise direction. As the speed of the comet is increased so that its orbiting velocity is three-fourths the pulse repetition frequency, it appears to be traveling counterclockwise. It appears to be moving not at all when its orbiting velocity equals the pulse repetition frequency. At five-fourths the pulse repetition frequency, it appears to be orbiting at the same speed as when it was traveling at the much slower speed of one-fourth the pulse repetition frequency.

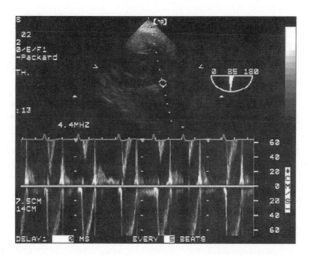

FIG. 5.10. Alias artifact. Alias artifact appears once velocities exceed the Nyquist limit. In this example, the pulsed wave Doppler sample volume is located in the left ventricular outflow tract, and when the peak velocities of the spectral signal exceed 70 cm/s, aliasing occurs and they appear on the opposite side of the baseline, a condition known as *wraparound*.

1. The first clinical principle is to select the view that places the transducer closest to the sample volume. Lessening the target distance increases the pulse repetition frequency, thus increasing the velocity that can be assessed.
2. The second clinical principle is to select a low transmitted frequency. The lower transmitted frequency has two major advantages:
   a. The modulated echo (f_r) will be of a lower frequency for any given blood velocity because $f_r = f_t + \Delta f$. Therefore, increased velocities can be measured without the aliasing that would be caused by a Doppler signal with a higher transmitted frequency.
   b. Lower frequencies provide a stronger signal because they are less attenuated by tissue. This is important because Doppler signals are much weaker than those used for imaging. Figure 5.11 illustrates the importance of target distance and transmitted frequency to the velocity performance of a Doppler system.
3. The third clinical principle is to set the baseline of the spectral display to provide the greatest range of velocities in the direction of interest. Figure 5.12 illustrates the practical implications of baseline adjustment.

Echocardiography technology has also tried to address the velocity limitation of pulsed wave Doppler systems with the development of *high-frequency pulsed Doppler*. This approach sacrifices some of the spatial resolution of the pulsed wave system in exchange for the ability to measure significantly faster flows. The principle of high-frequency pulsed Doppler is to emit a second or third pulse signal before the first signal has returned. In this way, the pulse repetition frequency is doubled or tripled, and it becomes possible to calculate a greater maximal velocity. However, with high-frequency pulsed Doppler, the operator cannot be sure that the reflected echoes have come from the intended target rather than from other targets located more proximally.

Despite technologic advancements, the Nyquist limit remains a major impediment to the measurement of high-velocity blood flows, such as those across stenotic valves and in congenital cardiac lesions, with pulsed wave Doppler. This limitation has led to an alternative approach for the Doppler assessment of high-velocity blood flows, which is continuous wave Doppler.

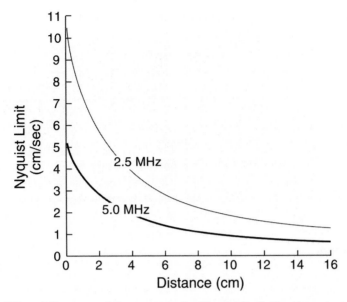

FIG. 5.11. Effect of distance and frequency on the Nyquist limit. Two important variables under the echocardiographer's control that can be used to minimize the potential for aliasing in Doppler signals are target distance and transmitted frequency. As the transducer is moved closer to the target or the transmitted frequency is lowered, the pulsed wave Nyquist limit rises substantially, allowing higher-velocity signals to be measured accurately.

Continuous Wave Doppler

The continuous wave Doppler technique avoids the maximal velocity limitation of pulsed wave systems. The transducer of a continuous wave system is composed of two crystals, one continuously transmitting and the other continuously receiving the reflected ultrasound signal. With continuous reception of the Doppler signal, the Nyquist limit is not applicable, and blood flows with very high velocities can be recorded accurately. A continuous wave transducer can measure velocities in excess of 7 m/s and thus is useful in measuring the high-velocity flows associated with stenotic valvular disease. Other differences between the pulsed wave and continuous wave techniques are important. Because the continuous wave signal is not time-gated like the pulsed wave technique, the continuous wave mode receives reflected signals from blood flow throughout its beam path. Unlike the clean envelope achieved with pulsed wave Doppler, the spectral display of continuous wave Doppler is typically shaded with the multitude of velocities recorded along the beam path (Fig. 5.13). Consequently, the use of continuous wave Doppler is limited primarily to detecting the highest velocities along the beam path, represented by the edge of the spectral envelope.

Color Flow Mapping

Color flow mapping provides a dramatic display of both blood flow and cardiac anatomy (see color figures following page 212). To achieve these remarkable images, the technique combines two-dimensional ultrasonic imaging and pulsed wave Doppler methods. The pulsed wave Doppler used for color flow mapping differs from that previously discussed in two important ways. First, instead of recording from a single, operator-selected sample volume,

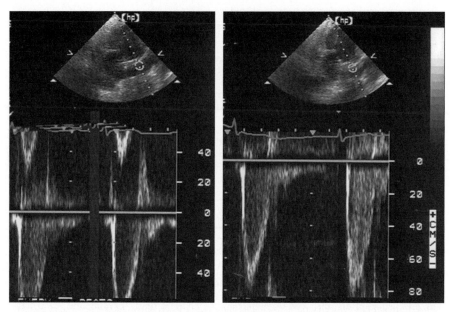

FIG. 5.12. Effect of baseline setting on pulsed wave Doppler aliasing. **Left:** With the velocity baseline set in the midportion of the display, the signal aliases at 50 cm/s. **Right:** The baseline has been adjusted to the upper portion of the display, which increases the Nyquist limit to more than 80 cm/s for flow away from the transducer and captures the spectral signal without aliasing.

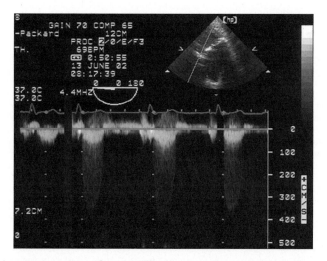

FIG. 5.13. Continuous wave spectral signal. Whereas pulsed wave Doppler obtains targeted sample volume recordings, the continuous wave system detects blood flow along the entire beam path. **Top:** In this example, the Doppler beam was positioned from the deep transgastric long-axis view. **Bottom:** The resulting spectral signal shows two distinct peaks, a pattern often referred to as a *double envelope*. The major peak at 400 cm/s is the high-velocity jet caused by aortic stenosis recorded from that portion of the beam in the aorta. The minor peak of 100 cm/s represents the blood velocity in the left ventricular outflow tract.

color flow mapping performs multiple pulsed wave sample determinations of velocity along the depth of each scan line. Multiple sample volume recordings are obtained along each scan line as the beam is swept through the sector. This approach provides flow data matched with the structural data obtained by two-dimensional imaging. The second difference is that the Doppler velocity data from each sample volume is color-coded and superimposed on top of the gray scale two-dimensional image. *In the most widely accepted color code, red indicates flow toward the transducer and blue indicates flow away from the transducer.* In addition to flow direction, flow velocity alters the color map. Increasing flow velocities are displayed by various hues; high-velocity flow toward the transducer is displayed as yellow, and high-velocity flow away from the transducer is displayed as cyan (see color figures following page 212). Flow with directional variance, as in areas of turbulence, is displayed as green.

The ability to provide a real-time, integrated display of flow and structural information makes color flow Doppler useful for assessing valvular function, aortic dissection, and congenital heart abnormalities. However, several important caveats to its use in the clinical setting must be noted. Because it relies on pulsed wave Doppler measurements, color flow mapping is susceptible to alias artifacts. In fact, *color flow will alias at a lower velocity than a conventional pulsed wave device because part of the signal must be used for image generation, and this effectively decreases the pulse repetition frequency.* Aliasing in the color flow map is illustrated in Figure 5.14 (see also Color Plate 5 following page 212). At the extreme of accurate velocity measurement (e.g., bright yellow for flow toward the transducer), progressively increasing flow rates appear cyan, then dark blue, and then dark red. In a high-velocity jet, several cycles of color alias can occur, which appear as a tiger stripe pattern in hues of red and blue. Because of the complex acquisition of multiple Doppler samples and the sharing of acquisition time with the imaging processor, the velocities displayed by the color flow mapper lack the fidelity of a conventional pulsed wave device. Color flow mapping cannot measure blood flow velocity nor track alterations in velocity through the cardiac cycle with the precision of a conventional Doppler device. *Because of these limitations, the color flow mapper is often used to identify a flow abnormality that is subsequently characterized by a conventional Doppler approach.*

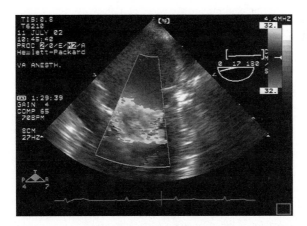

FIG. 5.14. Aliasing of color display. Blood flow through the mitral valve (midesophageal four-chamber view) during early diastole results in aliasing in the color flow mapper. Flow velocity accelerates in the left atrium as blood is funneled to the mitral valve orifice, shown as the color code of dark blue transitioning to light blue, and reaches 32 cm/s (the Nyquist limit), as seen on the color bar. As a result, aliasing signals are coded bright yellow, then red, as the velocity reaches a maximum at the level of the leaflet tips. Once in the left ventricle, the blood flow decelerates to fall below the Nyquist limit and is again appropriately coded blue by the echocardiographic system. (See Color Plate 5 following page 212.)

SUMMARY

Doppler echocardiography has greatly expanded the diagnostic capabilities of clinical echocardiography. Quantitative measurements of blood velocity derived from the spectral display of pulsed wave and continuous wave Doppler signals are widely used to characterize systolic and diastolic cardiac performance and valve function. Color flow mapping allows the visualization of cardiac blood flow. The broad clinical applications of Doppler echocardiography are described in detail in the next chapters. The clinician must remain mindful of the underlying principles of good technique to obtain optimal Doppler signals and avoid incorrect diagnoses related to erroneous measurements.

SUGGESTED READINGS

Hatle L, Angelsen B. *Doppler ultrasound in cardiology.* Philadelphia: Lea & Febiger, 1985.
Nishimura RA, Miller FA, Callahan MJ, et al. Doppler echocardiography: theory, instrumentation, technique, and application. *Mayo Clin Proc* 1985;60:321–343.
Quinones MA, Otto CM, Stoddard M, et al. Recommendations for the quantification of Doppler echocardiography: a report from the Doppler Quantification Task Force of the Nomenclature and Standards Committee of the American Society of Echocardiography. *J Am Soc Echocardiogr* 2002;15:167–184.
Weyman A. *Principles and practice of echocardiography.* Philadelphia: Lea & Febiger, 1994.

QUESTIONS

1. All of the following statements about Doppler echocardiography are true **except**
   a. The received Doppler signal is stronger than the two-dimensional signal.
   b. Christian Doppler was a Swedish echocardiographer.
   c. Doppler velocity measurements are based on changes in signal frequency.
   d. Doppler velocity measurements are based on reflections from plasma.
2. In clinical practice, the Doppler frequency shift is
   a. Typically 2.5 to 7.5 MHz
   b. Less than 1 MHz
   c. Not relevant to the Nyquist limit
   d. Negative for flow directed perpendicular to the ultrasound beam
3. The Doppler frequency shift is affected by all of the following **except**
   a. Transmitted frequency
   b. Blood velocity
   c. Incident angle of the ultrasound beam
   d. Distance of the target from the transducer
4. Fast Fourier analysis is applied to
   a. Pulsed wave but not continuous wave Doppler signals
   b. Identify the Doppler frequency shift
   c. Identify the component frequencies of the Doppler frequency shift
   d. Extract noise from weaker Doppler signals
5. All of the following statements are true of pulsed wave Doppler **except**
   a. It requires two separate crystals.
   b. It is useful to identify blood flow in a particular area.
   c. It has a limited maximal velocity that can be measured.
   d. It is the basis for color flow Doppler.
6. Techniques useful to correct an alias signal include all of the following **except**
   a. Adjusting the baseline
   b. Positioning the transducer closer to the target
   c. Increasing the transmitted frequency
   d. Using high-frequency pulsed Doppler

7. The Nyquist limit is directly related to
   a. Blood flow velocity
   b. Pressure gradient
   c. Pulse repetition frequency
   d. Red cell mass
8. Which of the following statements about color flow Doppler is true?
   a. It is susceptible to aliasing.
   b. It is a good choice for measuring high-velocity blood flow.
   c. It is based on continuous wave technology.
   d. It provides nonquantitative information.
9. Demodulation
   a. Filters out noise in the Doppler signal
   b. Identifies the Doppler shift
   c. Is not necessary for color flow Doppler
   d. Is not necessary for continuous wave Doppler
10. A spectral display with sharp, dense edges
    a. Is diagnostic of stenotic lesions
    b. Suggests echoes from a strong reflector, such as a nearby calcified valve
    c. Ensures that the beam is parallel to the blood flow
    d. Suggests proper interrogation of blood flow

6

Quantitative Doppler and Hemodynamics

Andrew Maslow and Albert C. Perrino, Jr.

When you can measure what you are speaking about, and express it in numbers, you
know something about it; but when you cannot express it in numbers, your knowledge
is of a meagre and unsatisfactory kind.

—*Lord Kelvin*

Hemodynamics is the study of blood flow and its associated forces. The objective of this
chapter is to describe the use of Doppler echocardiography for the quantitative assessment
of hemodynamics. Although two-dimensional echocardiography displays cardiac dimensions
and motion, it does not readily assess cardiac blood flow and pressures. Doppler echocardiography provides excellent assessments of hemodynamics that compare favorably with
more invasive measurements. Accordingly, a quantitative Doppler assessment of blood flow,
chamber pressures, valvular disease, pulmonary vascular resistance, ventricular function
(systolic and diastolic), and anatomic defects is an essential component of the echocardiographic examination.

The accuracy of the Doppler evaluation depends on the ability to minimize interference
from neighboring blood flows and align the ultrasound beam parallel to the blood flow of
interest. Traditionally, transthoracic echocardiography was a superior approach because it
offered multiple windows and angles from which blood flow could be interrogated. The introduction of multiplane transesophageal echocardiography (TEE) has increased the number
of imaging windows and angles from which the heart can be evaluated with TEE and has
greatly facilitated accurate hemodynamic evaluation.

VOLUMETRIC FLOW CALCULATIONS

Doppler Measurements of Stroke Volume and Cardiac Output

Principles. In many instances, knowledge of the *volume* of blood flow is desired. Cardiac
output and stroke volume are familiar examples. It is important not to confuse blood flow
velocity, which is the speed at which blood flows (expressed in centimeters per second), with
volumetric flow, which is the amount of blood that flows (expressed in cubic centimeters per
second). The volumetric flow (Q) at any point in time equals the blood flow velocity (v) times
the cross-sectional area (CSA) of the conduit.

$$Q = v \times CSA$$

To determine the volumetric flow with echocardiography, a Doppler measurement of the
instantaneous blood flow velocities and a two-dimensional measurement of the CSA are
required.

In the clinical setting, the volume of blood produced during each cardiac cycle, known
as the *stroke volume (SV)*, is an important parameter of cardiac performance. To calculate
the SV, the instantaneous velocities during systole are traced from the spectral display, and
the internal software package of the echocardiographic system calculates the time-velocity
integral (TVI), which is expressed in centimeters (Fig 6.1). Conceptually, the TVI represents
the cumulative distance, commonly referred to as the *stroke distance*, that the red cells have
traveled during the systolic ejection phase. When the stroke distance is multiplied by the CSA
(in square centimeters) of the conduit (e.g., aorta, mitral valve, pulmonary artery) through

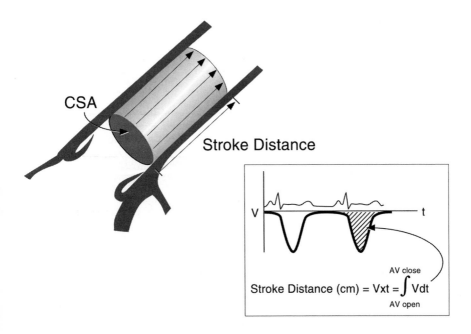

Stroke Volume (cc) = Stroke Distance × CSA

FIG. 6.1. Determination of stroke volume. Volumetric flow can be determined from a combination of area and velocity measurements. In this example, flow through the ascending aorta is used to determine the stroke volume. Integrating the Doppler-derived flow velocities over time (known as the *time-velocity integral*) during a single cardiac cycle calculates the stroke distance. The cross-sectional area measurement is obtained with two-dimensional echocardiography. The product of these two measurements, conceptualized as a cylinder, is the stroke volume.

which the blood has traveled, the SV (in cubic centimeters) is obtained (1–7). Cardiac output (CO), which expresses volumetric flow in cubic centimeters per minute, is estimated from the product of the SV and the heart rate.

Echocardiographic technique for Doppler measurements of stroke volume. The SV and CO are best measured with TEE at the left ventricular outflow tract (LVOT) or aortic valve (1–7). These locations offer several advantages to the clinical echocardiographer. First, the entire ejected SV traverses these structures, whereas it does not in more distant vessels, so that the total SV can be calculated. Second, Doppler interrogation typically assesses blood flow from only a small fraction of the total CSA of the vessel, and therefore SV calculations assume that the measured velocity reflects the mean flow velocity throughout the cross section of the vessel. This assumption is most accurate when blood flow is laminar and has the same velocity across the entire vessel, a situation known as a *blunt* or *flat flow profile* (Fig. 6.2). Because the blood is accelerated along the truncated LVOT during systole, the velocity profile has a blunt, uniform pattern rather than the parabolic pattern seen in the ascending aorta or pulmonary artery. Consequently, the LVOT and aortic valve are attractive because the risk for sampling blood velocities that are not reflective of the average blood flow velocity is reduced. Third, the LVOT and ascending aorta are more circular and the CSA changes less during the cardiac cycle. Multiplane TEE offers excellent windows at these sites for both Doppler blood flow measurements and two-dimensional

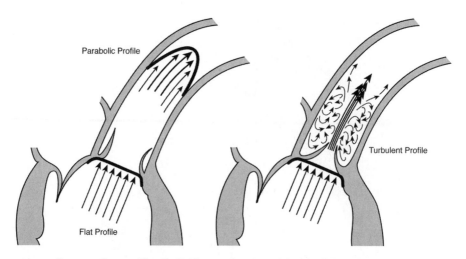

FIG. 6.2. Common flow profiles. **Left:** The acceleration of the blood flow as it enters the truncated left ventricular outflow tract leads to a "flat" profile in which velocities are uniform. As blood travels in the ascending aorta, the effects of wall friction and a curved conduit result in an asymmetric and parabolic flow profile. **Right:** When blood is forced through a narrow opening, laminar flow is replaced with turbulence. In this illustration, aortic stenosis has created a narrow, high-velocity jet encased by turbulent flow.

echocardiographic measurements of the CSA. Several clinical studies have confirmed that the CO measurements obtained by TEE compare favorably with those obtained by thermodilution (1–3,5–7).

LVOT or transaortic valvular flows are most reliably obtained from the transgastric (TG) long-axis and the deep TG long-axis views because the blood flow is nearly parallel to the ultrasound beam. It is critical to interrogate blood flow carefully through minor alterations in the probe position and multiplane angle to obtain the optimal Doppler spectral signal. The maximal velocity profile with a dense spectral signal is sought.

Calculation of the left ventricular outflow tract stroke volume
1. The pulsed wave Doppler sample volume is positioned in the LVOT immediately proximal to the aortic valve (TG long-axis and deep TG long-axis views).
2. The CSA for the LVOT is best obtained from the midesophageal (ME) LVOT view. The CSA is calculated from a measurement of the LVOT diameter as follows: $CSA_{LVOT} = \pi(\text{diameter}/2)^2$.

Calculation of the transaortic valve stroke volume
1. The continuous wave Doppler beam is directed through the aortic valve orifice from the TG long-axis or deep TG long-axis view (Fig. 6.3).
2. The CSA of the valve is best estimated by planimetry of the equilateral triangle–shaped orifice observed in mid systole (6). The aortic valve is viewed in cross section from the ME aortic valve short-axis window, and frame-by-frame review is used to capture the valve in mid systole. Planimetry of the triangle-shaped orifice yields the effective CSA.

Calculation of the stroke volume of the right side of the heart: Alternatively, right-sided flows and diameters can be analyzed from the main pulmonary artery (PA) or the mitral valve (MV). Pulsed wave or continuous wave Doppler analysis proceeds after the main PA

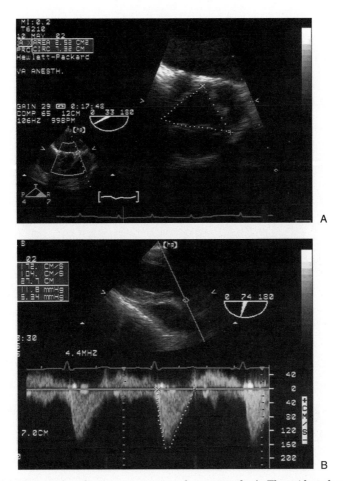

FIG. 6.3. Calculation of cardiac output: aortic valve approach. **A:** The midesophageal aortic valve short-axis image is displayed. The average cross-sectional area of the aortic valve during systolic flow is determined by planimetry of the triangular opening observed during midsystole, which yields a measurement of 2.5 cm^2. **B:** The transgastric long-axis view is displayed with continuous wave Doppler directed through the aortic valve orifice. The outer envelope of the spectral signal is traced to provide a calculated stroke distance of 27.7 cm. The heart rate is 94/min. Stroke Volume = 2.5 cm^2 × 27.7 cm = 69.2 cm^3; Cardiac Output = 69.2 cm^3 × 94/min = 6505 cm^3/min.

is imaged from high esophageal windows at the level of the superior mediastinal vessels (Fig. 6.4) or the right ventricular outflow tract (RVOT) is imaged from TG windows at 110- to 150-degree rotation of the transducer and rightward turn of the TEE probe (Fig. 6.5). In all cases, the maximal velocity profile is sought. Flow across the MV is measured by placing the sample volume at the level of the mitral annulus to obtain the transmitral TVI, which is then multiplied by the area of the MV annulus. Compared with the diameters of the LVOT and ascending aorta, the diameters of the main PA and MV fluctuate more during the cardiac cycle, and these measurements are less reliable than those from the LVOT and aortic valve (4). In addition, the MV orifice is not circular, and its size changes during diastole.

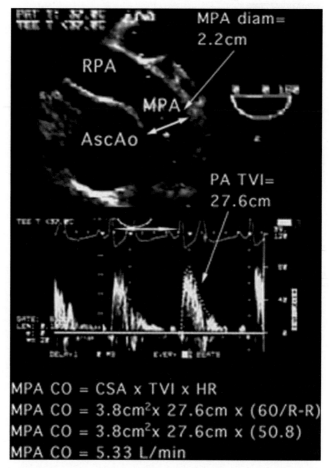

FIG. 6.4. Calculation of cardiac output: pulmonary artery approach. **Top:** Midesophageal ascending aorta short-axis view. The pulsed wave Doppler beam is aligned as close to parallel as possible to the blood flow in the pulmonary artery, and the diameter of the main pulmonary artery is measured at the site where the pulsed wave sample volume is placed. In this case, the diameter of the main pulmonary artery is 2.2 cm. With the formula $\pi(D/2)^2$, the cross-sectional area is calculated to be 3.8 cm^2. **Bottom:** Manual tracing of the spectral display of pulmonary blood velocities shows a time-velocity integral of 27.6 cm. When multiplied by the cross-sectional area and the heart rate, the cardiac output is calculated to be 5.33 L/min. MPA, main pulmonary artery; RPA, right pulmonary artery; AscAo, ascending aorta; CO, cardiac output; Diam, diameter; TVI, time-velocity integral; R-R, time interval between two R waves on the electrocardiogram.

Regurgitant Volume

Regurgitant volume is the quantity of blood that flows back through a regurgitant lesion in a single cardiac cycle. The total SV traversing a regurgitant valve during systole is greater than that in a normal valve. For a regurgitant valve, the total SV equals the regurgitant volume plus the SV delivered to the peripheral circulation. The regurgitant volume can be

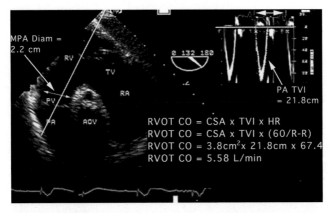

FIG. 6.5. Calculation of cardiac output: right ventricular outflow tract approach. **Left:** Transgastric right ventricular inflow/outflow view. The Doppler beam is aligned as close to parallel as possible to the blood flow through the right ventricular outflow tract, and the diameter is measured at the site where the pulsed wave sample volume is placed. In this case, the diameter of the main pulmonary artery is 2.2 cm. **Right:** Pulsed wave Doppler is used to obtain the right ventricular outflow tract time-velocity integral. With the formula $\pi(D/2)^2$, the cross-sectional area is calculated to be 3.8 cm^2. When this value is multiplied by the time-velocity integral and the heart rate, the cardiac output is calculated to be 5.58 L/min. RVOT, right ventricular outflow tract; PA, pulmonary artery; RV, right ventricle; TV, tricuspid valve; RA, right atrium; PV, pulmonic valve; Aov, aortic valve; CO, cardiac output; Diam, diameter; TVI, time-velocity integral; R-R, time interval between two R waves on the electrocardiogram.

calculated as the difference between the total forward flow through the regurgitant valve and the total forward flow through a reference valve.

$$\text{Regurgitant Volume} = \text{forward flow through regurgitant valve} - \text{forward flow through reference valve}$$

In the case of mitral regurgitation (in the absence of significant aortic valve disease), the SV across the aortic valve can be used as the true SV.

$$\text{Regurgitant volume}_{MV} = \text{forward flow through MV} - \text{flow through AV}$$

$$\text{RV}_{MV}(cc) = \text{SV}_{MV} - \text{SV}_{AV}$$

However, there is a significant potential for error in the mitral flow measurements because the MV orifice is not circular (4), and its diameter changes during the cardiac cycle. Similarly, the aortic regurgitant volume can be calculated as follows:

$$\text{Regurgitant volume}_{AV} = \text{forward flow through AV} - \text{flow through MV}$$

The regurgitant fraction is simply the ratio of the regurgitant volume to the total SV through the diseased valve and is typically expressed as a percentage:

$$\text{Regurgitant fraction (\%)} = \text{regurgitant volume/forward flow}$$

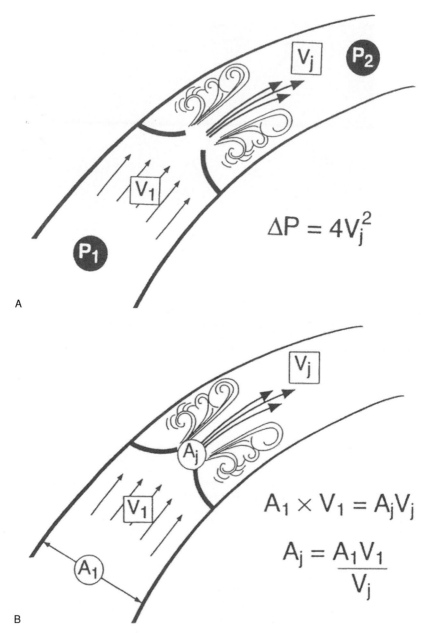

FIG. 6.6. Calculating the pressure gradient and valve area. **A:** Bernoulli equation. The simplified Bernoulli equation states that the pressure drop ($P_2 - P_1 = \Delta P$) across a stenotic orifice is four times the square of the velocity of the high-velocity jet. P_1, blood pressure proximal to stenosis; V_1, flow velocity proximal to stenosis; P_2, blood pressure distal to stenosis; V_j, flow velocity through stenosis. **B:** Continuity equation. The continuity equation is often described as the principle of "what goes in must come out." Accordingly, flow proximal to the stenosis ($A_1 \times v_1$) should equal flow through the stenosis ($A_j \times v_j$). A_1, cross-sectional area proximal to stenosis; V_1, flow velocity proximal to stenosis; A_j, cross-sectional area of stenosis; v_j, flow velocity through stenosis.

Alternative techniques to measure the severity of valvular regurgitation are discussed in Chapters 8 and 11.

Intracardiac Shunts

The ratio of pulmonic to systemic SV, Q_p/Q_s, is important in assessing the severity of shunts and in guiding treatment. Intracardiac shunts are assessed by calculating the SV (9). By measuring the left-sided (LVOT or aortic valve) and right-sided (PA or RVOT) SVs, one can determine Q_p/Q_s:

$$Q_p/Q_s = SV_{\text{Right Heart (eg PA, RVOT)}} / SV_{\text{Left Heart (eg LVOT, A}_{ov})}$$

These measurements are often combined with two-dimensional and color Doppler data to provide a complete assessment of congenital lesions.

Valve Area: The Continuity Equation

The principle of conservation of mass is the basis of the *continuity equation*, which is commonly used to measure the aortic valve area (10) (Fig 6.6B). The continuity equation simply states that the volume of blood passing through one site (e.g., the LVOT) is equal to the mass or volume of blood passing through another site (e.g., the aortic valve). Of course, there must be no intervening channels for this principle to apply. By using the principle of volumetric flow, discussed earlier, the continuity equation can be applied clinically.

$$\text{Volumetric Flow}_1 = \text{Volumetric Flow}_2$$

$$CSA_1 \times TVI_1 = CSA_2 \times TVI_2$$

$$CSA_1 = CSA_2 \times TVI_2/TVI_1$$

To calculate the area of the aortic valve (AoV):

$$\text{Area}_{\text{AoV}} = \text{Area}_{\text{LVOT}} \times (V_{\text{LVOT}}/V_{\text{AoV}})$$

$$\text{Area}_{\text{AoV}} = \pi(D_{\text{LVOT}}/2)^2 \times (V_{\text{LVOT}}/V_{\text{AoV}})$$

where D_{LVOT} is the diameter of the LVOT and v_{LVOT} is the velocity in the LVOT.

TEE assessments of LVOT and aortic flows and of LVOT diameter were described earlier in the section "Doppler Measurements of Stroke Volume and Cardiac Output." The continuity equation is the basis for assessments based on the proximal isovelocity surface area method (11–13), which is described in detail in Chapter 9.

INTRACARDIAC PRESSURES AND PRESSURE GRADIENTS: THE BERNOULLI EQUATION

Pressure gradients are used to estimate intracavitary pressures and to assess conditions such as valvular disease (e.g., aortic stenosis), septal defects, outflow tract abnormalities (e.g., LVOT obstruction), and major vessel pathology (e.g., coarctation). As blood flows across a narrowed or stenotic orifice, blood flow velocity increases. The increase in velocity is related to the degree of narrowing. The Bernoulli equation describes the relation between the increases in blood flow velocity and the pressure gradient across the narrowed orifice (14):

$$\Delta P = 1/2\rho(v_2{}^2 - v_1{}^2) + \rho(dv/dt)dx + R(v)$$

| Convection acceleration | Flow acceleration | Viscous friction |

where P is the pressure gradient across the area of interest (mm Hg), ρ is the density of blood (1.06×10^3 kg/m^3), v_1 is the peak velocity of blood flow proximal to area of interest (m/s), and v_2 is the peak velocity of blood flow across the area of interest (m/s).

In clinical practice, the Bernoulli equation is simplified by ignoring the effects of flow acceleration, viscous friction, and the velocity proximal to the area of interest (v_1) because:

1. Peak flows are of interest in clinical measurements. During peak flow, the flow acceleration is virtually nonexistent and thus can be ignored.
2. Viscous friction contributes significantly only in discrete orifices with an area of less than 0.25 cm^2. Blood flow is thought to be constant for orifices with an area greater than this, so that viscous friction is also eliminated in the Bernoulli calculation.
3. For clinically significant lesions, v_2 is substantially greater than v_1, such that $v_2^2 - v_1^2$ is approximated by just v_2^2.

The elimination of these factors yields the simplified Bernoulli equation:

$$\text{Simplified Bernoulli Equation: } \Delta P = 4v_2^2$$

Thus, a pressure gradient is obtained in clinical echocardiography by the straightforward process of measuring the peak velocity of blood flow across the lesion of interest (Fig. 6.6A).

To calculate the pressure gradient, the pulsed wave Doppler sample volume or continuous wave Doppler beam is directed across the region of interest. The measured peak velocity is then entered into the simplified Bernoulli equation ($\Delta P = 4v_2^2$) to estimate the pressure gradient. When blood flow velocities are high (≥ 1.4 m/s), continuous wave Doppler is preferred to avoid the aliasing that may occur with pulsed wave Doppler. It is imperative that the Doppler beam be positioned so that it interrogates the jet with the highest velocity; otherwise, the pressure gradient will be significantly underestimated. To obtain the highest velocity flow, interrogation from multiple windows is preferred. Also, accuracy is improved by assessing multiple flow profiles (3–5 for a regular rhythm and 10 for an irregular rhythm) at end-expiration. *The simplified Bernoulli equation is the basis for most pressure gradient calculations in clinical echocardiography.*

Assessment of Valvular Disease

The Bernoulli equation is most commonly used to measure the pressure gradient across a stenotic valve. This application is illustrated in Figure 6.6A. The assessment of valvular stenosis is discussed extensively in Chapters 9 and 12.

In addition, the rate of decline in the pressure gradient across the valve is related to the severity of disease (15). The *pressure half-time* is the time required for the peak transvalvular pressure gradient to decrease by 50%. Typically, a larger orifice has a shorter pressure half-time because pressure can equalize more quickly. The assessment of mitral stenosis and aortic insufficiency can be aided by pressure half-time measurements (see Chapters 9 and 12).

Measurement of Intracavitary Pressures

Intracavitary and pulmonary arterial pressures can be measured by combining a Doppler-derived pressure gradient from a regurgitant jet and a known (or estimated) pressure either proximal or distal to the chamber of interest (Table 6.1). Because accuracy depends on alignment of the ultrasound beam with the blood flow, velocities of central regurgitant jets are more accurately assessed than those of eccentric jets.

Right ventricular systolic pressure and pulmonary artery systolic pressure. With the simplified Bernoulli equation, the peak velocity of the tricuspid regurgitant (TR) jet is used to calculate the pressure gradient between the right ventricle (RV) and right atrium (RA) (16). The peak TR velocity is obtained by placing the continuous wave Doppler beam parallel

TABLE 6.1. CALCULATION OF CARDIOPULMONARY PRESSURES

Pressure	Equation
RVSP or PASP	$= 4(v_{TR})^2 + RAP$
PAMP	$= 4(v_{early\ PI})^2 + RAP$
PADP	$= 4(v_{late\ PI})^2 + RAP$
LAP	$= SBP - 4(v_{MR})^2$
LVEDP	$= DBP - 4(v_{AIend})^2$

RVSP, right ventricular systolic pressure; PASP and PADP, pulmonary artery systolic and diastolic pressures; PAMP, pulmonary artery mean pressure; LAP, left atrial pressure; LVEDP, left ventricular end-diastolic pressure; v, peak velocity; TR, tricuspid regurgitation; PI, pulmonic valve insufficiency; MR, mitral regurgitation; AI, aortic insufficiency; RAP, right atrial pressure; SBP, systolic blood pressure; DBP, diastolic blood pressure.

to the regurgitant jet. By adding a known or estimated RA pressure (RAP) or central venous pressure (CVP) to the RV-RA pressure gradient, the RV systolic pressure is estimated. In patients without significant pulmonic valve stenosis or RVOT obstruction, the RV systolic pressure (RVSP) and PA systolic pressure (PASP) are similar (Fig. 6.7).

$$RVSP \text{ or } PASP \text{ mmHg} = 4v_{TR}^2 + RAP \text{ mmHg}$$

The TEE examination is performed by using the ME RV inflow view with the transducer rotated from 0 to 110 degrees. Interference from left atrial (LA) flows is minimized in many

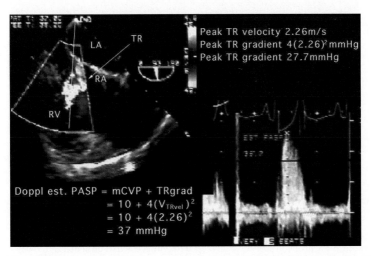

FIG. 6.7. The pulmonary artery systolic pressure is estimated from the peak velocity of the tricuspid regurgitant velocity profile (*arrow*). This was obtained from the midesophageal right ventricular inflow window. The peak velocity was 2.3 m/s. The simplified Bernoulli equation ($4v_2^2$) was used to calculate the trans-tricuspid, or ventriculoatrial, gradient, which was added to a known central venous pressure of 10 mm Hg to obtain a pulmonary artery systolic pressure of 37 mm Hg. TR, tricuspid regurgitation; LA, left atrium; RA, right atrium; RV, right ventricle; PASP, pulmonary artery systolic pressure; mCVP, known mean central venous pressure; TRvel, peak tricuspid regurgitation velocity; Trgrad, peak tricuspid regurgitation gradient.

patients by advancing the probe to the level of the coronary sinus, so that the position of the Doppler beam is posterior to the LA.

Pulmonary artery mean pressure and pulmonary artery diastolic pressure. These pressures are determined from the pulmonic valve regurgitation (PI) flow profile (16,17) (Fig. 6.8). After the continuous wave Doppler beam is placed parallel to the regurgitant jet, the peak early diastolic velocity is obtained to measure the early diastolic gradient between the PA and RV. Because RA pressure is equal to RV pressure in early diastole, this gradient is added to a known or estimated RA pressure to yield the PA mean pressure (PAMP).

$$PAMP = 4(v_{early_{PI}})^2 + CVP$$

The PA diastolic pressure (PADP) can be estimated by using the late peak velocity from the same flow profile.

$$PADP = 4(v_{late_{PI}})^2 + CVP$$

The pulmonic valve regurgitant flow is interrogated by using gastric views with rotation of the transducer from 110 to 150 degrees combined with rightward rotation of the TEE probe.

Left atrial and left ventricular pressures. These pressures are derived by applying the Bernoulli equation or by examining the flow patterns across the MV and pulmonary veins (18–23) (Fig. 6.9; see Color Plate 6 following page 212).

To measure the LA pressure (LAP), the peak velocity of the mitral regurgitation (MR) flow profile is obtained. The calculated pressure gradient is then subtracted from a known

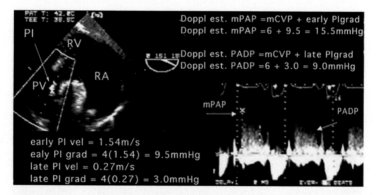

FIG. 6.8. Pulmonary artery mean and diastolic pressures. These can be obtained from the early and late pulmonary insufficiency velocities and calculated gradients by using the simplified Bernoulli equation (*early and late pulmonary insufficiency gradient*). From the transgastric right ventricular inflow and outflow window (transducer rotated from 110 to 145 degrees and the transesophageal echocardiographic probe rotated to the right), the pulmonic valve regurgitation can be analyzed with pulsed wave or continuous wave Doppler. The *arrow* on the left marks the early peak velocity, from which the mean pulmonary artery pressure can be calculated with the simplified Bernoulli equation. The *arrow* on the right marks the late peak velocity, from which the pulmonary artery diastolic pressure can be calculated. In this case, the Doppler-measured early and late pulmonary insufficiency gradients (9.5 and 3.0 mm Hg, respectively) were added to a mean central venous pressure of 6 mm Hg to yield a mean pulmonary artery pressure of 15.5 mm Hg and a pulmonary artery diastolic pressure of 9.0 mm Hg. AV, aortic valve; PV, pulmonic valve; TV, tricuspid valve; RVOT, right ventricular outflow tract; RA, right atrium; mCVP, mean central venous pressure; mPAP, mean pulmonary artery pressure; PADP, pulmonary artery diastolic pressure; PIgrad, pulmonary insufficiency gradient; PIvel, pulmonary insufficiency velocity.

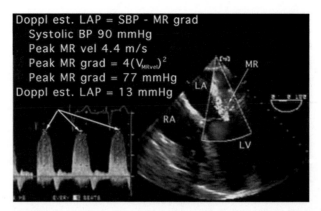

Doppl est. LAP = SBP - MR grad
Systolic BP 90 mmHg
Peak MR vel 4.4 m/s
Peak MR grad = $4(V_{MRvel})^2$
Peak MR grad = 77 mmHg
Doppl est. LAP = 13 mmHg

FIG. 6.9. The left atrial pressure can be estimated by using the mitral regurgitation velocity profile. The peak ventriculoatrial pressure gradient, measured by using the peak velocity of the mitral regurgitation profile (*arrow*) and the simplified Bernoulli equation, is subtracted from the known systolic blood pressure. In this case, the systolic blood pressure was 122 mm Hg, and the peak velocity was 5.18 m/s (107 mm Hg). The Doppler-estimated left atrial pressure was 15 mm Hg. The known pulmonary capillary wedge pressure was 14 mm Hg. LAP, left atrial pressure; MR, mitral regurgitation; RA, right atrial pressure; LV, left ventricle; vel, velocity; grad, gradient; SBP, systolic blood pressure; V_{Mrvel}, peak velocity of the mitral regurgitant flow profile. (See Color Plate 6 following page 212.)

systemic systolic blood pressure (SBP), which is similar to left ventricular (LV) systolic pressures in the absence of aortic valve disease or obstructive outflow tract pathologies.

$$LAP = SBP - 4(v_{MR})^2$$

Most often, standard ME views provide the best alignment of the ultrasound beam and MR flow.

Left ventricular end-diastolic pressure. The LV end-diastolic pressure (LVEDP) is assessed by using the aortic valve regurgitation (AI) velocity profile (19) (Fig. 6.10; see Color Plate 7 following page 212). The end-diastolic velocity is obtained by placing the continuous wave Doppler beam parallel to the regurgitant jet. The calculated aortic-ventricular gradient, measured from the peak end-diastolic velocity, is subtracted from the systemic diastolic pressure (DBP) to yield the LVEDP.

$$LVEDP = DBP - 4(v_{AIend})^2$$

The AI flow profile is obtained by using TG windows of the aortic valve and LVOT, in particular the deep and long-axis views.

LA and LV pressures can also be estimated from the transmitral and pulmonary venous velocity patterns (20–26). This approach is discussed in detail in Chapter 7.

HEART RHYTHM

Pulsed wave Doppler echocardiography is valuable in assessing heart rhythm. In particular, Doppler analysis of transmitral flow and flow in the LA appendage may be useful in assessing rate, rhythm, and atrial function. As discussed in detail in Chapter 7, normal transmitral flow analysis demonstrates early (E wave) and late (A wave) atrial contraction components. The latter describes the contribution of the atrial contraction to the ventricular preload. The

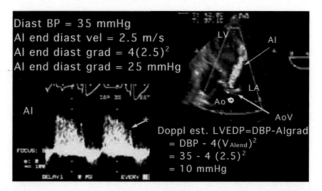

Diast BP = 35 mmHg
AI end diast vel = 2.5 m/s
AI end diast grad = $4(2.5)^2$
AI end diast grad = 25 mmHg

Doppl est. LVEDP=DBP-AIgrad
= DBP - $4(V_{AIend})^2$
= 35 - $4 (2.5)^2$
= 10 mmHg

FIG. 6.10. The left ventricular end-diastolic pressure can be estimated by using the aortic valve insufficiency velocity profile. The aortic-ventricular gradient, measured from the end-diastolic velocity of the aortic insufficiency regurgitation profile (*arrow*) and the simplified Bernoulli equation, is subtracted from the systemic pressure. In this case, the diastolic pressure was 45 mm Hg, and the late peak velocity was 2.91 m/s (gradient = 34 mm Hg). The estimated left ventricular end-diastolic pressure is 11 mm Hg (45 − 35 mm Hg). Diast BP, systemic diastolic blood pressure; AI, aortic insufficiency; diast, diastolic; vel, velocity; grad, gradient; LVEDP, left ventricular end-diastolic pressure; V_{AIend}, end-diastolic velocity of the aortic insufficiency jet; Ao, ascending aorta; LA, left atrium; LV, left ventricle. (See Color Plate 7 following page 212.)

presence of both waves indicates that a sinus or atrioventricular rhythm is present. The velocity profile of the LA appendage may also help to diagnose an atrial dysrhythmia. The normal LA appendage profile contains a single positive deflection during atrial contraction.

SUMMARY

Quantitative hemodynamic assessment with Doppler echocardiography offers a range of measurements: valve area, pressure gradients, chamber pressures, blood flow, resistances, and rate/rhythm. These measurements are essential in assessing valvular disease. The echocardiographer should establish a systematic approach to quantitative Doppler that is clinically useful and can be performed reliably and easily on-line. In combination with the two-dimensional echocardiographic examination, these quantitative techniques provide extensive information about cardiac performance.

REFERENCES

1. Savino JS, Troianos CA, Aukburg S, et al. Measurements of pulmonary blood flow with transesophageal two-dimensional and Doppler echocardiography. *Anesthesiology* 1991;75:445–451.
2. Gorcsan III J, Diana P, Ball BS, et al. Intraoperative determination of cardiac output by transesophageal continuous wave Doppler. *Am Heart J* 1992;123:171–176.
3. Maslow AD, Haering J, Comunale M, et al. Measurement of cardiac output by pulsed wave Doppler of the right ventricular outflow tract. *Anesth Analg* 1996;83:466–471.
4. Stewart WJ, Jiang L, Mich R, et al. Variable effects of changes in flow rate through the aortic, pulmonary, and mitral valves on valve area and flow velocity: impact on quantitative Doppler flow calculations. *J Am Coll Cardiol* 1985;6:653–662.
5. Muhiuden IA, Kuecherer HF, Lee E, et al. Intraoperative estimation of cardiac output by transesophageal pulsed Doppler echocardiography. *Anesthesiology* 1991;74:9–14.

6. Darmon PL, Hillel Z, Mogtader, et al. Cardiac output by transesophageal echocardiography using continuous-wave Doppler across the aortic valve. *Anesthesiology* 1994;80:796–805.
7. Perrino AC, Harris SN, Luther MA. Intraoperative determination of cardiac output using multiplane transesophageal echocardiography: a comparison to thermodilution. *Anesthesiology* 1998;89:350–357.
8. Ebeid MR, Ferrer PL, Robinson B, et al. Doppler echocardiographic evaluation of pulmonary vascular resistance in children with congenital heart disease. *J Am Soc Echocardiogr* 1996;9:822–831.
9. Valdes-Cruz LM, Horowitz S, Mesel E, et al. A pulsed Doppler echocardiographic method for calculating pulmonary and systemic blood flow in atrial level shunts: validation studies in animals and initial human experience. *Circulation* 1984;69:80–86.
10. Blumberg FC, Pfeifer M, Holmer SR, et al. Quantification of aortic stenosis in mechanically ventilated patients using multiplane transesophageal Doppler echocardiography. *Chest* 1998;114:94–97.
11. Bargiggia GS, Tronconi L, Sahn DJ, et al. A new method for quantitation of mitral regurgitation based on color flow Doppler imaging of flow convergence proximal to regurgitant orifice. *Circulation* 1991;84:1481–1489.
12. Rodriguez L, Thomas JD, Monterroso V, et al. Validation of the proximal flow convergence method: calculation of orifice area in patients with mitral stenosis. *Circulation* 1993;88:1157–1165.
13. Rittoo D, Sutherland GR, Shaw TR. Quantification of left-to-right atrial shunting defect size after balloon mitral commissurotomy using biplane transesophageal echocardiography, color flow Doppler mapping, and the principle of proximal flow convergence. *Circulation* 1993;87:1591–1603.
14. Nishimura RA, Miller FA, Callahan MJ, et al. Doppler echocardiography: theory, instrumentation, technique, and application. *Mayo Clin Proc* 1985;60:321–343.
15. Nakatani S, Masuyama T, Kodama K, et al. Value and limitations of Doppler echocardiography in the quantification of stenotic mitral valve area: comparison of the pressure half-time and the continuity equation methods. *Circulation* 1988;77:78–85.
16. Come PC. Echocardiographic recognition of pulmonary arterial disease and determination of its cause. *Am J Med* 1988;84:384–393.
17. Lee RT, Lord CP, Plappert T, et al. Prospective Doppler echocardiographic evaluation of pulmonary artery diastolic pressure in the medical intensive care unit. *Am J Cardiol* 1989;64:1366–1377.
18. Gorcsan III J, Snow FR, Paulsen W, et al. Noninvasive estimation of left atrial pressure in patients with congestive heart failure and mitral regurgitation by Doppler echocardiography. *Am Heart J* 1991;121:858–863.
19. Nishimura RA, Tajik AJ. Determination of left-sided pressure gradients by utilizing Doppler aortic and mitral regurgitation signals: validation by simultaneous dual catheter and Doppler studies. *J Am Coll Cardiol* 1988;11:317–321.
20. Oh JK, Appleton CP, Hatle LK, et al. The noninvasive assessment of left ventricular diastolic function with two-dimensional and Doppler echocardiography. *J Am Soc Echocardiogr* 1997;10:246–270.
21. Nishimura RA, Housmans PR, Hatle LK, et al. Assessment of diastolic function of the heart: background and current applications of Doppler echocardiography. Part 2. Clinical studies. *Mayo Clin Proc* 1989;64:181–294.
22. Nagueh SF, Kopelen HA, Quinones MA. Assessment of left ventricular filling pressures by Doppler in the presence of atrial fibrillation. *Circulation* 1996;94:2138–2145.
23. Temporelli PL, Scapellato F, Corra U, et al. Estimation of pulmonary wedge pressure by transmitral Doppler in patients with chronic heart failure and atrial fibrillation. *Am J Cardiol* 1999;83:724–727.
24. Moller JE, Poulsen SH, Songderfaard E, et al. Preload dependence of color M-mode Doppler flow propagation velocity in controls and in patients with left ventricular dysfunction. *J Am Soc Echocardiogr* 2000;13:902–909.
25. Garcia MJ, Ares MA, Asher C, et al. An index of early left ventricular filling that combined with pulsed Doppler peak E velocity may estimate capillary wedge pressure. *J Am Coll Cardiol* 1997;29:448–454.

26. Gonzalez-Viachez F, Ares M, Ayuela J, et al. Combined use of pulsed and color M-mode Doppler echocardiography for the estimation of pulmonary capillary wedge pressure: an empirical approach based on an analytical relation. *J Am Coll Cardiol* 1999;34: 515–523.

QUESTIONS

1. All the statements below are true **except**
   a. Intracardiac pressures can be estimated with Doppler echocardiography.
   b. Intracardiac pressures can be indirectly measured with Doppler echocardiography.
   c. Intracardiac pressures can be assessed with the Bernoulli equation.
   d. Intracardiac pressures can be directly measured with Doppler echocardiography.
   e. Intracardiac pressures can be estimated by using blood flow profiles obtained with Doppler echocardiography.
2. The Doppler assessment of SV
   a. Is performed accurately regardless of the orifice shape
   b. Is best measured across the MV
   c. Can be used to assess pulmonary-to-systemic blood flow
   d. Is measured only with pulsed wave Doppler echocardiography
   e. Does not require two-dimensional echocardiographic measurements
3. The following statements regarding Doppler measurement of intracardiac pressures are true **except**
   a. The PA diastolic and mean pressures can be obtained from the pulmonary valve insufficiency flow profile.
   b. The PA systolic pressure and RV systolic pressure may be equal.
   c. Pressure gradients are related to known pressures either proximal or distal to the chamber of interest.
   d. LV diastolic pressure is measured by using the MV regurgitant flow profile.
   e. If the proximal velocity (v_1) is high, then the result obtained with the simplified Bernoulli equation may not be accurate.
4. Doppler measurements of flow velocities must be repeated and averaged to account for
   a. Operator error
   b. Cor triatriatum
   c. Beat-to-beat variability
   d. Higher transducer frequencies used in TEE
   e. Use of continuous wave Doppler
5. The order of accuracy (best to least) in the measurement of SV is
   a. PA, LVOT, pulmonary vein
   b. LVOT, MV, pulmonary vein
   c. LVOT, pulmonary vein, MV
   d. LVOT, PA, MV
   e. MV, PA, LVOT
6. The direct measurement of central pressures
   a. Involves the use of regurgitant flows
   b. Involves the peak end-diastolic velocity of the pulmonic valve regurgitant profile
   c. Cannot be done with echocardiography
   d. Requires a known or estimated pressure
   e. Involves two-dimensional echocardiography but not Doppler echocardiography

A 72-year-old, with a known atrial septal defect (Qp:Qs = 1.8) and mild right ventricular (RV) dysfunction, is undergoing abdominal aortic aneurysm surgery. On release of the aortic cross-clamp, the heart rate (HR) increases to 100 bpm, the blood pressure decreases to 80/40 (mean 53) mm Hg, and the arterial saturation falls to 91%. The central venous pressure was 15 mm Hg. The TEE exam reveals: Normal left ventricular (LV) systolic function, moderate RV dysfunction, moderate tricuspid regurgitation (TR peak velocity 3 m/s), mild mitral regurgitation (MR peak velocity 4 m/s), and mild aortic valve (AV) insufficiency (end AI peak velocity 2.5 m/s; early AI peak velocity 3 m/s). The LV outflow tract (LVOT) diameter is

2.0 cm, the time-velocity integral (TVI) is 10 cm, and the peak velocity is 1.0 m/s. The trans-aortic valve peak velocity is 1.4 m/s. The main pulmonary artery (MPA) diameter is 2.2 cm, and the TVI is 10 cm.

7. After release of the aortic cross-clamp which of the following are true?
   A. The estimated PA systolic pressure is approximately 50 mm Hg.
   B. The AV area is approximately 2.2 cm^2.
   C. The Doppler estimate of LV end diastolic pressure is 15 mm Hg.
   D. The Doppler estimate of LV end diastolic pressure is 4 mm Hg.
      a. **A, B,** and **C**
      b. **A** and **C**
      c. **B** and **D**
      d. **D**
      e. **A, B, C,** and **D**
8. All of the following statements regarding the case in Question #7 are true **except**
   a. The systemic cardiac output is 3.14 L/min.
   b. The systemic stroke volume is 31.4 mL/beat.
   c. The Qp/Qs is approximately 1.2.
   d. The main pulmonary artery cardiac output is 3.00 L/min.
   e. Arterial desaturation and altered hemodynamics may be due increased RV dysfunction and right to left shunt across the atrial septal defect.

A 12-year-old girl undergoing corrective spine surgery for kyphoscoliosis has a decrease in the systemic BP to 65/40 (mean 48) mm Hg, and an increase in the HR from 90 to 120 bpm. The central venous pressure is 10 mm Hg. TEE exam reveals hyperdynamic RV and LV function, and normal valve function. The LVOT diameter is 2.0 cm, and the TVI is 15 cm. The peak velocity of the tricuspid regurgitation flow profile is 2 m/s.

9. Which of the following statements is false?
   a. The patient may be experiencing anaphylaxis.
   b. The PA diastolic pressure cannot be obtained from the data presented.
   c. The cardiac output is 5.65 L/min.
   d. The estimated PA systolic pressure is approximately 26 mm Hg.
   e. The patient has had a pulmonary embolism.

A 75-year-old man experiences hypotension after induction of anesthesia (BP 65/40 mm Hg; HR 90 bpm). A TEE exam reveals normal LV function and moderate RV hypokinesis. The LV cavity is small. There is moderate AI and mild MR. The LVOT diameter is 2.0 cm with a peak velocity of 1.0 m/s. The peak velocity across the AV is 4.0 m/s and the TVI is 30 cm.

10. Which of the following statements is true?
    A. The left ventricular outflow tract area is 3.14 cm2.
    B. The aortic valve area is 0.78 cm2.
    C. The systemic cardiac output is 2.11 L/min.
    D. The systemic stroke volume is 23.4 mL/beat.
       a. **A, B,** and **C**
       b. **A** and **C**
       c. **B** and **D**
       d. **D**
       e. **A, B, C,** and **D**

Evaluation of Ventricular Diastolic Function

Stanton K. Shernan and Michael R. Zile

In comparison with systole, the diastolic phase of the cardiac cycle has only recently become appropriately recognized as an important, independent component of overall cardiac performance. Diastole is no longer perceived simply as a passive stage of ventricular filling interposed between each contraction. Adequate ventricular filling actually depends on a complex interaction between ventricular relaxation, compliance, and systolic function, in addition to an important late diastolic contribution from atrial contraction.

Following the advent of cardiac catheterization in the 1960s, the quantification of ventricular mechanics and ventricular diastolic properties accelerated with the introduction of pulsed wave Doppler echocardiography in the early 1980s. With its relative feasibility, safety, and practicality, echocardiography has helped to delineate diastolic dysfunction during the last several decades as a major pathophysiologic component of several cardiac disorders, including acute and chronic congestive heart failure (1). In addition, Doppler echocardiographic modalities have been used to predict functional class and prognosis (2). Echocardiographic studies have also suggested that diastolic dysfunction may contribute to perioperative hemodynamic instability and adverse outcomes following cardiac surgery (3). This chapter presents a practical approach to understanding the importance and utility of traditional and newer echocardiographic modalities in assessing ventricular filling and diastolic dysfunction.

CLINICAL RELEVANCE OF DIASTOLIC DYSFUNCTION

Congestive heart failure is the most common diagnosis among inpatients in the United States and accounts for 720,000 hospital admissions annually (4). Nearly half of patients with congestive heart failure have diastolic dysfunction and a normal ejection fraction (5). Diastolic dysfunction increases with age, especially in elderly persons with hypertensive heart disease (5). Although the prognosis for patients with diastolic heart failure is more favorable than that for patients with systolic dysfunction, mortality is nonetheless increased fourfold in comparisons with age- and gender-matched normal subjects (6). Thus, diastolic dysfunction poses an important and clinically relevant challenge to health care practitioners.

The relatively high prevalence of diastolic heart failure in the community is also a concern for the perioperative intensivist because many affected patients are brought to the operating room for cardiovascular procedures. Preoperative diastolic dysfunction has been reported in 30% to 70% of cardiac surgical patients and is independently associated with difficult weaning from cardiopulmonary bypass (CPB), an increased need for inotropic support, and increased morbidity (3,7). Following CPB, acute or progressive diastolic dysfunction associated with ischemia-reperfusion injury, hypothermia, metabolic disturbances, or myocardial edema may develop and persist for several minutes to days (8). Identifying high-risk patients preoperatively and monitoring their diastolic function intraoperatively may allow for the institution of prophylactic therapeutic strategies, including the administration of pharmacologic agents with direct or indirect lusitropic properties (9) that can facilitate weaning from CPB and reduce perioperative morbidity.

BASICS OF DIASTOLIC PHYSIOLOGY

The diastolic phase of the cardiac cycle is defined as the period from aortic valve closure to mitral valve (MV) closure (Fig. 7.1). Diastole can be subdivided into an initial isovolumic relaxation period that is followed by early rapid left ventricular (LV) inflow, responsible for

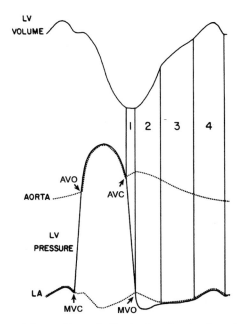

FIG. 7.1. Diastolic phase of the cardiac cycle. During isovolumic relaxation (*1*), left ventricular (*LV*) pressure decreases rapidly after aortic valve closure (*AVC*). When LV pressure decreases below the left atrial (*LA*) pressure, the mitral valve opens (*MVO*), initiating early, rapid LV filling (*2*). Equilibration of LV and LA pressures results in diminished transmitral flow during diastasis (*3*) until atrial contraction (*4*), which normally contributes less than 20% of the total LV end-diastolic volume. Diastole terminates with MV closure (*MVC*) before isovolumic contraction and AV opening (*AVO*), which permits LV ejection. (From Plotnick GD. Changes in diastolic function—difficult to measure, harder to interpret. *Am Heart J* 1989;118:637–641, with permission.)

80% to 90% of diastolic filling, diastasis, and finally atrial systole (10). LV filling during diastole depends on a complex interaction of numerous factors, including ventricular relaxation, diastolic suction, viscous-elastic forces of the myocardium, pericardial restraint, ventricular interaction, MV dynamics, load heterogeneity, intrathoracic pressure, heart rate/rhythm, and atrial function (11).

Diastolic dysfunction is often defined clinically as an impaired capacity of the ventricles to fill at low pressure and usually involves an abnormality in ventricular relaxation or chamber compliance. **LV relaxation** is associated with the resequestration of calcium from the cytosol to the sarcoplasmic reticulum via a complex energy-dependent process that is required to deactivate the contractile elements and subsequently allow the myofibrils return to their original, precontraction length (12). Ventricular relaxation is classically evaluated with high-fidelity, manometer-tipped catheters that measure the rate and duration of the LV pressure decrease after systolic contraction during isovolumic relaxation (13) (Fig. 7.2A). The time constant of relaxation (τ) is a clinically and experimentally acceptable technique for assessing isovolumic relaxation, although limitations have been described (12). **LV chamber compliance** depends on the passive properties of the ventricle and is determined from the exponential relationship between the change in volume and the change in pressure during diastolic filling (dV/dP) (Fig. 7.2B) (13).

The contribution of the left atrium (LA) to the LV end-diastolic volume (LVEDV) can also be an important determinant of filling. The LA serves not only as a blood reservoir and passive conduit but also as an active pump during contraction at end-diastole. The contribution of

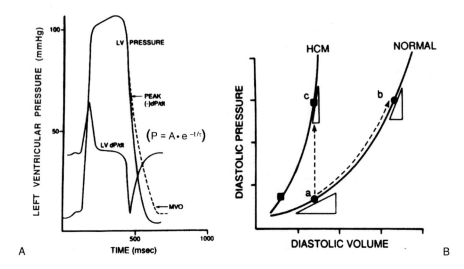

FIG. 7.2. A: Left ventricular (*LV*) relaxation can be invasively evaluated by measuring the minimal value of the first derivative of ventricular pressure with respect to time ($-dp/dt_{min}$), or preferably by calculating the time constant (τ) of the isovolumic LV pressure decline according to the equation shown. An increase in τ (*dashed line*) generally indicates impaired LV relaxation (myocardial ischemia, hypertrophic heart disease, negative inotropes), which can be associated with decreased LV filling and diminished cardiac performance. *P*, LV pressure; *A*, LV pressure at $-dp/dt_{min}$; *t*, time after $-dp/dt_{min}$; *e*, natural logarithm; *MVO*, mitral valve opening. (Modified from Zile M, Smith V. Relaxation and diastolic properties of the heart. In: Fozzard H, Haber E, Jennings R, et al., eds. *The heart and cardiovascular system: scientific foundations,* 2nd ed. New York: Raven Press, 1991:1353–1367, with permission.) **B:** LV pressure-volume (*P-V*) relationships. LV compliance (*dV/dP*) is described by the tangent drawn to the P-V curve at a particular point. A decrease in LV compliance results in an increase in LV filling pressure, depicted as either a shift of the P-V curve upward and to the left when myocardial stiffness increases (point a → c), or to a steeper portion of the curve when volume increases (point a → b). (Reproduced from Zile M, Smith V. Relaxation and diastolic properties of the heart. In: Fozzard H, Haber E, Jennings R, et al., eds. *The heart and cardiovascular system: scientific foundations,* 2nd ed. New York: Raven Press, 1991:1353–1367, with permission.)

the LA to LV diastolic filling is usually less than 20% in young healthy persons but may approach 50% in persons in whom decreased LV filling is associated with early diastolic dysfunction.

ECHOCARDIOGRAPHIC EVALUATION OF LEFT VENTRICULAR DIASTOLIC FUNCTION

Conventional direct assessment of diastolic function requires invasive measurements (high-fidelity intraventricular micromanometry catheters) or sophisticated technology (three-dimensional sonomicrometry, cardiac magnetic resonance imaging, ultrafast computed tomography) (12). Pulmonary artery catheterization can be useful for assessing global cardiac performance; however, in the evaluation of diastolic function, it is limited by an inability to measure LV pressure and volume or transmitral flow directly. In contrast, echocardiography provides a relatively safe, practical, and noninvasive means of evaluating diastolic function.

Two-Dimensional and M-Mode Echocardiography

Indirect evidence of diastolic dysfunction can be obtained during a comprehensive two-dimensional echocardiographic examination by assessing the LV ejection fraction and LVEDV. Echocardiographic evidence of LV hypertrophy without dilation and with normal systolic function indicates the presence of diastolic heart failure in a symptomatic patient. LA enlargement (>4 cm) is often associated with elevated LV filling pressures (14).

Doppler Echocardiographic Evaluation of Left Ventricular Filling: Transmitral Inflow

The use of Doppler echocardiography to measure transmitral blood flow velocities provides valuable information in the assessment of diastolic function. The pulsed wave Doppler recording of transmitral blood flow velocities is obtained by placing the sample volume at the MV leaflet tips (Fig. 7.3). A typical Doppler transmitral blood flow velocity profile has a biphasic pattern. An initial peak flow velocity (E-wave) occurs during early diastolic filling, and a later peak flow velocity (A-wave) occurs during atrial systole. Blood flow during the interposed period of diastasis is usually minimal because little LV filling occurs during this phase. Several indices of diastolic function have been derived from the Doppler transmitral blood flow velocity profile and correlated with more classic measures of diastolic function, including angiography, radionuclide techniques, and direct measures of intraventricular pressure (12,15) (Table 7.1).

TABLE 7.1. LEFT AND RIGHT VENTRICULAR DOPPLER ECHOCARDIOGRAPHIC INDICES OF DIASTOLIC FUNCTION FILLING DYNAMICS IN NORMAL SUBJECTS

	Age 21–49 y	Age ≥ 50 y
Left ventricular inflow		
Peak E (cm/s)	72 (44–100)	62 (34–90)
Peak A (cm/s)	40 (20–60)	59 (31–87)
E/A ratio	1.9 (0.7–3.1)	1.1 (0.5–1.7)
DT (ms)	179 (139–219)	210 (138–282)
IVRT (ms)	76 (54–98)	90 (56–124)
Pulmonary vein		
Peak S (cm/s)	48 (30–66)	71 (53–89)
Peak D (cm/s)	50 (30–70)	38 (20–56)
S/D ratio	1.0 (0.5–1.5)	1.7 (0.8–2.6)
Peak A (cm/s)	19 (11–27)	23 (−5 to 51)
Right ventricular inflow		
Peak E (cm/s)	51 (37–65)	41 (25–57)
Peak A (cm/s)	27 (11–43)	33 (17–49)
E/A	2.0 (1.0–3.0)	1.3 (0.5–2.1)
DT (cm/s)	188 (144–232)	198 (152–244)
Superior vena cava		
Peak S (cm/s)	41 (23–59)	42 (18–66)
Peak D (cm/s)	22 (12–32)	22 (12–32)
Peak A (cm/s)	13 (7–19)	16 (10–22)

Normal reference values for Doppler echocardiographic indices of ventricular diastolic function in two age groups of normal subjects. Data presented are mean values (confidence interval).

A, late diastolic atrial flow velocity associated with atrial contraction; D, diastolic flow velocity; DT, deceleration time; E, early diastolic flow velocity; IVRT, isovolumic relaxation time; S, systolic flow velocity.

From Cohen G, Pietrolungo J, Thomas J, et al. A practical guide to assessment of ventricular diastolic function using Doppler echocardiography. *J Am Coll Cardiol* 1996;27:1754, with permission.

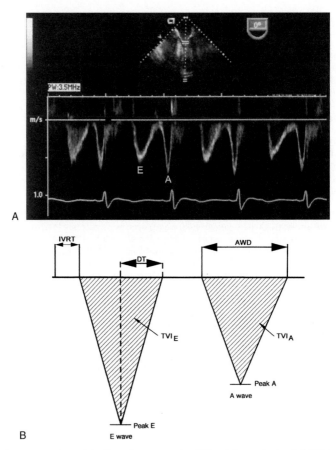

FIG. 7.3. A: Determination of the Doppler transmitral blood flow velocity (*TMDF*) profile with transesophageal echocardiography. The profile is obtained by placing a pulsed wave Doppler sample volume (1–2 mm) at the tips of the mitral valve (*MV*). The initial rapid phase of early left ventricular (*LV*) filling (*E*) is followed by a variable period of minimal flow (diastasis) and finally late diastolic filling during atrial contraction (*A*). **B:** Schematic of the TMDF profile depicting relevant indices of diastolic function. Several indices of LV diastolic function can be obtained from the profile: the E- and A-wave peak velocities and ratio; the E- and A-wave time-velocity integrals (*TVI*, the area under each Doppler envelope) and corresponding E/A TVI ratio; the A-wave duration (*AWD*); the E-wave deceleration time (*DT*, the time interval from the peak E-wave velocity to the zero baseline); and the isovolumic relaxation time (*IVRT*, the time from the cessation of systolic ventricular outflow to the onset of transmitral LV inflow).

PHYSIOLOGY OF TRANSMITRAL FLOW VELOCITIES

Doppler transmitral blood flow velocities are determined by the transmitral pressure gradient, which in turn depends on several variables, including heart rate and rhythm, early filling loads, atrial contractility, MV disease, ventricular septal interactions, the intrinsic LV lusitropic state, and ventricular compliance (6). With normal aging, delayed LV relaxation at any given LV pressure creates a lower initial transmitral pressure gradient. This results in proportionally less early filling (lower peak E-wave velocity) and a greater amount of compensatory late filling (higher peak A-wave velocity), accounting for 35% to 40% of LV diastolic inflow. Conversely, the more efficient LV relaxation and elastic recoil of young adults is associated with predominantly early LV filling, corresponding to a greater initial transmitral pressure gradient and a smaller contribution (10%–15%) from atrial contraction. Alternatively, elevation of the transmitral pressure gradient in patients with decreased LV compliance is primarily a consequence of progressively increasing LA pressure. Thus, alterations in LV relaxation and compliance, along with consequential changes in LA pressure, alter the transmitral pressure gradient and resulting Doppler transmitral blood flow velocity profiles. The isovolumic relaxation time (IVRT), which is the time from the cessation of systolic ventricular outflow to the onset of LV inflow, is also affected by alterations of diastolic function. A shortened IVRT (<60 ms) indicates premature MV opening and can be observed in patients with elevated LA pressure. Delayed MV opening (IVRT > 110 ms) occurs with impaired LV relaxation. The deceleration time (the interval from the peak E-wave velocity to the zero baseline) generally reflects the mean LA pressure and LV compliance (16). A relatively short deceleration time (<140 ms) can be seen in patients with reduced LV compliance, whereas a prolonged deceleration time is associated with poor LV relaxation.

PATHOLOGIC TRANSMITRAL FLOW VELOCITIES

Impaired Relaxation Filling Pattern

Changes in LV relaxation and compliance contribute to the spectrum of Doppler LV filling patterns seen in progressive diastolic dysfunction. The initial abnormality of diastolic filling in most disorders of cardiac physiology is impaired myocardial relaxation exceeding that expected with aging alone. Impaired LV relaxation occurs in myocardial ischemia/infarction, LV hypertrophy, hypertrophic cardiomyopathy, and the early stages of infiltrative disorders (17). The Doppler transmitral blood flow velocity profile associated with **impaired relaxation** is typically characterized by a prolonged IVRT and a decreased initial transmitral pressure gradient (18) (Fig. 7.4). Consequently, the peak E-wave velocity decreases relative to the peak A-wave velocity when LV relaxation is impaired (E/A < 1) because the MV tends to open before relaxation is complete. In addition, the duration of LV relaxation is prolonged and results in a prolonged deceleration time (11) because the LA-LV pressure gradient takes longer to equilibrate. A subsequent compensatory increase in flow during atrial contraction accounts for the increased peak A-wave velocity, time-velocity integral (TVI), and duration because of the relatively high atrial preload. *Thus, the Doppler transmitral blood flow velocity profile in impaired relaxation is characterized by "E/A reversal" (decreased peak E-wave velocity and increased peak A-wave velocity), a prolonged IVRT, and a prolonged deceleration time.*

Restrictive Filling Pattern

Diastolic dysfunction associated with markedly decreased LV compliance and severely increased LA pressure is often described as a "restrictive" LV filling disorder (17). The Doppler transmitral blood flow velocity profile associated with a **restrictive pattern** of LV diastolic dysfunction is characterized by an elevated peak E-wave velocity relative to the A-wave velocity as a consequence of the elevated LA pressure (18) (Fig. 7.4). Even though impaired relaxation coexists with decreased compliance when diastolic dysfunction has progressed, the consequential increase in LV end-diastolic pressure (LVEDP) results in a markedly elevated LA pressure and an elevated peak E-wave velocity, consistent with very rapid filling during early diastole. The IVRT is shortened because the MV opens prematurely as a consequence of the elevated LA pressure. The deceleration time is also abnormally short because early transmitral flow into the poorly compliant LV results in

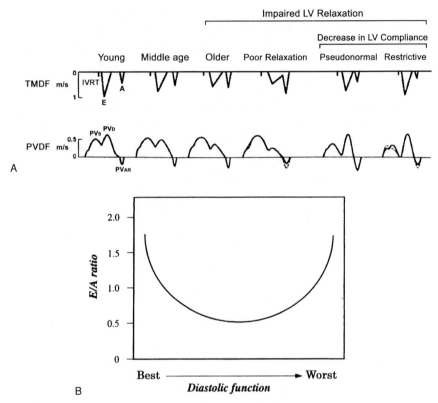

FIG. 7.4. A: The impact of progressive left ventricular (*LV*) diastolic dysfunction on Doppler transmitral (*TMDF*) and pulmonary venous (*PVDF*) blood flow velocity profiles. Note that all pulsed Doppler indices of the TMDF and PVDF profiles present a parabolic distribution during the progression from normal diastolic function to advanced diastolic dysfunction. The transmitral pressure gradient is initially elevated in normal, young individuals as a consequence of vigorous LV relaxation and elastic recoil; it diminishes when relaxation becomes impaired and finally increases again when left atrial pressure increases secondary to an elevated LV end-diastolic pressure in the restrictive pattern of LV diastolic dysfunction. Corresponding changes are noted in the PVDF profile. E, E-wave; A, A-wave; IVRT, LV isovolumic relaxation time; PV_{AR}, late diastolic retrograde velocity; PV_{S1}, first systolic component; PV_{S2}, second systolic component; PV_D, diastolic component. (Modified from Appleton C, Hatle L. The natural history of left ventricular filling abnormalities: assessment by two-dimensional and Doppler echocardiography. *Echocardiography* 1992;9:437–457, with permission.) **B:** Parabolic distribution of transmitral E/A velocity ratios associated with progressive diastolic dysfunction.

rapid equilibration of the LA and LV pressures, which may even be associated with diastolic mitral regurgitation (17). Finally, the peak A-wave velocity and duration tend to be compromised by poor atrial contractility and the rapid increase in LV pressure, which can prematurely terminate late mitral inflow. *Thus, a restrictive Doppler transmitral blood flow velocity profile is characterized by a elevated peak E-wave velocity and a decreased peak A-wave velocity (E/A ratio > 2.0), along with a shortened IVRT and deceleration time.*

Pseudonormalized Filling Pattern

Typically, diastolic dysfunction progresses from impaired relaxation to restrictive pathophysiology. During this transition, the Doppler transmitral blood flow velocity profile may assume a **pseudonormalized pattern** that resembles normal LV filling (18) (Fig. 7.4A). The pseudonormalized filling pattern represents a moderate stage of diastolic dysfunction in which a "normal" early transmitral pressure gradient is generated by the balance between compromised LV relaxation and gradually increasing filling pressures as LV compliance decreases. Consequently, for varying degrees of diastolic dysfunction, the spectrum of E/A velocity ratios assumes a parabolic shape, beginning with a vigorous LV relaxation pattern seen in young, athletic individuals and terminating with a similar-appearing restrictive pattern consistent with severe diastolic dysfunction (Fig. 7.4B). *The intermediate, pseudonormalized stage of diastolic dysfunction is therefore characterized by normal values for the peak E-wave and A-wave velocities, IVRT, and deceleration time. Reducing the preload with reverse Trendelenburg positioning, partial CPB, or a Valsalva maneuver (19) or by administering nitroglycerin may also reveal underlying impaired LV relaxation in a patient with pseudonormalized transmitral inflow (20).* Normal individuals usually respond to preload reduction with a more proportional decrease in both E-wave and A-wave velocities (17). Preload reduction may also be useful in grading the severity of diastolic dysfunction (20). For example, a restrictive pattern is considered "irreversible, end-stage" if it does not pseudonormalize in response to preload reduction (10).

Doppler Echocardiographic Evaluation of Left Atrial Filling: Pulmonary Venous Flow

The evaluation of LA filling can provide important insights into LV diastolic function, especially when combined with data obtained from the transmitral blood flow velocity profile. A typical Doppler pulmonary venous (PV) blood flow velocity profile consists of an antegrade systolic velocity, which may appear monophasic or biphasic, especially in the presence of low LA pressure, probably because of the temporal dissociation of atrial relaxation and mitral annular motion (21) (Fig. 7.5; see Color Plate 8 following page 212). The first systolic component, PV_{S1}, depends on LA relaxation and the subsequent decrease in pressure. The later peak, PV_{S2}, reflects right ventricular (RV) stroke volume, LA compliance, the effects of early ventricular systole on LA pressure, and any concomitant mitral regurgitation. An additional large antegrade velocity occurs during diastole (PV_D) following early transmitral inflow while the LA serves as an open conduit between the PV and LV. The late diastolic retrograde velocity, also known as *pulmonary venous atrial flow reversal (PV_{AR})*, occurs during LA systole and depends on LA contractility, heart rate, and compliance of the LA, PV, and LV (6).

Normally, the PV systolic peak amplitude and TVI are equal to or slightly greater than the corresponding PV_D values (15) (Table 7.1). A reduced systolic fraction (systolic TVI divided by the sum of systolic and diastolic TVI) of less than 40% has been correlated with increased mean LA pressure (22). In addition, the normal PV_{AR} duration ($\sim$90–115 ms) is the same or less than the transmitral A-wave duration ($\sim$120–140 ms) (16). In general, LA contraction should result in a net forward flow of blood volume toward a normal, compliant LV that is greater than any retrograde flow back toward the PV. A PV_{AR} velocity that exceeds the mitral A-wave by more than 35 cm/s or a PV_{AR} duration more than 30 ms longer than the transmitral A-wave duration usually indicates an age-independent elevation in LVEDP (23).

The Doppler analysis of PV blood flow velocity complements the assessment of transmitral blood flow velocity in the evaluation of various stages of diastolic dysfunction (Fig. 7.4). The Doppler PV blood flow velocity profile consistent with impaired LV relaxation is characterized by a reduced PV_D velocity that parallels the mitral E-wave velocity and a compensatory increase in the PV_S velocity, resulting in a pattern of *systolic predominance*. Conversely, the systolic antegrade velocity is reduced when LV filling is restrictive because of the elevated LA pressure and decreased LV compliance, resulting in a pattern of *systolic blunting*. A greater proportion of antegrade flow occurs during diastole, although the PV_D deceleration time is usually shortened, analogous to the rapid deceleration of the transmitral E-wave velocity. The PV_{AR} velocity and duration may be prolonged in the presence of restrictive pathophysiology

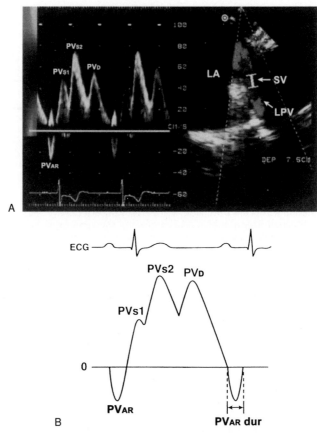

FIG. 7.5. A: Doppler pulmonary venous blood flow (*PVDF*) velocity profile. Left atrial (*LA*) filling can be assessed by placing a pulsed wave Doppler sample volume (2–4 mm) approximately 1.0 cm into a pulmonary vein (*PV*) orifice where it joins the LA. (See Color Plate 8 following page 212.) **B:** Schematic of the PVDF profile depicting relevant indices of diastolic function. Indices of left ventricular (*LV*) diastolic function obtained from the PVDF profile include the peak systolic/diastolic velocity ratio as well as the peak A-wave reversal velocity and duration. LAA, left atrial appendage; LUPV, left upper pulmonary vein; PV_{AR}, late diastolic retrograde velocity; PV_{AR} dur, PV_{AR}-wave duration; PV_{S1}, first systolic component; PV_{S2}, second systolic component; PV_D, diastolic component; SV, sample volume; LPV, left pulmonary vein.

because of decreased LV compliance and an associated increase in LA pressure, which can promote retrograde flow. Alternatively, the PV_{AR} velocity may be diminished in patients with severe, irreversible restrictive filling because of atrial mechanical failure (24). The pseudonormalized Doppler PV blood flow velocity profile is often characterized by a pattern of relative systolic blunting and a prolonged PV_{AR} duration and velocity in comparison with the transmitral A-wave duration, depending on the LA pressure and degree of reduced LV compliance (Fig. 7.4). In this scenario, the Doppler PV blood flow velocity pattern may be helpful in distinguishing a pseudonormal from a normal Doppler transmitral blood flow velocity profile. However, in normal young adults and athletes who do not rely on a significant LA contribution for LV filling, the LA behaves more like a "passive conduit," and PV blunting may be commonly observed (24).

Influence of Physiologic Variables on Left Atrial and Left Ventricular Doppler Flow Profiles

The Doppler transmitral and pulmonary venous blood flow velocity profiles are considered useful for evaluating LV diastolic function in both nonsurgical and surgical patient populations. The utility of these echocardiographic parameters throughout the perioperative period is limited, however, by the unavoidable effects of changes in preload, afterload, heart rate, and rhythm on peak velocities and the proportions of early and late filling (25). Increases in preload are often associated with a more proportional increase in the transmitral peak E-wave velocity, a shortened IVRT, and a steeper deceleration time. The opposite changes occur with decreases in preload. Mitral regurgitation may produce a Doppler transmitral blood flow velocity profile with an increased E-wave velocity as a consequence of the elevated LA pressure and increased volume flow rate across the MV. Isolated LV systolic dysfunction may be also be associated with an increased transmitral peak E-wave velocity and reduced A-wave because diastolic filling occurs at a steeper portion of the LV pressure-volume curve (26). Finally, the location of the pulsed wave Doppler sample volume and respiratory pattern can also affect the transmitral blood flow velocity profile (27).

Tachycardia causes a fusion of the transmitral E- and A-wave velocities and a pseudo-increase in the A-wave velocity and duration, especially if the E- and A-wave velocity is more than 20 cm/s (6). Dysrhythmias and pacing may also be associated with unique alterations in the Doppler transmitral and PV blood flow velocity profiles. For example, atrial flutter may present with "flutter waves" in the Doppler transmitral blood flow velocity profile. In patients with atrial fibrillation, the transmitral and PV_{AR} waves are absent, and the E-wave peak velocity and deceleration time vary with the length of the cardiac cycle. Atrial fibrillation may also be associated with a loss of PV_{S1} and a decrease in PV_{S2} relative to the dominant PV_D (28). The peak acceleration rate of the E-wave velocity (29), shortening of the transmitral E-wave deceleration time, and duration and initial deceleration slope time of PV_D may still correlate with increased LV filling pressure in the presence of atrial fibrillation (28).

Newer Echocardiographic Techniques for Assessing Left Ventricular Diastolic Function

Assessment of mitral annular motion with Doppler tissue imaging. Newer echocardiographic techniques for assessing LV diastolic function have been described that reportedly are less vulnerable to the effects of acute changes in loading conditions. Mitral annular motion is evaluated with Doppler tissue imaging, a technique that uses a low-velocity, high-amplitude signal to eliminate the high velocities associated with blood flow and provides a signal with a high degree of temporal and velocity range resolution (30). In the initial studies of the evaluation of mitral annular motion with Doppler tissue imaging, transthoracic echocardiography and a four- or two-chamber apical acoustic window were used. A midesophageal four-chamber view obtained with a transesophageal echocardiographic probe is also appropriate for positioning a pulsed wave Doppler sample volume (2.5–5.0 mm) on the lateral corner of the mitral annulus (Fig. 7.6). Alternatively, the septal side of the mitral annulus can be evaluated, although the tissue velocities tend to be lower and blood flow velocities in the LV outflow tract may obscure the Doppler tissue profile (31). The pulsed wave Doppler beam should be aligned as close to parallel as possible to the longitudinal axial motion of the LV. It is important to realize that these recorded velocities not only represent the rate of myocardial fiber shortening and lengthening in a specifically selected segment at the level of the mitral annulus, but also are influenced by velocities associated with the translation and rotation of cardiac structures (32). The lowest wall filter and minimal optimal gain should be used to eliminate blood flow velocity signals produced by transmitral flow. Finally, the Nyquist limit, sweep speed, and size of the Doppler profile should be adjusted for optimal visualization.

The mitral annular Doppler tissue imaging profile has a systolic component that has been shown to correlate with the ejection fraction (31), and a biphasic diastolic component that appears as an exact mirror image of the Doppler transmitral blood flow velocity profile except that the magnitude of the tissue velocities is much lower (8–15 cm/s). The initial early

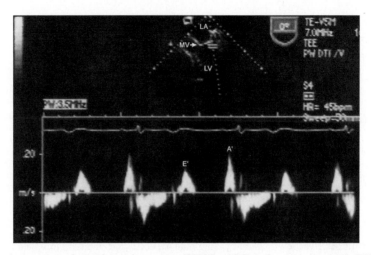

FIG. 7.6. Assessment of mitral annular motion (MAM) with Doppler tissue imaging (DTI). The pulsed wave Doppler sample volume is positioned at the level of the lateral mitral valve (MV) annulus to obtain the DTI profile. The mitral annular DTI profile has a biphasic diastolic component that includes an initial early (E′) and a later (A′) diastolic tissue velocity. The later diastolic tissue velocity (A′) reflects left atrial systolic function. LA, left atrium; LV, left ventricle.

diastolic tissue velocity (E′) begins simultaneously with mitral inflow, yet its peak precedes the peak transmitral E-wave velocity and ends before LV inflow termination (33). In the absence of gross geometric distortion and severe regional wall motion abnormalities, E′ reflects tissue velocities associated with changes in the LV volume and is primarily influenced by the rate of myocardial relaxation and elastic recoil. In a normal subject, the peak E′ velocity is greater than the later diastolic tissue velocity (A′), which tends to reflect LA systolic function (34).

E′ has been demonstrated to correlate with τ, supporting its value as an index of LV relaxation (30). E′ and E′/A′ have also been shown to decline with age and are reduced in pathologic LV hypertrophy, similar to transmitral inflow velocities (31,32). The concordance between mitral annular motion assessed by Doppler tissue imaging and mitral inflow velocities, however, is disrupted in progressive diastolic dysfunction when poor relaxation coexists with an elevated filling pressure. In patients with an elevated LVEDP who present with a pseudonormal (32) or restrictive Doppler transmitral inflow velocity profile (33), E′ remains reduced, suggesting relative preload independence (Fig. 7.7). *E′ has actually been shown to be the best discriminator between normal and pseudonormal profiles in comparison with single or combined indices of Doppler transmitral or PV blood flow velocity profiles* (30). Furthermore, neither peak E′ velocity nor the E′/A′ velocity ratio changes significantly after preload alteration with an infusion of saline solution or nitroglycerin (34). Thus, E′ is a relatively preload-insensitive measure of LV diastolic function that may be particularly useful in the perioperative period, when loading conditions can vary considerably.

Color M-mode transmitral propagation velocity. The onset of active LV relaxation is asynchronous, initially starting in apical myocardial segments that serve as a prominent source of recoil during early diastole (35). Early LV relaxation generates a suction force that creates an intraventricular pressure gradient initiated at the level of the mitral orifice. This pressure gradient is maintained in the mid LV during early diastole and is responsible for accelerating flow and promoting sequential filling toward the apex (35).

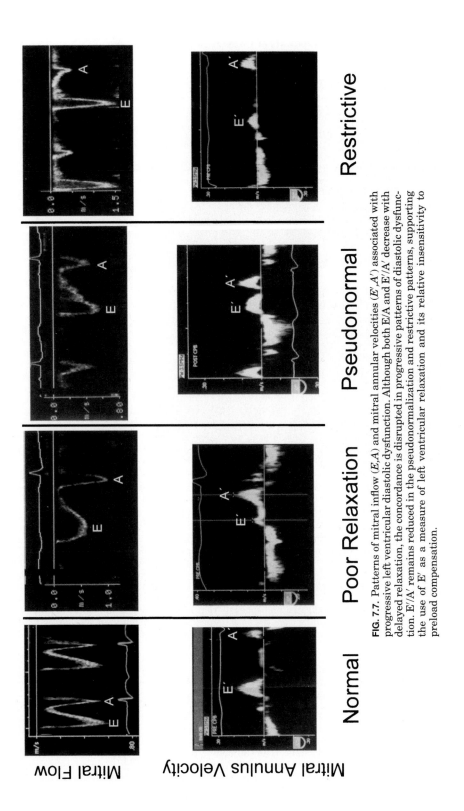

FIG. 7.7. Patterns of mitral inflow (E,A) and mitral annular velocities (E',A') associated with progressive left ventricular diastolic dysfunction. Although both E/A and E'/A' decrease with delayed relaxation, the concordance is disrupted in progressive patterns of diastolic dysfunction. E'/A' remains reduced in the pseudonormalization and restrictive patterns, supporting the use of E' as a measure of left ventricular relaxation and its relative insensitivity to preload compensation.

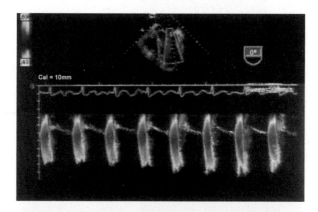

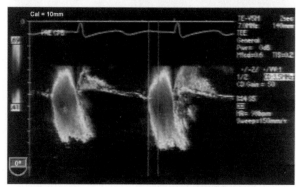

FIG. 7.8. Transmitral color M-mode Doppler flow propagation velocity (Vp) is obtained by placing the M-mode cursor through the center of the mitral inflow region in a transesophageal midesophageal four-chamber view and measuring the slope of the first aliasing velocity. (See Color Plate 9 following page 212.)

The propagation rate of LV peak inflow velocity, which is driven by rapid ventricular relaxation, can be evaluated with color M-mode Doppler echocardiography. Whereas standard pulsed wave Doppler permits only a temporal distribution of blood flow velocities in a single spatial location, color M-mode Doppler echocardiography provides a spatial-temporal distribution of these velocities that can be used to delineate the slope of the propagating wave front (Vp) from the mitral orifice toward the LV apex (32). The velocity at which flow propagates within the ventricle (Vp) can be determined from the slope of the color wave front (Fig. 7.8; see Color Plate 9 following page 212). A significant negative correlation between Vp and τ has been demonstrated and suggests that rapid LV relaxation (short τ) promotes faster propagation of LV filling from the base to the apex (36). In addition, patients with elevated LV minimal pressure and LVEDP have lower Vp values (35). Thus, Vp may represent a useful technique for evaluating LV diastolic function.

Color M-mode Doppler images of LV filling are often obtained with the use of transthoracic apical long-axis acoustic windows. A midesophageal, four-chamber transesophageal echocardiographic view also permits visualization of Vp when an M-mode Doppler beam is aligned parallel to the Doppler color flow display of transmitral inflow (Fig. 7.8; see Color Plate 9 following page 212). Vp can be measured from the first aliasing velocity slope beginning at the mitral annulus and ideally extending 3 to 4 cm into the LV toward the apex (32). Visualization of the color wave front can be optimized by shifting the baseline toward the direction of flow, maximizing sweep speed, and adjusting the depth.

In young healthy individuals, color M-mode Vp has been reported between 55 and 100 cm/s (36). Impaired LV relaxation results in a diminished ventricular minimal pressure, so that the propagation of early filling is compromised (Fig 7.9; see Color Plate 10 following

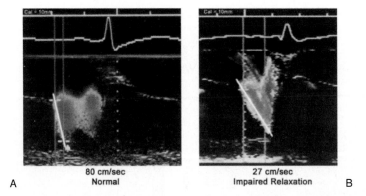

A   80 cm/sec   27 cm/sec   B
       Normal   Impaired Relaxation

FIG. 7.9. In comparison with the transmitral color M-mode (motion mode) propagation veloc-ity (Vp) in a normal subject (**A**), Vp is reduced in a patient with impaired left ventricular relaxation (**B**). (See Color Plate 10 following page 212.)

page 212). In contrast to standard Doppler indices of filling, Vp is relatively independent of preload yet responds to changes in lusitropic conditions (37) and systolic performance (38). Consequently, whereas Doppler transmitral and PV blood flow velocity profiles tend to show a parabolic distribution from normal through progressive diastolic dysfunction, Vp remains reduced in pseudonormal or restrictive LV filling. Furthermore, altering the preload by means of various techniques (partial CPB, inferior vena cava occlusion, intravenous nitro-glycerin, amyl nitrate inhalation, Valsalva maneuver, Trendelenburg positioning, leg lifting) is associated with changes in transmitral peak E-wave velocity, E-wave/A-wave velocity ra-tios, and E-wave deceleration, but it has little effect on Vp (38–40). Interestingly, the ratio of peak E-wave velocity to propagation velocity (E/Vp) may be useful to predict LA pres-sure (38) and also relates directly to LV filling pressures in patients with atrial fibrillation (29). *Thus, like E′, Vp is a relatively preload-insensitive measure of LV diastolic function that may be particularly useful in the perioperative period, when loading conditions can vary considerably* (7).

RIGHT VENTRICULAR DIASTOLIC FUNCTION

RV diastolic function can be assessed indirectly by a comprehensive two-dimensional echocardiographic examination of RV mass or volume. A thorough assessment of RV diastolic function, however, requires a Doppler echocardiographic evaluation of trans-tricuspid blood flow velocities (Fig. 7.10A). Doppler trans-tricuspid flow velocities are affected by the same physiologic variables that affect LV filling, although they tend to be lower because of the larger size of the tricuspid valve annulus. Direct comparisons of RV and LV inflow velocities also reveal differences in timing and reciprocal respiratory variations. During spontaneous inspiration, negative intrapleural pressure results in an increase in right atrial (RA) volume and RV diastolic filling velocities up to 20% greater than at end-expiration (26). LA and LV filling is actually reduced during spontaneous inspiration relative to end-expiration. These reciprocal patterns of respiratory variation become exaggerated in patients with diastolic dysfunction. Although it has not been thoroughly investigated, positive-pressure ventilation would presumably have an effect on Doppler trans-tricuspid blood flow velocity patterns opposite to that of spontaneous ventilation.

An echocardiographic evaluation of RV diastolic function also includes an assessment of RA inflow velocities and the hepatic venous, inferior vena cava, and superior vena cava Doppler profiles, all of which have similar contours and components. The hepatic veins join the intrahepatic inferior vena cava tangentially and can be visualized by advancing and turning the transesophageal echocardiographic probe rightward from a midesophageal

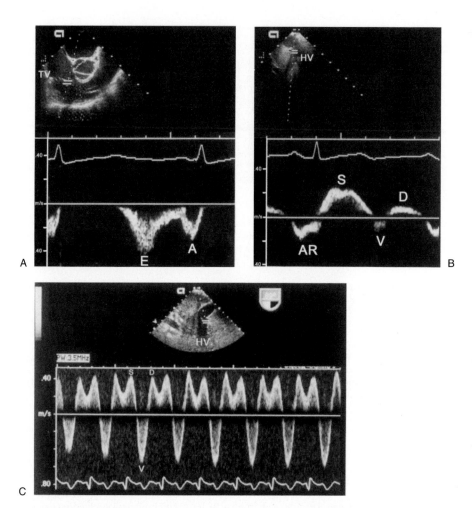

FIG. 7.10. A: Normal trans-tricuspid Doppler flow velocity profile. **B:** Normal hepatic venous Doppler flow velocity profiles. **C:** Prominent hepatic flow reversal at end-systole (*V*) in a patient with decreased right ventricular compliance. *E*, early diastolic velocity; *A*, late diastolic velocity; *AR*, atrial contraction flow reversal; *S*, antegrade early systolic flow; *D*, antegrade flow during right ventricular filling; *HV*, hepatic vein; *TV*, tricuspid valve.

bicaval acoustic view. The normal hepatic venous Doppler profile (Fig. 7.10A) is characterized by the following: (a) a small reversal of flow following atrial contraction (*AR-wave*); (b) an antegrade systolic phase during atrial filling from the superior vena cava and inferior vena cava (*S-wave*) that is influenced by tricuspid valve annular motion, RA relaxation, and tricuspid regurgitation; (c) a second small flow reversal at end-systole (*V-wave*) that is influenced by RV and RA compliance; and (d) a second antegrade filling phase while the RA acts as a passive conduit during RV filling (*D-wave*) (26).

Diastolic RV dysfunction can manifest with the same relative changes in trans-tricuspid peak E- and A-wave velocities, E-wave/A-wave ratios, and deceleration time that occur in the Doppler transmitral blood flow velocity profiles associated with alterations in LV relaxation and compliance (41,42). The ratio of the total hepatic reverse flow integral to the total forward flow integral ($TVI_A + TVI_V/TVI_S + TVI_D$) increases with either RV diastolic dysfunction or significant tricuspid regurgitation, but it appears to be more affected by the former (43). In addition, a marked shortening of the trans-tricuspid deceleration time and the diastolic predominance of hepatic venous flow with prominent V- and A-wave reversals during spontaneous inspiration indicate significant decreases in RV compliance and increased diastolic filling pressures (6) (Fig. 7.10B). Changes in the diameter of the inferior vena cava during spontaneous inspiration also reflect RA pressure. In general, low RA pressure (0–5 mm Hg) is associated with a small diameter of the inferior vena cava (<1.5 cm) and a spontaneous inspiratory collapse of more than 50% of the original diameter. In contrast, significant increases in RA pressure (>20 mm Hg) are associated with a dilated inferior vena cava and hepatic veins, with little respiratory variation (26). Diastolic RV dysfunction (lower tricuspid valve peak E-wave velocity, lower E/A ratios, and prolonged RV IVRT) has also been demonstrated in patients with pulmonary hypertension and in those with symptomatic congestive heart failure, even in the absence of pulmonary hypertension, suggesting a potential role for ventricular interdependence in impaired RV filling (44).

PERICARDIAL DISEASE: CONSTRICTIVE PERICARDITIS AND PERICARDIAL TAMPONADE

Pericardial pathology, including constrictive pericarditis and pericardial tamponade resulting from effusions, can impede diastolic flow. Although chest radiography and magnetic resonance imaging may be helpful in diagnosing pericardial disease, echocardiography continues to be essential for delineating the associated pathophysiology. Two-dimensional echocardiography can be helpful in diagnosing constrictive pericarditis by identifying a thickened, fibrotic, and calcified echogenic pericardium together with abnormal ventricular septal motion, flattening of the LV posterior wall during diastole, and a dilated inferior vena cava (45). Alternatively, two-dimensional echocardiographic identification of pericardial effusions usually reveals an echo-free space that may contain thrombi. Although small (<25 mL), loculated effusions can be difficult to visualize, larger effusions associated with pericardial tamponade pathophysiology are usually accompanied by additional two-dimensional echocardiographic and M-mode features, including persistence of the effusion throughout the cardiac cycle, a characteristic "swinging motion" of the heart, early diastolic RV collapse, late diastolic to early systolic RA inversion, and abnormal ventricular septal motion (45).

The diagnosis of constrictive pericarditis and pericardial tamponade includes the identification of significant respiratory variation in atrial and ventricular Doppler inflow profiles. Normally, during spontaneous respiration, intrathoracic pressures are transmitted equally to the pericardial space and intracardiac chambers. The transmission of intrathoracic pressure, however, is prevented by the thickened, noncompliant pericardium in patients with constrictive pericarditis and by significant pericardial effusions. Consequently, LA and LV filling pressure gradients are decreased during spontaneous *inspiration,* resulting in diminished PV forward diastolic velocities, delayed MV opening, prolonged IVRT, and decreased mitral E-wave velocity (28,46). Similarly, relative increases in LA and LV filling pressure gradients during spontaneous *expiration* are responsible for corresponding increases in Doppler LA and LV inflow velocities. The exaggeration of ventricular interdependence in constrictive pericarditis and pericardial tamponade is responsible for reciprocal changes in right-sided intracardiac flows that result in increased tricuspid E-wave velocities during spontaneous inspiration. In addition, hepatic venous forward velocities decrease and reverse flows increase during expiration (47). Because the direction of the intrathoracic pressure changes associated with positive-pressure ventilation is opposite to the direction of the changes that occur with spontaneous breathing, mechanical ventilation reverses the respiratory variation pattern of LA and LV inflow velocities seen in constrictive pericarditis (48). Thus, the demonstration of respiratory variation in Doppler atrial and ventricular inflow profiles can be a useful technique to establish the diagnosis of hemodynamically significant pericardial pathology.

The distinction between restriction and constriction based on Doppler LV and LA inflow velocities alone can be difficult because both disorders may present with profiles resembling

TABLE 7.2. DOPPLER ECHOCARDIOGRAPHIC VALUES FOR INDICES OF LEFT
VENTRICULAR DIASTOLIC DYSFUNCTION

	Normal (young)	Normal (adult)	Impaired relaxation	Pseudonormal filling	Restrictive filling
E/A (cm/s)	>1	>1	<1	1–2	>2
DT (msc)	<220	<220	>220	150–200	<150
IVRT (ms)	<100	<100	>100	60–100	<60
S/D	<1	≥1	≥1	<1	<1
PV$_{AR}$ (cm/s)	<35	<35	<35	≥35[a]	≥25[a]
Vp (cm/s)	>55	>45	<45	<45	<45
E' (cm/s)	>10	>8	<8	<8	<8

[a]Unless atrial mechanical failure is present.

E/A, early-to-late left ventricular (LV) filling ratio; DT, early LV filling deceleration time; IVRT, isovolumic relaxation time; S/D, systolic-to-diastolic pulmonary venous flow ratio; PV$_{AR}$, pulmonary venous peak atrial contraction reversal velocity; V$_P$, transmitral color M-mode propagation velocity; E', peak early diastolic mitral annular velocity.

From Garcia M, Thomas J, Klein A. New Doppler echocardiographic applications for the study of diastolic function. *J Am Coll Cardiol* 1998;32:872, with permission.

restrictive LV diastolic filling (46). However, discordant pressure changes between the LV and RV during respiration are unusual in restrictive cardiomyopathy. Consequently, constrictive pericarditis can be differentiated from restrictive cardiomyopathy by the demonstration of respiratory variation in Doppler transmitral and PV blood flow velocities (49). Furthermore, patients with constrictive pericarditis and preserved systolic function have a more rapid Vp (50) and a normal or elevated E' (51) in comparison with patients who have restrictive cardiomyopathy.

SUMMARY

Normal diastolic function is required for optimal cardiac performance. Impaired ventricular filling and increased chamber stiffness are responsible for a significant component of the pathophysiology associated with congestive heart failure. Diastolic dysfunction is prevalent among cardiovascular surgical patients and may contribute to perioperative morbidity. Echocardiography provides an effective, noninvasive means for determining the presence, extent, and causes of diastolic dysfunction (Table 7.2). Although conventional Doppler echocardiographic measurements of atrial and ventricular inflow velocities are still an important component of a thorough examination, newer techniques, including Doppler tissue imaging of the mitral annulus and color M-mode transmitral propagation velocity, may be less sensitive to changes in loading conditions. It is hoped that in the near future, more sensitive, cost-effective echocardiographic techniques for diagnosing diastolic dysfunction will be available to facilitate the development of perioperative therapeutic interventions.

REFERENCES

1. Grossman W. Diastolic dysfunction in congestive heart failure. *N Engl J Med* 1991;22:1557–1564.
2. Pinamonti B, Lenarda A, Sinagra G, et al. Restrictive left ventricular filling pattern in dilated cardiomyopathy assessed by Doppler echocardiography: clinical, echocardiographic, and hemodynamic correlations and prognostic implications. *J Am Coll Cardiol* 1993;22:808–815.

3. Bernard F, Denault A, Babin D, et al. Diastolic dysfunction is predictive of difficult weaning from cardiopulmonary bypass. *Anesth Analg* 2001;92:291–298.
4. Yusef S, Thom T, Abbott RD. Changes in hypertension treatment and congestive heart failure mortality in the United States. *Hypertension* 1989;13[Suppl]:174–179.
5. Vasan R, Larson M, Benjamin E, et al. Congestive heart failure in subjects with normal versus reduced left ventricular ejection fraction: prevalence and mortality in a population-based cohort. *J Am Coll Cardiol* 1999;33:1948–1955.
6. Appleton C, Firstenberg M, Garcia M, et al. The echo-Doppler evaluation of left ventricular diastolic function: a current perspective. *Cardiol Clin* 2000;18:513–546.
7. Djainani G, Ti L, Mackensen B, et al. Color M-mode propagation velocity identifies patients with diastolic dysfunction during coronary bypass surgery. *Anesth Analg* 2001; 92:SCA74.
8. De Hert S, Rodrigus I, Haenen L, et al. Recovery of systolic and diastolic left ventricular function early after cardiopulmonary bypass. *Anesthesiology* 1996;85:1063–1075.
9. Doolan L, Jones E, Kalman J, et al. A placebo-controlled trial verifying the efficacy of milrinone in weaning high-risk patients from cardiopulmonary bypass. *J Cardiothorac Vasc Anesth* 1997;11:37–41.
10. Plotnick GD. Changes in diastolic function—difficult to measure, harder to interpret. *Am Heart J* 1989;118:637–641.
11. Nishimura R, Tajik A. Evaluation of diastolic filling of left ventricle in health and disease: Doppler echocardiography is the clinician's Rosetta stone. *J Am Coll Cardiol* 1997;30: 8–18.
12. Pagel P, Grossman W, Haering J, et al. Left ventricular diastolic function in the normal and diseased heart: perspectives for the anesthesiologist. *Anesthesiology* 1993;79: 836–854.
13. Zile M, Smith V. Relaxation and diastolic properties of the heart. In: Fozzard H, Haber E, Jennings R, et al., eds. *The heart and cardiovascular system: scientific foundations,* 2nd ed. New York: Raven Press, 1991:1353–1367.
14. Appleton C, Galloway J, Gonzalez M, et al. Estimation of left ventricular filling pressures using two-dimensional and Doppler echocardiography in adult patients with cardiac disease: additional value of analyzing left atrial size, left atrial ejection fraction and the difference in duration of pulmonary venous and mitral flow velocity at atrial contraction. *J Am Coll Cardiol* 1993;22:1972–1982.
15. Cohen G, Pietrolungo J, Thomas J, et al. A practical guide to assessment of ventricular diastolic function using Doppler echocardiography. *J Am Coll Cardiol* 1996;27: 1753–1760.
16. Little W, Ohno M, Kitzman D, et al. Determination of left ventricular chamber stiffness from the time for deceleration of early left ventricular filling. *Circulation* 1995;92: 1933–1939.
17. Oh J, Appleton C, Hatle L, et al. The noninvasive assessment of left ventricular diastolic function with two-dimensional and Doppler echocardiography. *J Am Soc Echocardiogr* 1997;10:246–270.
18. Appleton C, Hatle L. The natural history of left ventricular filling abnormalities: assessment by two-dimensional and Doppler echocardiography. *Echocardiography* 1992;9: 437–457.
19. Dumesnil J, Gaudreault G, Honos G, et al. Use of Valsalva maneuver to unmask left ventricular diastolic function abnormalities by Doppler echocardiography in patients with coronary artery disease or systemic hypertension. *Am J Cardiol* 1991;68: 515–519.
20. Hurrell D, Nishimura R, Ilstrup D, et al. Utility of preload alteration in assessment of left ventricular filling pressure by Doppler echocardiography: a simultaneous catheterization and Doppler echocardiographic study. *J Am Coll Cardiol* 1997;30: 459–467.
21. Nishimura R, Abel M, Hatle L, et al. Relation of pulmonary vein to mitral flow velocities by transesophageal Doppler echocardiography: effect of different loading conditions. *Circulation* 1990;81:488–497.
22. Kuecherer H, Muhiudeen I, Kusumoto F, et al. Estimation of mean left atrial pressure from transesophageal pulsed Doppler echocardiography of pulmonary venous flow. *Circulation* 1990;82:1127–1139.

23. Yamamoto K, Nishimura R, Burnett J, et al. Assessment of end-diastolic pressure by Doppler echocardiography: contribution of duration of pulmonary venous versus mitral flow velocity curves at atrial contraction. *J Am Soc Echocardiogr* 1997;10: 52–59.
24. Appleton C, Hatle L, Popp R. Relation of transmitral flow velocity patterns to left ventricular diastolic function: new insights from a combined hemodynamic and Doppler echocardiographic study. *J Am Coll Cardiol* 1988;12:426–440.
25. Nishimura R, Abel M, Hatle L, et al. Assessment of diastolic function of the heart: background and current applications of Doppler echocardiography: part II. Clinical studies. *Mayo Clin Proc* 1989;64:181–204.
26. Otto C. Echocardiographic evaluation of ventricular diastolic filling and function. In: Otto C, ed. *Textbook of clinical echocardiography,* 2nd ed. Philadelphia: WB Saunders, 2000:132–152.
27. Oka Y, Kato M, Strom J. Mitral valve. In: Oka Y, Goldiner P, eds. *Transesophageal echocardiography.* Philadelphia: JB Lippincott, 1992:99–151.
28. Oh JK, Seward JB, Tajik AJ. Assessment of diastolic function. In: *The echo manual,* 2nd ed. Philadelphia: Lippincott Williams & Wilkins, 1999:45–57.
29. Nagueh S, Kopelen H, Quinones M. Assessment of left ventricular filling pressures by Doppler in the presence of atrial fibrillation. *Circulation* 1996;94:2138–2145.
30. Farias C, Rodriguez L, Garcia M, et al. Assessment of diastolic function by tissue Doppler echocardiography: comparison with standard transmitral and pulmonary venous flow. *J Am Soc Echocardiogr* 1999;12:609–617.
31. Nagueh S, Middleton K, Kopelen H, et al. Doppler tissue imaging: a noninvasive technique for evaluation of left ventricular relaxation and estimation of filling pressures. *J Am Coll Cardiol* 1997;30:1527–1533.
32. Garcia M, Thomas J, Klein A. New Doppler echocardiographic applications for the study of diastolic function. *J Am Coll Cardiol* 1998;32:865–875.
33. Garcia M, Rodriguez L, Ares M, et al. Differentiation of constrictive pericarditis from restrictive cardiomyopathy: assessment of left ventricular diastolic velocities in longitudinal axis by Doppler tissue imaging. *J Am Coll Cardiol* 1996;27:108–114.
34. Sohn D, Chai I, Lee D, et al. Assessment of mitral annulus velocity by Doppler tissue imaging in the evaluation of left ventricular diastolic function. *J Am Coll Cardiol* 1997;30:474–480.
35. Takatsuji H, Mikami T, Urasawa K, et al. A new approach for evaluation of left ventricular diastolic function: spatial and temporal analysis of left ventricular filling flow propagation by color M-mode Doppler echocardiography. *J Am Coll Cardiol* 1996;27: 363–371.
36. Brun P, Tribouilloy C, Duval A, et al. Left ventricular flow propagation velocity during early filling is related to wall relaxation: a color M-mode Doppler analysis. *J Am Coll Cardiol* 1992;20:420–432.
37. Garcia M, Smedira N, Greenberg N, et al. Color M-mode Doppler flow propagation velocity is a preload insensitive index of left ventricular relaxation: animal and human validation. *J Am Coll Cardiol* 2000;35:201–208.
38. Garcia M, Ares M, Asher C, et al. An index of early left ventricular filling that combined with pulsed Doppler peak E velocity may estimate capillary wedge pressure. *J Am Coll Cardiol* 1997;29:448–454.
39. Moller J, Poulsen S, Sondergaard E, et al. Preload dependence of color M-mode Doppler flow propagation velocity in controls and in patients with left ventricular dysfunction. *J Am Soc Echocardiogr* 2000;13:902–909.
40. Garcia M, Palac R, Malenka D, et al. Color M-mode Doppler flow propagation velocity is a relatively preload-independent index of left ventricular filling. *J Am Soc Echocardiogr* 1999;12:129–137.
41. Klein A, Hatle L, Burstow D, et al. Comprehensive Doppler assessment of right ventricular diastolic function in cardiac amyloidosis. *J Am Coll Cardiol* 1990;15:99–108.
42. Spencer K, Weinert L, Lang R. Effect of age, heart rate and tricuspid regurgitation on the Doppler echocardiographic evaluation of right ventricular diastolic function. *Cardiology* 1999;92:59–64.
43. Nomura T, Lebowitz L, Koide Y, et al. Evaluation of hepatic venous flow using

transesophageal echocardiography in coronary artery bypass surgery: an index of right ventricular function. *J Thorac Cardiovasc Anesth* 1995;9:9–17.

44. Yu C, Sanderson J, Chan S, et al. Right ventricular diastolic dysfunction in heart failure. *Circulation* 1996;93:1509–1514.

45. Feigenbaum H. Pericardial disease. In: Feigenbaum H, ed. *Echocardiography*, 5th ed. Baltimore: Williams & Wilkins, 1994:556–588.

46. Klein A, Cohen G, Pietrolungo J, et al. Differentiation of constrictive pericarditis from restrictive cardiomyopathy by Doppler transesophageal echocardiographic measurements of respiratory variations in pulmonary venous flow. *J Am Coll Cardiol* 1993;22:1935–1943.

47. Burstow D, Oh J, Bailey K, et al. Cardiac tamponade: characteristic Doppler observations. *Mayo Clin Proc* 1989;64:312–324.

48. Abdalla I, Murray D, Awad H, et al. Reversal of the pattern of respiratory variation of Doppler inflow velocities in constrictive pericarditis during mechanical ventilation. *J Am Soc Echocardiogr* 2000;13:827–831.

49. Schiavone W, Calafiore P, Salcedo E. Transesophageal Doppler echocardiographic demonstration of pulmonary venous flow velocity in restrictive cardiomyopathy and constrictive pericarditis. *Am J Cardiol* 1989;63:1286–1288.

50. Rodriguez L, Ares M, Vandervoort P, et al. Does color M-mode flow propagation differentiate between patients with restrictive vs. constrictive physiology? *J Am Coll Cardiol* 1996;27:268A. Abstract.

51. Rajagopalan N, Garcia M, Rodriguez L, et al. Comparison of Doppler echocardiographic methods to differentiate constrictive pericarditis from restrictive cardiomyopathy. *J Am Coll Cardiol* 1998;31:164A. Abstract.

QUESTIONS

1. Which of the following patterns of LV diastolic dysfunction occurs most commonly in acute myocardial ischemia?
   a. Restrictive
   b. Pseudonormal
   c. Constrictive
   d. Poor relaxation

2. During spontaneous inspiration, patients with pericardial tamponade are most likely to demonstrate which of the following changes in the peak E-wave velocity of the Doppler trans-tricuspid and transmitral flow profiles?

Peak E-wave Velocity	
Trans-tricuspid	Transmitral
a. Increase	Decrease
b. Decrease	Decrease
c. Decrease	Increase
d. Increase	Increase

3. In comparison with the poor relaxation pattern of LV diastolic dysfunction, the restrictive pattern is characterized by which of the following changes in the Doppler transmitral flow velocity IVRT and E-wave deceleration time?

Transmitral Doppler Flow Velocity	
Isovolumic Relaxation Time	E-wave Deceleration Time
a. Increase	Increase
b. Increase	Decrease
c. Decrease	Increase
d. Decrease	Decrease

4. An increased pulmonary AR-wave/mitral A-wave duration ratio is consistent with which of the following conditions?
   a. Increased LA compliance
   b. Decreased LA pressure
   c. Increased LVEDP
   d. Decreased PV compliance
5. A Doppler PV blood flow velocity profile with a biphasic systolic component has an initial antegrade velocity (PV_{S1}) that is most closely related to which of the following cardiac cycle components?
   a. LA relaxation
   b. LV contraction
   c. LA contraction
   d. LV compliance
6. In comparison with normal adult values, the restrictive pattern of LV diastolic function exhibits which one of the following sets of relative changes in Doppler echocardiographic velocities?

Pulmonary Vein Systolic/Diastolic Velocity Ratio	Mitral Annular Doppler Tissue Imaging Peak E Velocity (E′)	Transmitral Color M-Mode Propagation Velocity (Vp)
a. Increased	Increased	Decreased
b. Decreased	Decreased	Decreased
c. Increased	Increased	Increased
d. Decreased	Decreased	Increased

7. Which of the following Doppler echocardiographic measurements is the best predictor of increased LV filling pressure in patients with atrial fibrillation?
   a. Increased PV_{AR}/MV_A duration ratio
   b. Decreased PV diastolic flow
   c. Increased transmitral peak E-wave velocity
   d. Decreased transmitral E-wave deceleration time
8. The use of a Valsalva maneuver will convert a pseudonormalized LV inflow pattern to which of the following transmitral Doppler flow velocity patterns?
   a. Normal
   b. Restrictive
   c. Poor relaxation
   d. Constrictive.
9. The transmitral color M-mode propagation velocity (Vp) is most likely to decrease during which of the following conditions?
   a. Administration of esmolol
   b. Reverse Trendelenburg positioning
   c. Administration of nitroglycerin
   d. Valsalva maneuver
10. Which of the following echocardiographic measurements made during spontaneous inspiration is most consistent with a diagnosis of decreased RV compliance and increased filling pressures?
    a. Prolonged trans-tricuspid E-wave deceleration time
    b. Diastolic predominance of hepatic venous flow
    c. Diminished hepatic AR-wave TVI
    d. More than 50% inspiratory collapse of the inferior vena cava

PART III

TRANSESOPHAGEAL ECHOCARDIOGRAPHY IN VALVULAR DISEASE AND SURGERY

8

Mitral Regurgitation

A. Stephane Lambert

Mitral regurgitation (MR) is a common disease, and its evaluation by transesophageal echocardiography (TEE) presents a major challenge to intraoperative echocardiographers, yet few applications of intraoperative TEE have as much impact on the course of surgery and on patient outcome as the evaluation of MR.

ANATOMY

The mitral valve (MV) is bicuspid and consists of a large anterior leaflet and a smaller posterior leaflet (see color tip following page 212 for figures of heart valves). The anterior leaflet covers about two thirds of the surface of the valve. Although the posterior leaflet covers only one third of the surface of the valve, it wraps around the anterior leaflet and accounts for about two thirds of the circumference of the valve. The leaflets join at the anterolateral and posteromedial commissures. The posterior leaflet is divided into three scallops. The coaptation between the two leaflets in systole is semicircular, not linear. It is important to keep this feature in mind so that the various TEE planes of the MV can be understood. The valve is encircled by a fibrous ring, the mitral annulus; this plays an important role in proper valve closure by reducing its diameter in systole. The MV is attached to two papillary muscles, anterolateral and posteromedial, through chordae tendineae. Chordae tendineae extend from each papillary muscle to both mitral leaflets. During systole, the papillary muscles contract to keep the chordae tendineae taut and prevent prolapse of the leaflets into the left atrium. The anterior leaflet of the MV is attached to the same fibrous structure as the left and noncoronary cusps of the aortic valve, an area sometimes referred to as the *fibrous body* or *crux* of the heart.

NOMENCLATURE SCHEMES

Three basic nomenclature schemes are used (1) (Fig. 8.1). Each institution or group of practitioners has its preferred scheme, and the reader is advised to acquire a basic understanding of all of them to avoid confusion. For example, *P2* refers to a different area of the valve in the Carpentier and Duran nomenclatures.

　　1. *Classic.* The classic anatomic nomenclature refers to the three scallops of the posterior leaflet of the MV as *anterolateral, middle,* and *posteromedial* (2). The anterolateral scallop is closest to the left atrial appendage.
　　2. *Carpentier.* A second popular nomenclature, attributed to Carpentier et al. (3), defines the three scallops of the posterior leaflet as *P1, P2,* and *P3;* P1 is closest to the left atrial appendage. It also defines the three corresponding areas of the anterior leaflet as *A1* (opposite P1), *A2* (opposite P2), and *A3* (opposite P3). *The Carpentier nomenclature is the most popular and is used throughout this book.*
　　3. *Duran.* The Duran nomenclature (4) refers to the three scallops of the posterior leaflet as *P1, PM* (middle), and *P2;* again, P1 is closest to the left atrial appendage. In this nomenclature, the anterior leaflet is divided into only two areas, *A1* and *A2,* opposite the corresponding scallops of the posterior leaflet. In addition, the two commissural areas of the valve are defined as *C1* (between A1 and P1) and *C2* (between A2 and P2).

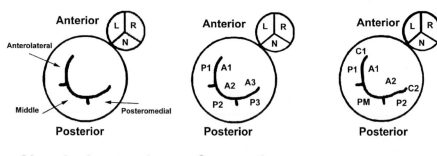

Classic Anatomic   Carpentier   Duran

FIG. 8.1. Schematic representation of the various systems of nomenclature of the mitral valve. The mitral valve is shown in its relation to the aortic valve. (Adapted from Lambert AS, Miller JP, Merrick SH, et al. Improved evaluation of the location and mechanism of mitral valve regurgitation with a systematic transesophageal echocardiography examination. *Anesth Analg* 1999;88:1205–1212, with permission.)

ETIOLOGY AND MECHANISM OF MITRAL REGURGITATION

MR is generally classified according to its etiology (Table 8.1). In addition, it is often useful to identify the pathophysiologic mechanism leading to the regurgitation: normal, excessive, or restricted leaflet motion (5,6) (Fig. 8.2).

1. ***Normal leaflet motion.*** If leaflet motion is normal, the most common causes of MR are ischemic papillary muscle dysfunction and annular dilation. In such cases, the MR is often central but may also be eccentric.

2. ***Excessive leaflet motion.*** The spectrum of severity of excessive leaflet motion is illustrated in Figure 8.3. *Billowing* refers to a condition in which part of a mitral leaflet projects above the annulus in systole, but the coaptation point remains below the mitral annulus. The term *prolapse* is used to describe the excursion of a leaflet tip above the level of the mitral annulus during systole. The term *flail* is reserved for a condition in which a leaflet edge flows freely into the left atrium as a result of one or more ruptured chordae tendineae.

TABLE 8.1. CAUSES OF MITRAL REGURGITATION

Congenital
  Endocardial cushion defect
  Associated with other pathologies (e.g., corrected transposition)
Myxomatous degeneration
Rheumatic (often accompanied by mitral stenosis)
Endocarditis
  Bacterial, viral, other
Papillary muscle disease
  Rupture
  Ischemia
Cardiomyopathy
  Dilated (ischemic, idiopathic, alcohol- or drug-related)
  Hypertrophic
Systemic lupus
Rheumatoid arthritis
Ankylosing spondylitis

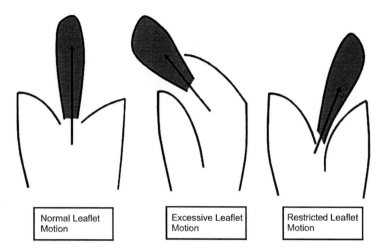

FIG. 8.2. Mitral valve leaflet motion. Leaflet motion can be normal with or without annular dilation, excessive, or restricted. The usual direction of the mitral regurgitant jet in each case is also depicted.

The distinction between severe prolapse and flail is sometimes difficult because the ruptured chordae may not be visible by echocardiography. It is also somewhat academic because the hemodynamic consequences and surgical treatment of the two are often the same.

3. ***Restricted leaflet motion.*** Restricted leaflet motion is commonly the result of fibrosis or calcification, and it sometimes coexists with a degree of mitral stenosis. An ischemic (i.e., stiff) papillary muscle may also restrict leaflet motion and cause failure of coaptation.

INTRAOPERATIVE EXAMINATION OF THE REGURGITANT MITRAL VALVE

The intraoperative evaluation of MR requires the echocardiographer to address three essential questions:

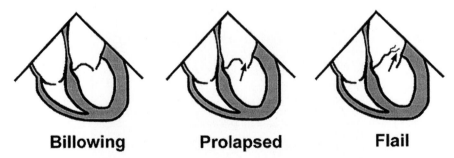

FIG. 8.3. Excessive leaflet motion. Billowing is an extension of part of a leaflet above the level of the mitral annulus in systole. In prolapse, the tip of the leaflet protrudes above the annulus in systole. Flail is a condition in which the edge of the leaflet is free-flowing in the left atrium. Ruptured chordae tendineae can sometimes also be seen.

1. How severe is the MR?
2. What is the mechanism of the MR and where on the MV is the lesion?
3. Can the valve be repaired?

Step 1: Grading the Severity of Mitral Regurgitation

1. *Two-dimensional examination.* The basic two-dimensional examination (see Chapter 2) often provides clues that significant MR is present. The clues may be direct, such as a large coaptation defect or a structural anomaly of a leaflet (Fig. 8.4), or they may be indirect indicators of the hemodynamic effects of severe MR, such as volume overload of the left ventricle and left atrium or signs of pulmonary hypertension (enlarged, hypertrophic right ventricle, dilated pulmonary artery, tricuspid regurgitation). These abnormalities should alert the clinician to undertake a more detailed two-dimensional examination of the MV for the precise localization of lesions, as is discussed later.

2. *Color flow Doppler examination.* Color flow Doppler remains the easiest and best method to screen for MR because of its high sensitivity and specificity. It also provides a semiquantitative assessment of the severity of MR. MR is graded as trivial, mild, moderate, or severe. These correspond to the 1+, 2+, 3+, and 4+ scores reported from angiography. The size and depth of penetration of the regurgitant jet provide a rough estimate of the severity of regurgitation.

a. *Color map of the regurgitant jet area.* The ratio of the regurgitant jet area to the total left atrial area has been reported to correlate well with the severity of MR (7). A ratio

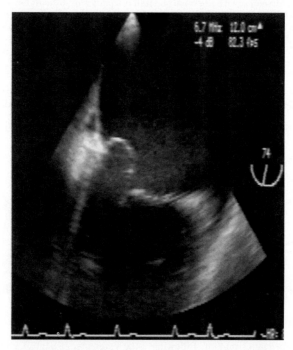

FIG. 8.4. Severe prolapse of the posteromedial segment of the posterior mitral leaflet. This is a two-dimensional transesophageal echocardiographic image in the midesophageal commissural view. Note that the whole segment extends above the mitral annulus into the left atrium. Doppler examination in this case revealed severe mitral regurgitation.

TABLE 8.2. GRADING OF MITRAL REGURGITATION

Method	Mild	Moderate	Severe
MR jet area atrial area	20%–30%	30%–40%	>40%
Vena contracta width			>5.5 mm
MR jet area	<3 cm^2	3.0–6.0 cm^2	>6 cm^2
Pulmonary vein flow	Blunted S wave	S wave < D wave	Systolic reversal
MR fraction	20%–30%	30%–50%	>55%
Mitral orifice (PISA)	<10 mm^2	10–25 mm^2	>25–35 mm^2

MR, mitral regurgitant; PISA, proximal isovelocity surface area.

greater than 40% suggests severe MR (Table 8.2). However, this technique has significant limitations (8–10), and the severity of MR should not be determined only by the size of the Doppler jet.

   The direction of the jet has important clinical implications. *Central jets typically result from annular dilation or ischemic papillary muscle dysfunction. Eccentric jets are almost always caused by a structural abnormality of the mitral apparatus and are consequently unlikely to improve after revascularization* (Fig. 8.5; see Color Plate 11 following page 212). In the case of a leaflet prolapse, the Doppler jet is directed away from the diseased leaflet. In the case of a restricted leaflet, the jet is directed toward the diseased leaflet (Fig. 8.2). Eccentric regurgitant jets always warrant close examination. Moreover, jets with enough energy to "hug the wall" of the atrium for some distance should be considered significant until proven otherwise (11).

b. *Width of the vena contracta.* The base of the jet, also known as *vena contracta,* can be measured, and diameters of 5.5 mm or more have been shown to correlate with severe MR on cardiac catheterization (12) (Fig. 8.6; see Color Plate 12 following page 212).

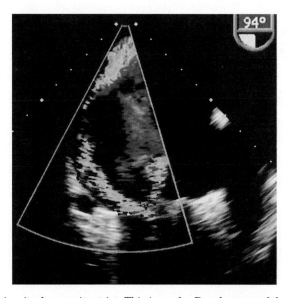

FIG. 8.5. Eccentric mitral regurgitant jet. This is a color Doppler scan of the mitral valve in the midesophageal four-chamber view. Note the severe mitral regurgitant jet, which "hugs" the posterior wall of the left atrium all the way to the top. Wall-hugging jets should be considered severe until proven otherwise. (See Color Plate 11 following page 212.)

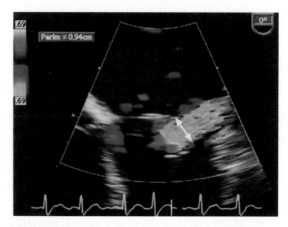

FIG. 8.6. Measurement of the vena contracta. This is a color Doppler scan of the mitral valve in the midesophageal four-chamber view. The diameter of the base of the mitral regurgitant jet correlates with the severity of regurgitation. (See Color Plate 12 following page 212.)

It is important to remember that any color Doppler assessment will be affected by the various settings of the echocardiography machine (e.g., aliasing velocity, pulse repetition frequency, frame rate), as is discussed in greater detail in Chapters 5 and 20. For example, excessive color gain settings will lead to a blooming of the regurgitant jet and an overestimation of MR.

3. *Spectral Doppler examination.* Spectral Doppler adds to the semiquantitative assessment of the valve. The number of particles (i.e., blood cells) that interact with the Doppler beam determines the density of the signal by continuous wave Doppler. A dense MR jet with a sharp border on continuous wave Doppler suggests that a large fraction of the left ventricular output is flowing back into the left atrium in systole. The evaluation of pulmonary venous flow by pulsed wave Doppler is also very important and should be a routine part of any assessment of MR. The normal pulsed wave Doppler pattern of pulmonary vein flow is forward in both systole and diastole (Fig. 8.7A). *Blunting or reversal of the systolic component is one of the most reliable signs of hemodynamically significant MR* (13) (Table 8.2; Fig. 8.7B).

The more precise, but less often used, quantitative assessments of MR require mathematical calculations, which are described in a later section of this chapter.

Step 2: What Is the Mechanism of the Lesion and Where on the Mitral Valve Is It Located?

Once significant MR has been diagnosed, the next step in the examination is to determine its mechanism and the precise location of the lesion. This is critical to the formulation of an appropriate surgical plan. A systematic and detailed two-dimensional echocardiographic examination of the MV involving a sequence of six views is performed (1,14) (Fig. 8.8). The goal is to obtain redundant views of all parts of the valve and to identify each mitral segment by using internal cardiac landmarks that are easily recognized. The recommended sequence of cross sections is as follows:

1. The examination begins in the midesophageal (ME) four-chamber view at an imaging plane 0 degree. The anterior mitral leaflet is medial, adjacent to the aortic valve, and the posterior leaflet is lateral. Anteflexion of the probe, so that the left ventricular outflow tract

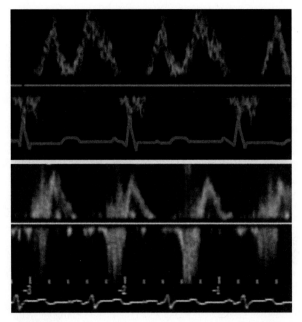

FIG. 8.7. Pulsed wave Doppler scan of the pulmonary venous flow. **Top:** Normal pattern. **Bottom:** Typical pattern of systolic reversal seen in severe mitral regurgitation.

(LVOT) is within the scan, demonstrates the anterior segments of the valve (A1A2, P1P2). Retroflexion of the probe, with the LVOT absent from the plane of scanning, allows examination of the posterior segments of the valve (A2A3, P2P3). This author does not believe that one can discriminate between P1 and P2 or between P2 and P3 with only 0-degree views.

2. Rotation of the imaging plane to about 90 degrees allows one to obtain the ME two-chamber view. Here, scanning the entire valve from right to left (by rotating the shaft of the probe) allows one to obtain three reproducible cross sections (Fig. 8.9). Further definition of P1, P2, P3, A3, and A2 is possible with these views.

3. The transducer should then be adjusted to obtain the best possible cut through the commissures. This view usually is obtained at between 60 and 90 degrees and is sometimes called the *ME commissural view* (15) (see Appendix 1). The presence and severity of disease at the level of the commissures can be determined here.

4. Rotating the imaging plane to about 150 degrees (ME long-axis view) provides a cross section through the middle of the MV, which allows reliable identification of A2 and P2 (see Appendix 1).

5. Finally, the short-axis view of the MV with color Doppler provides additional information on the origin of the regurgitant jet(s) (Fig. 8.8).

With experience, this detailed examination can be performed very quickly. Learning to recognize the variants of normal will help the echocardiographer to appreciate the wide spectrum of pathologies.

Step 3: Can the Valve Be Repaired?

MV repair has many proven advantages over valve replacement (16,17), but its feasibility depends on the location, extent, and mechanism of the MR. Repair is often undertaken for

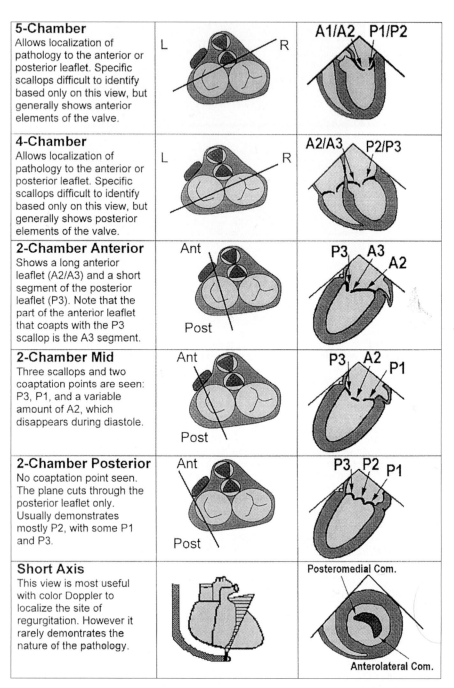

5-Chamber Allows localization of pathology to the anterior or posterior leaflet. Specific scallops difficult to identify based only on this view, but generally shows anterior elements of the valve.		A1/A2 P1/P2
4-Chamber Allows localization of pathology to the anterior or posterior leaflet. Specific scallops difficult to identify based only on this view, but generally shows posterior elements of the valve.		A2/A3 P2/P3
2-Chamber Anterior Shows a long anterior leaflet (A2/A3) and a short segment of the posterior leaflet (P3). Note that the part of the anterior leaflet that coapts with the P3 scallop is the A3 segment.	Ant Post	P3 A3 A2
2-Chamber Mid Three scallops and two coaptation points are seen: P3, P1, and a variable amount of A2, which disappears during diastole.	Ant Post	P3 A2 P1
2-Chamber Posterior No coaptation point seen. The plane cuts through the posterior leaflet only. Usually demonstrates mostly P2, with some P1 and P3.	Ant Post	P3 P2 P1
Short Axis This view is most useful with color Doppler to localize the site of regurgitation. However it rarely demontrates the nature of the pathology.		Posteromedial Com. Anterolateral Com.

FIG. 8.8. Systemic transesophageal echocardiographic examination of the mitral valve. (From Lambert AS, Miller JP, Merrick SH, et al. Improved evaluation of the location and mechanism of mitral valve regurgitation with a systematic transesophageal echocardiography examination. *Anesth Analg* 1999;88:1205–1212, with permission.)

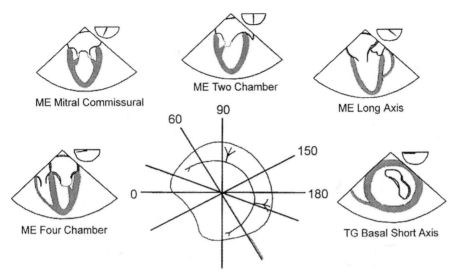

FIG. 8.9. Cross sections of the mitral valve as described in the American Society of Echocardiography/Society of Cardiovascular Anesthesiologists guidelines for performing comprehensive intraoperative transesophageal echocardiographic examinations. (Adapted from Shanewise JS, Cheung AT, Aronson S, et al. ASE/SCA guidelines for performing a comprehensive intraoperative multiplane transesophageal echocardiography examination: recommendations of the American Society of Echocardiography Council for Intraoperative Echocardiography and the Society of Cardiovascular Anesthesiologists Task Force for Certification in Perioperative Transesophageal Echocardiography. *Anesth Analg* 1999;89:870–884, with permission.)

lesions of prolapse of the posterior middle scallop (P2) because it tends to be easy, whereas lesions that involve the anterior leaflet or both leaflets, as well as calcified or fibrotic leaflets, are generally more challenging (16,18,19). Ultimately, the determination of whether a valve can be repaired depends on the surgeon, and it is important for echocardiographers to get to know their surgical colleagues. (See Chapter 10 for more details.)

QUANTITATIVE EVALUATION OF THE MITRAL VALVE

The regurgitant volume, regurgitant fraction, and regurgitant orifice area can all be calculated with TEE. All of these parameters rely on the continuity principle.

1. *Calculation of regurgitant volume.* The regurgitant volume is the amount of blood that is regurgitated into the left atrium during ventricular systole. The regurgitant volume is determined by subtracting the forward stroke volume across the LVOT in systole (area$_{LVOT}$ × time-velocity integral$_{LVOT}$) from the volume that crosses the MV in diastole (area$_{MV}$ × time-velocity integral$_{MV}$). This determination is limited because the MV opening is oval, not round, and its area varies throughout diastole. Because of these features, calculation of the area of the MV based on a fixed circular model is inaccurate. Alternatively, one can substitute the stroke volume in the proximal pulmonary artery because this is a round structure with a relatively constant diameter throughout the cardiac cycle.

2. *Calculation of regurgitant fraction.* The regurgitant fraction is the ratio of the regurgitant volume to the volume that flows forward across the MV in diastole (the total stroke volume).

3. *Calculation of the regurgitant orifice area.* Calculation of the regurgitant orifice area requires use of the proximal isovelocity surface area (PISA) method. Conceptually, PISA

is a modification of the continuity equation and assumes that as blood cells are forced into a narrow regurgitant orifice, they accelerate along a series of concentric hemispheres. By simply calculating the surface area of the hemisphere where the velocity equals the Nyquist limit and measuring the maximal velocity of the MR jet, one can extrapolate the area of the regurgitant orifice. This method is used in the evaluation of mitral stenosis and is described in detail in Chapter 9.

The regurgitant volume, regurgitant fraction, and regurgitant orifice area are important research tools. They are sometimes calculated in the echocardiography laboratory to better quantify the severity of MR lesions and are summarized in Table 8.2. *Unfortunately, the calculations are time-consuming and tend to be impractical in the setting of a busy operating room.*

PITFALLS IN THE EVALUATION OF MITRAL REGURGITATION

Most clinicians would agree that it is better to have no information than erroneous information. Patients with severe MR often have a dilated heart and a distorted cardiac anatomy. For this reason, the TEE examination can be very challenging because the appearance of the various TEE cross sections of the MV is altered. *In the operating room, general anesthesia can have major effects on preload, afterload, and contractility, which in turn affect the severity of MR.* Finally, if myocardial ischemia is present at the time of the examination, it can also affect the regurgitation. All of these factors must be taken into consideration when evaluating the MV.

SUMMARY

Intraoperative TEE has become an integral part of the surgical decision-making process in MV surgery. A thorough and systematic approach to the examination of the MV allows one to define the pathology and precisely determine its location on the valve.

REFERENCES

1. Lambert AS, Miller JP, Merrick SH, et al. Improved evaluation of the location and mechanism of mitral valve regurgitation with a systematic transesophageal echocardiography examination. *Anesth Analg* 1999;88:1205–1212.
2. Cheitlin MD, Finkbeiner WE. Cardiac anatomy. In: Chatterjee K, Cheitlin MD, Karliner J, et al., eds. *Cardiology, an illustrated text.* Philadelphia: JB Lippincott, 1991:1.9–1.10.
3. Carpentier AF, Lessana A, Relland JY, et al. The "physio-ring": an advanced concept in mitral valve annuloplasty. *Ann Thorac Surg* 1995;60:1177–1185.
4. Kumar N, Kumar M, Duran CM. A revised terminology for recording surgical findings of the mitral valve. *J Heart Valve Dis* 1995;4:70–75.
5. Carpentier AF. Cardiac valve surgery—the "French correction." *J Thorac Cardiovasc Surg* 1983;86:323–327.
6. Stewart WJ, Currie PJ, Salcedo EE, et al. Evaluation of mitral leaflet motion by echocardiography and jet direction by Doppler color flow mapping to determine the mechanisms of mitral regurgitation. *J Am Coll Cardiol* 1992;20:1353–1361.
7. Helmcke F, Nanda NC, Hsiung MC, et al. Color Doppler assessment of mitral regurgitation with orthogonal planes. *Circulation* 1987;75:175–183.
8. Cape EG, Yoganathan AP, Weyman AE, et al. Adjacent solid boundaries alter the size of regurgitant jets on Doppler color flow maps. *J Am Coll Cardiol* 1991;17:1094–1102.
9. Simpson IA, Valdes-Cruz LM, Sahn DJ, et al. Doppler color flow mapping of simulated in vitro regurgitant jets: evaluation of the effects of orifice size and hemodynamic variables. *J Am Coll Cardiol* 1989;13:1195–1207.

10. Stevenson J. Two-dimensional color Doppler estimation of the severity of atrioventricular valve regurgitation: important effects of instrument gain setting, pulse repetition frequency and carrier frequency. *J Am Soc Echocardiogr* 1989;2:1–10.
11. Schiller NB, Foster E, Redberg RF. Transesophageal echocardiography in the evaluation of mitral regurgitation. The twenty-four signs of severe mitral regurgitation. *Cardiol Clin* 1993;11:399–408.
12. Tribouilloy C, Shen WF, Quere JP, et al. Assessment of severity of mitral regurgitation by measuring regurgitant jet width at its origin with transesophageal Doppler color flow imaging. *Circulation* 1992;85:1248–1253.
13. Pu M, Griffin BP, Vandervoort PM, et al. The value of assessing pulmonary venous flow velocity for predicting severity of mitral regurgitation: a quantitative assessment integrating left ventricular function. *J Am Soc Echocardiogr* 1999;12:736–743.
14. Foster GP, Isselbacher EM, Rose GA, et al. Accurate localization of mitral regurgitant defects using multiplane transesophageal echocardiography. *Ann Thorac Surg* 1998;65:1025–1031.
15. Shanewise JS, Cheung AT, Aronson S, et al. ASE/SCA guidelines for performing a comprehensive intraoperative multiplane transesophageal echocardiography examination: recommendations of the American Society of Echocardiography Council for Intraoperative Echocardiography and the Society of Cardiovascular Anesthesiologists Task Force for Certification in Perioperative Transesophageal Echocardiography. *Anesth Analg* 1999;89:870–884.
16. David TE, Armstrong S, Sun Z, et al. Late results of mitral valve repair for mitral regurgitation due to degenerative disease. *Ann Thorac Surg* 1993;56:7–12.
17. Spencer FC, Galloway AC, Grossi EA, et al. Recent developments and evolving techniques of mitral valve reconstruction. *Ann Thorac Surg* 1998;65:307–313.
18. Alvarez JM, Gray D, Choong C, et al. Repair of the anterior mitral leaflet. *Aust N Z J Med* 1993;23:279–284.
19. Cosgrove DM, Stewart WJ. Mitral valvuloplasty. *Curr Probl Cardiol* 1989;14:359–415.

QUESTIONS

1. Which of the following, in the Carpentier nomenclature, corresponds to the middle scallop of the posterior leaflet?
   a. P1
   b. P2
   c. P3
   d. A2
2. Which of the following, in the Carpentier nomenclature, does **not** receive chordae tendineae from the anterolateral papillary muscle?
   a. P2
   b. P1
   c. P3
   d. A1
3. Which of the following is anatomically closest to the left atrial appendage (Carpentier nomenclature)?
   a. P1
   b. A2
   c. A3
   d. P3
4. Which of the following statements is **true**?
   a. Billowing is a condition in which part of a mitral leaflet projects above the annulus in systole, but the coaptation point remains below the mitral annulus.
   b. Prolapse is the excursion of a leaflet tip above the level of the mitral annulus during systole.
   c. Flail is a condition in which a leaflet edge flows freely into the left atrium, usually as a result of rupture of one or more chordae tendineae.
   d. All of these statements are true.

5. Which of the following does not have a direct effect on the apparent severity of MR by color Doppler?
   a. Size of the regurgitant orifice
   b. Nyquist limit
   c. Systemic blood pressure
   d. Right ventricular systolic pressure
6. What is the name given to the base of the MR jet by color Doppler?
   a. Convergence area
   b. Vena contracta
   c. Isovelocity surface area
   d. Aliasing area
7. Which standard TEE cross section typically shows the P1, A2, and P3 scallops?
   a. ME bicommissural view
   b. ME four-chamber view
   c. ME two-chamber view
   d. ME long-axis view
8. Which one of the following disease processes of the MV is **generally accepted** to be the easiest to repair?
   a. A2 flail
   b. A2-P2 prolapse
   c. P2 prolapse
   d. P3 flail
9. What is the significance of a wall-hugging (eccentric) jet?
   a. It tends to be associated with a structural defect of one of the leaflets.
   b. It is usually the result of annular dilation.
   c. It generally is relieved by correction of the underlying myocardial ischemia.
   d. It is of no clinical significance.
10. Which of the following statements regarding the spectral Doppler assessment of MR is **false**?
    a. The density of the continuous wave Doppler signal correlates with the severity of MR.
    b. The peak velocity of the continuous wave Doppler signal correlates with the severity of MR.
    c. Reversal of systolic pulmonary venous flow suggests hemodynamically significant MR.
    d. The normal pattern of pulmonary venous flow is forward in systole and forward in diastole.

Mitral Valve Stenosis

Colleen Gorman Koch

The 19th century physician Jean Nicholas Corvisart established the diagnostic value of percussion in the physical diagnosis of cardiac disorders. He described the diastolic thrill of mitral stenosis (MS) as "a peculiar rushing like water, difficult to be described, sensible to the hand applied over the precordial region, a rushing which proceeds apparently from the embarrassment which the blood undergoes in passing through an opening which is no longer proportioned to the quantity of fluid which it ought to discharge" (1). As early as 1898, D. W. Samways discussed the potential for performing cardiac surgery in the most severe cases of MS in an article entitled "Cardiac Peristalsis: Its Nature and Effects," published in *The Lancet* (2). In the modern era of heart disease, cardiac catheterization has provided hemodynamic information and assessed the severity of MS. Popovic et al. (3) investigated time-related trends in the use of preoperative invasive hemodynamic measurements in 1,985 patients with isolated valvular stenosis. During an 8-year study period, cardiac catheterization before valve surgery remained a common practice; however, it was performed primarily to ascertain coronary anatomy. The need for invasive hemodynamic measurements acquired during catheterization dramatically decreased, superseded by noninvasive hemodynamic measurements obtained with echocardiography (3). *Currently, two-dimensional and Doppler echocardiography have supplanted cardiac catheterization in providing a complete evaluation of patients with MS (4).*

MITRAL VALVE ANATOMY

Morphologically, the mitral valve (MV) apparatus is composed of the left atrial (LA) wall, mitral annulus, anterior and posterior MV leaflets, chordal tendons, anterolateral and posteromedial papillary muscles, and left ventricular (LV) myocardium (5,6). The valvular tissue can be divided into two commissural regions, the anterolateral commissure and the posteromedial commissure, and two leaflet areas, the anterior and posterior MV leaflets. The anterior mitral leaflet is somewhat triangular in shape, with an attachment to approximately one third of the circumference of the mitral annulus. It is attached to the fibrous skeleton of the heart, as are the left coronary cusp and half of the noncoronary cusp of the aortic valve. The attachment of the posterior mitral leaflet to the mitral annulus is lengthier than that of the anterior mitral leaflet. Clefts along the free margin of the posterior leaflet allow the identification of individual scallops (5). Although the anterior mitral leaflet base-to-margin dimension is longer than that of the posterior mitral leaflet, and although the basal attachments are different for each leaflet, the two leaflets are nearly identical in overall surface area. Chordal tendons from each papillary muscle attach to both of the MV leaflets. On average, 120 chordal tendons attach to the undersurface of the MV leaflets. The chordal tendons subdivide as they project from the papillary muscles toward the MV leaflets. The spaces between the chordae serve as secondary orifices between the LA and LV (6).

The normal MV orifice area is approximately 4 to 6 cm^2. An orifice area in the range of 2 cm^2 causes a minimal elevation in the transvalvular pressure gradient, whereas a valve area of less than 1.4 cm^2 is associated with a significant transvalvular pressure gradient and the clinical presentation of MS (7–9).

ETIOLOGY OF MITRAL STENOSIS

The causes of MS include the following: rheumatic heart disease, LA myxoma, severe mitral annular calcification, thrombus formation, parachute MV deformity, congenital MS,

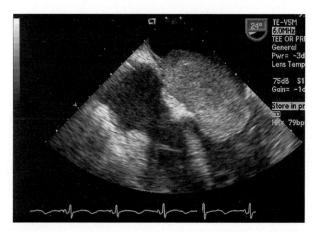

FIG. 9.1. A transesophageal echocardiographic midesophageal four-chamber image displays a 3 × 6-cm left atrial myxoma causing symptomatic mitral stenosis. The atrial myxoma is visualized prolapsed through the mitral valve into the left ventricular cavity during diastole.

supravalvular mitral ring, and cor triatriatum (6,10). Figures 9.1 and 9.2 depict a large LA myxoma obstructing mitral inflow.

The most common cause of MS in adult patients is still rheumatic heart disease (6,9,10). Pathologic features of rheumatic MS include fusion of the commissures; contracture, scarring, and diffuse thickening of the leaflet tissue and subvalvular apparatus; and calcium deposition within the mitral leaflets. This process results in a diminished size of the effective valvular orifice, in addition to valve rigidity as a consequence of the leaflet fibrosis and calcification. As the valve area becomes more restricted, increases in the transvalvular pressure gradient and LA pressure may lead to pulmonary hypertension with tricuspid regurgitation and right ventricular dysfunction (6,8–10).

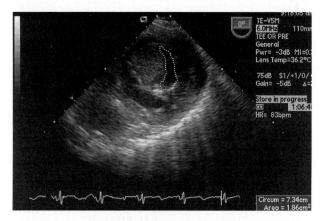

FIG. 9.2. An atrial myxoma displayed from a transgastric basal short-axis imaging plane occupies a large portion of the mitral orifice. The mitral valve orifice measures 1.86 cm^2 in diastole.

TRANSESOPHAGEAL ECHOCARDIOGRAPHIC EVALUATION OF MITRAL STENOSIS

A discussion of the complete diagnostic evaluation follows, and the chapter concludes with a concise summary of the recommended approach to an accurate diagnosis of MS.

Two-Dimensional Echocardiography

The anatomy of MS can be defined more clearly from multiple imaging planes of two-dimensional transesophageal echocardiography (TEE) than by any other diagnostic modality. Based on the pathophysiologic features of rheumatic MS, key features that must be identified echocardiographically include the following: degree of leaflet thickening, amount of calcium deposition, extent of subvalvular involvement, decrement in leaflet mobility, and overall changes in chamber dimensions and function (11). Related issues, such as involvement of other valve structures and pulmonary hypertension, can also be assessed.

Mitral leaflet tissue can display varying degrees of thickening and calcium deposition that cause the MV leaflets to appear "enhanced," or echo-bright. The "shadow" cast by calcium may obstruct the view of the distal anatomy; one of the strengths of TEE in this circumstance is the ability to view the structures from another plane, so that the operator can see beyond the "shadow." The standard midesophageal (ME) views (four-chamber, commissural, two-chamber, and long-axis) assist in evaluating the extent of disease. The chordal tendons can display varying degrees of thickening and contracture. The transgastric (TG) long-axis imaging plane provides the best information with regard to the extent of subvalvular involvement in the rheumatic process. The characteristic two-dimensional echocardiographic findings associated with rheumatic MS are represented in Figure 9.3. Rheumatic heart disease results in varying degrees of restricted mitral leaflet motion. In two-dimensional TEE, restricted leaflet motion is characterized by decreased leaflet excursion and by diastolic "doming" of the anterior mitral leaflet. The appearance of "doming" is the result of fusion of the anterior and posterior leaflets along the medial and lateral commissures. The leaflets are restricted or abnormally stenotic at the tips. The maximal amplitude of motion occurs in the mobile midsection, giving the anterior mitral leaflet an arched appearance, convex

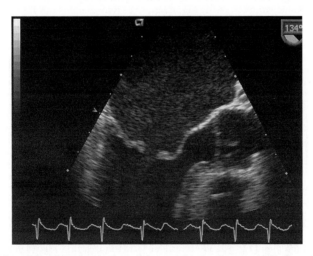

FIG. 9.3. A midesophageal long-axis view of rheumatic mitral stenosis displays the characteristic diastolic "doming" of the anterior mitral leaflet in diastole and an enlarged left atrium. The mitral leaflets are thickened, particularly at their margins, and appear echo-bright secondary to calcium deposition.

TABLE 9.1. ECHOCARDIOGRAPHIC SCORING SYSTEM

Grade	Mobility	Subvalvular thickening	Thickening	Calcification
1	Highly mobile valve with only leaflet tips restricted	Minimal thickening just below the mitral leaflets	Leaflets nearly normal in thickness (4–5 mm)	Single area of increased echo brightness
2	Leaflet mid and base portions have normal mobility	Thickening of chordal structures extending up to one third of chordal length	Mid leaflets normal, considerable thickening of margins (5–8 mm)	Scattered areas of brightness confined to leaflet margins
3	Valve continues to move forward in diastole, mainly from base	Thickening extending to the distal third of chords	Thickening extending through the entire leaflet (5–8 mm)	Brightness extending into midportion of the leaflets
4	No or minimal forward movement of the leaflets in diastole	Extensive thickening and shortening of all chordal structures extending down to papillary muscles	Considerable thickening of all leaflet tissue (>8–10 mm)	Extensive brightness throughout much of the leaflet tissue

From Wilkins G, Weyman A, Abascal A, et al. Percutaneous ballon dilatation of the mitral valve: an analysis of echocardiographic variables related to outcome and the mechanism of dilatation. *Br Heart J* 1988;60:300, with permission.

toward the LV outflow tract in diastole (12,13). Figure 9.3 demonstrates the characteristic "doming" or "hockey stick" deformity of the anterior mitral leaflet in diastole.

Echocardiographic scoring system. In 1988, Wilkins et al. (11) developed an echocardiographic scoring system to assess MV morphology and its relationship to the success of percutaneous balloon dilation of the MV. Each of the four components of the scoring system is graded on a scale of 0 to 4, such that total scores range from 0 to 16. The four components of the scoring system assess the MV for the pathologic changes characteristically associated with rheumatic heart disease: reduced leaflet mobility, leaflet thickening, subvalvular thickening, and calcification. These investigators reported that a high echocardiographic score (>11), which is representative of advanced leaflet deformity, was associated with a suboptimal outcome after balloon dilation of the MV. A low echocardiographic score (<9) was associated with an optimal outcome (11). Table 9.1 presents the scoring system and describes what each grade on the scale represents for each of the four components. Although this scoring system was developed for patients undergoing mitral balloon dilation, it can serve as a useful guide during the TEE examination of patients with rheumatic MS.

Standard chamber dimensions can be altered depending on the duration and degree of MS. Typically, an increase in the LA area is associated with chronic volume and pressure overload. Because of the low-flow state, LA spontaneous echo contrast or thrombus formation may be present. Daniel et al. (14) characterized LA spontaneous echo contrast as "dynamic clouds of echoes curling up slowly in a circular or spiral shape within the left atrium." They found that LA spontaneous echo contrast is useful in identifying those patients with MS who are at increased risk for thromboembolic events. TEE is more sensitive than transthoracic echocardiography in detecting LA spontaneous echo contrast. Because LA spontaneous echo contrast indicates blood stasis and may be a warning of thrombus formation, it is critical to scan the LA completely to exclude thrombus formation (14,15). Figure 9.4 displays a ME view of the LA with a thrombus in the LA appendage.

Diastolic properties of the LV are also affected in rheumatic MS. In patients with severe isolated rheumatic MS, Liu et al. (16) demonstrated reduced LV diastolic compliance. The

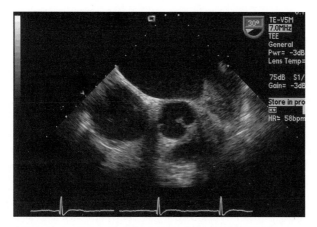

FIG. 9.4. A left atrial appendage thrombus (*arrow*) is visualized from a short-axis imaging plane of the left atrium.

reduction in compliance appeared to be related to a functional restriction resulting from chordal tethering to a rigid valve apparatus, a finding that was immediately reversed after balloon mitral valvuloplasty. LV systolic performance in patients with severe isolated MS was nearly identical to that in age-matched controls. Chronic elevation in LA pressure can cause structural alterations in the pulmonary vasculature, leading to pulmonary hypertension and ultimately right-sided heart failure (8,9). TEE evaluation of the right side of the heart may demonstrate varying degrees of right ventricular dysfunction and tricuspid regurgitation. *A comprehensive two-dimensional and Doppler TEE examination of the heart should be performed to exclude these associated findings and other valvular pathology.*

Physiologic Assessments

Determination of the pressure gradient. Normal flow velocity across the MV is less than 1.3 m/s. The pressure drop across a stenotic valve can be calculated from the instantaneous flow velocity by means of the simplified Bernoulli equation (17,18):

$$\text{Pressure Gradient (mm Hg)} = 4v^2$$

where v represents the instantaneous velocity.

The equation is modified from the original in that the terms that account for viscous friction and flow acceleration have been eliminated. Because the velocity distal to the obstruction is significantly greater than the velocity proximal to the obstruction, the proximal velocity term can be ignored (17,18). Continuous wave Doppler interrogation of the inflow velocities across the valve is performed with use of the ME four-chamber, two-chamber, or long-axis view. Following manual tracing of the diastolic spectral profile, the echocardiographic machine software provides a mean gradient in millimeters of mercury. Figure 9.5 (see also Color Plate 13 following page 212) displays a mean gradient measurement across the MV in a patient with MS obtained with continuous wave Doppler and the ME four-chamber view. *It is important to note that an increase in forward flow through the mitral orifice, such as occurs in severe mitral valvular regurgitation, can result in a high transmitral gradient even though the valve is only mildly stenotic. One therefore must be aware that the degree of MS can be overestimated in the face of significant mitral regurgitation* (4). Pressure gradients are underestimated if the angle between the sampling beam and the flow vector is large (>20 degrees) (17,19). Visualizing the inflow jet with color Doppler and aligning the sample beam with the

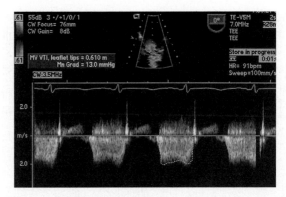

FIG. 9.5. A diastolic spectral profile of mitral inflow has been obtained with continuous wave Doppler in this patient with mitral stenosis. The profile has been traced out, and a mean pressure gradient of 13 mm Hg has been calculated with the software available within the machine. Note that the inflow velocities are close to 2 m/s. (See Color Plate 13 following page 212.)

color inflow can help to minimize this problem (19). In general, a mean gradient of more than 10 mm Hg across a stenotic valve is considered to indicate severe stenosis (20) (Table 9.2).

Calculations of valve area. The severity of MS is also estimated by determining the reduction in MV area. This can be done with the use of two-dimensional and Doppler echocardiographic techniques.

Planimetry valve area: Planimetry is a conceptually simple two-dimensional technique used to calculate the MV area. It involves directly visualizing the MV orifice in diastole from a TG basal short-axis imaging plane and tracing the orifice margins to acquire a valve area measurement in square centimeters (Fig. 9.6). The results obtained with technique have been shown to correlate well with valve area measurements acquired invasively (12,21,22). Figure 9.6 demonstrates the use of planimetry in calculating the MV area from the TG basal short-axis imaging plane in a patient with rheumatic MS. A number of operator "pitfalls" should be recognized when this technique is used to optimize its accuracy. Instrumentation factors are critical in obtaining adequate images for planimetry. For example, if the receiver gain settings are too low, the edges of the valve may be obscured, resulting in "echo dropout," and the valve area will be overestimated (12). The opposite occurs when the gain settings are set too high, with resultant image saturation and a falsely narrowed valve orifice (23). Inadequate imaging plane orientation is another important measurement error with this technique. The stenotic MV looks like a funnel in diastole, the narrowest part being the commissural tip of the valve. *It is critical to scan the MV orifice superiorly to inferiorly to acquire the smallest orifice area.* Measuring too superiorly, in the body of the leaflets, can overestimate the valve area (21–23). In patients who have undergone mitral valvuloplasty, the valve area may be underestimated because of the inability to measure the extent of the commissural fractures with planimetry.

TABLE 9.2. SEVERITY OF MITRAL STENOSIS

	Grade		
	Mild	**Moderate**	**Severe**
Mean gradient (mm Hg)	6	6–10	>10
PHT (ms)	100	200	>300
MVA (cm^2)	1.6–2.0	1.0–1.5	<1.0

PHT, pressure half-time; MVA, mitral valve area.

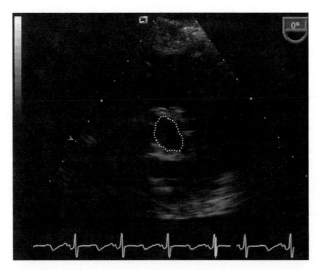

FIG. 9.6. The mitral valve orifice assumes a "fish mouth" appearance in a transgastric basal short-axis imaging plane in a patient with rheumatic mitral stenosis. Tracing of the orifice margins of the mitral valve during diastole resulted in a mitral valve area measurement of 1.25 cm^2.

Pressure half-time: The pressure half-time describes the pressure difference between the LA and LV and can be quantitatively related to the degree of MS. As MS becomes more severe, the rate of pressure decline between the LA and LV is proportionally slower, and consequently the gradient between the LA and LV is maintained for a longer period of time. The pressure half-time is the time required for the atrioventricular pressure difference to decrease from the maximum to one-half that value. To calculate the pressure half-time, the peak transmitral flow velocity is measured by Doppler, and the time it takes to decrease by a factor of the square root of 2 is traced and measured (20,24,25). Figure 9.7 (see also Color

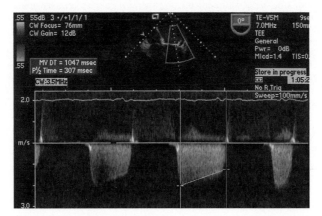

FIG. 9.7. A diastolic spectral profile of mitral inflow obtained with continuous wave Doppler. Severe mitral stenosis is confirmed by a pressure half-time measurement of 307 ms. (See Color Plate 14 following page 212.)

TABLE 9.3. METHODS OF DETERMINING MITRAL VALVE AREA

Planimetry	Trace frozen short-axis view in diastole
Pressure half-time (PHT, ms)	MVA = 220/PHT
Deceleration time (DT, ms)	MVA = 759/DT
Continuity equation	MVA = (LVOT Area × LVOT TVI)/(MV TVI)
PISA	MVA = $2\pi r^2 \times \alpha/180° \times$ Va/Vp

MS, milliseconds; MVA, mitral valve area (square centimeters); α, funnel angle; Va, aliasing velocity; Vp, peak transmitral velocity; LVOT, left ventricular outflow tract; TVI, time-velocity integral; PISA, proximal isovelocity surface area.

Plate 14 following page 212) displays the pressure half-time measurement in a patient with MS. The signal is acquired by aligning the continuous wave Doppler beam with the mitral inflow and acquiring a transmitral flow velocity signal. The machine software automatically calculates the pressure half-time after the operator labels the maximal and minimal velocities. The pressure half-time increases as the severity of MS increases (20,24–26). In a normal MV, the pressure half-time is generally less than 60 ms. In mild MS, the average pressure half-time is approximately 100 ms; in moderate MS, it is approximately 200 ms, and in severe MS, the average pressure half-time measurement is more than 300 ms (24,25,27) (Table 9.3).

Pressure half-time mitral valve area: The MV area can be calculated from the pressure half-time measurement by using the following formula, originally described by Hatle and Angelsen (27):

$$\text{MV Area}\,(\text{cm}^2) = 220\,/\,\text{Pressure Half-Time (ms)}$$

They noted that the rate of pressure decline across a stenotic MV depends on the cross-sectional area of the valvular orifice. Hence, the tighter the orifice (smaller cross-sectional area), the slower the rate of pressure decline.

The measurements obtained with the pressure half-time method are influenced by hemodynamic factors and depend on the compliance of the LA and LV. These factors must be taken into consideration when the pressure half-time method is applied to a stenotic MV. For example, *decreased LV compliance and severe aortic regurgitation can cause a rapid rise in the LV diastolic pressure, with a resultant shortening of the pressure half-time measurement and an overestimation of the MV area* (28,29). Braverman et al. (28) demonstrated the dependence of the pressure half-time method for calculating the MV area on hemodynamic variables such as peak transmitral gradient and atrioventricular compliance. Conditions such as previous mitral valvuloplasty, atrial septal defect, atrial tachycardia, and restrictive cardiomyopathy also affect the accuracy of the pressure half-time method (20,30–32).

Deceleration time. The deceleration time is another simple means of evaluating the MV area, in which decay of the mitral inflow profile through a stenotic MV is examined. The following formula describes the relationship of the deceleration time to the MV area (19):

$$\text{MV Area}\,(\text{cm}^2) = 759\,/\,\text{Deceleration Time (ms)}$$

The deceleration time is the interval between the peak velocity and the time at which the extrapolated inflow velocity reaches baseline. Figure 9.8 graphically displays the measurement of deceleration time. For profiles in which the decay is linear, the pressure half-time is equal to 29% of the deceleration time (20,26).

Advanced Concepts That May Be Helpful in Difficult Cases

Continuity equation. The continuity equation for calculating the area of a valve is based on the law of conservation of mass in hydrodynamics. In the absence of valvular regurgitation or

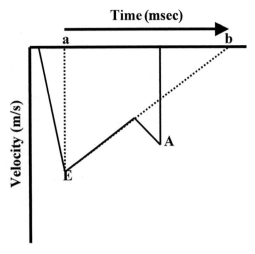

FIG. 9.8. The deceleration time is the interval between the peak velocity (a) and the time at which the extrapolated inflow velocity reaches baseline (b).

shunts, flow volume at the MV should equal that at another valve according to the following equation (26,29):

$$\text{Volumetric Flow} = \text{Area}_1 \times \text{Time-Velocity Integral}_1$$
$$= \text{Area}_2 \times \text{Time-Velocity Integral}_2$$

Therefore,

$$\text{Area}_2 = (\text{Area}_1 \times \text{Time-Velocity Integral}_1) / \text{Time-Velocity Integral}_2$$

Flow through the MV can be calculated based on measurements made by Doppler echocardiography as the product of the valve orifice area and the time-velocity integral of the mitral inflow. Area$_1$ × time-velocity integral$_1$ represents volumetric flow through the reference valve. The reference area (area$_1$) is a cross-sectional area measurement that assumes the geometric model of a circle: πr^2. The LV outflow tract or pulmonary artery is commonly used for the reference area and time-velocity integral measurements. The equation is rearranged to solve for the MS area, area$_2$, as previously discussed. *The continuity equation is theoretically independent of transvalvular pressure gradients, LV compliance, and changing hemodynamic conditions, such as the increased forward flow that occurs during exercise (28,29,32). The continuity equation does not apply in circumstances of regurgitation in the reference valve or the MV because the forward volumetric flows are not equal, so that significant error is introduced (29,33).*

Proximal isovelocity surface area method. The proximal isovelocity surface area (PISA) method, or flow convergence method, applies the continuity principle to color flow Doppler mapping in the region of the MV orifice where flow is converging from the LA. Figure 9.9 (see also Color Plate 15 following page 212) displays a color flow Doppler example of proximal flow convergence in a patient with rheumatic MS. When blood flow converges on an orifice that is small relative to the proximal chamber, it may be considered to form isovelocity "shells" with the shape of a hemisphere. The velocity of blood flow increases as blood approaches the small orifice, resulting in aliasing of the color flow signal and the creation of a large proximal flow convergence region or shell. As blood approaches the orifice, its increasing velocity is pictured by color flow imaging as progressively smaller shells. The radius of the first aliasing

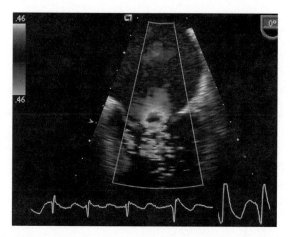

FIG. 9.9. Color Doppler imaging from this midesophageal four-chamber view of the mitral valve demonstrates proximal isovelocity surface area (PISA) or flow convergence on the left atrial side of the mitral valve. (See Color Plate 15 following page 212.)

velocity shell is measured from the tips of the MV leaflets to the aliasing boundary (19,34–37) (Fig. 9.10). The volumetric flow rate can be calculated as the product of the surface area of the hemisphere of flow and the aliasing velocity. The mitral inflow velocity profile (at the orifice) is obtained with continuous wave Doppler. The basic elements of the continuity equation can thus be identified by this straightforward color mapping, but the calculation of a valve area requires a correction for the true shape of the mitral orifice. Truly hemispheric shells would occur if the surface of the valve were flat with the leaflets apposed at 180 degrees. The angle α subtended by the mitral leaflets creates a funnel-shaped surface; an angle correction factor ($\alpha/180$ degrees) adjusts the hemispheric surface area pictured by color flow mapping to calculate the volumetric flow rate more accurately. The instantaneous volumetric flow rate (Q) in this region can be calculated as the product of the surface area of a hemisphere ($2\pi r^2$) and the aliasing velocity at the shell (Va):

$$Q = 2\pi r^2 \times \alpha/180 \text{ degrees} \times Va$$

Flow through this region should equal flow through the restricted orifice based on the continuity principle (34–36). Once the flow rate (Q) is calculated, the MV area can be obtained with the use of the continuity equation:

$$\text{MV Area (cm}^2) = Q/Vp \text{ (cm/s)}$$

where Q is the volumetric flow rate and Vp is the peak transmitral inflow velocity.

Figure 9.10 illustrates the use of the flow convergence method in the calculation of MV area.

The MV area can be measured accurately with this method in the presence of mitral insufficiency. Several investigators have validated the use of the flow convergence method in the calculation of MV area by direct comparisons with anatomic and calculated measurements of orifice size (34,36,38,39). Calculation of MV area by the flow convergence method can be time-consuming; however, its accuracy is not influenced by associated mitral or aortic regurgitation. This method of calculating MV area may be best under circumstances in which two-dimensional planimetry is technically limited, when the continuity equation cannot be applied with use of a reference volumetric flow, and when the pressure half-time method is affected by hemodynamic changes (35).

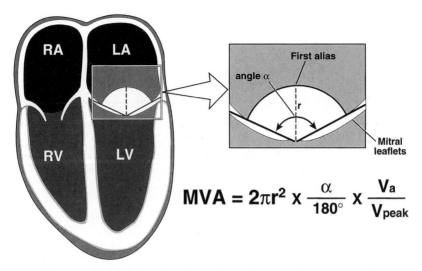

$$\text{MVA} = 2\pi r^2 \times \frac{\alpha}{180°} \times \frac{V_a}{V_{peak}}$$

FIG. 9.10. Midesophageal four-chamber view of the mitral valve demonstrates the measurements needed to calculate the mitral valve area by the proximal isovelocity surface area (PISA) method. $\alpha/180°$, angle correction factor; Va, aliasing velocity; Vp, peak transmitral inflow velocity; RA, right atrium; RV, right ventricle; LA, left atrium; LV, left ventricle; MVA, mitral valve area. (Adapted from Rodriguez L, Thomas JD, Monterroso V, et al. Validation of the proximal flow convergence method: calculation of orifice area in patients with mitral stenosis. *Circulation* 1993;88:1157–1165, with permission.)

A PRACTICAL APPROACH TO THE EVALUATION OF MITRAL STENOSIS

Step 1. A two-dimensional evaluation of the MV is performed with a focus on answering the following questions: What is the appearance of the valve—that is, is the valve disfigured? Are the leaflets of normal thickness and mobility? If not, further assessment of the valve is needed to determine whether it is stenotic or regurgitant (see Chapter 8). Planimetry of the MV in the TG basal short-axis view is initially performed to obtain a rough estimate of the MV area.

Step 2. After completion of the two-dimensional examination, MV inflow interrogation with continuous wave Doppler is performed. The diastolic mitral inflow velocity profile is traced (Fig. 9.5; see Color Plate 13 following page 212), and the mean pressure gradient is determined with the internal software of the echocardiography machine. In addition, the pressure half-time method is used to calculate the MV area (Fig. 9.7; see Color Plate 14 following page 212). Most TEE machines also extrapolate the flow decay and calculate the deceleration time.

If the measurements are in agreement according to Table 9.2, no further evaluation is required.

Step 3. The advanced methods (continuity equation and PISA) are reserved for those patients for whom the pressure half-time method is unreliable or unavailable.

SUMMARY

Table 9.3 summarizes the techniques used to calculate the MV area, and Table 9.2 presents the scores for the various degrees of MS obtained with each of these techniques. In general, an MV area of 1.6 to 2.0 cm^2 is considered to indicate mild MS, 1.0 to 1.5 cm^2 moderate MS, and less than 1.0 cm^2 severe MS (9,20). Each technique has its limitations. *Agreement between the various methods of evaluating the valve together with clinical correlation will enhance accuracy and overall judgment.*

REFERENCES

1. Acierno LJ. Physical examination. In: *The history of cardiology.* London: Parthenon Publishing Group, 1994:461–462.
2. Acierno LJ. Surgical modalities. In: *The history of cardiology.* London: Parthenon Publishing Group, 1994:627.
3. Popovic AD, Thomas JD, Neskovic A, et al. Time-related trends in the preoperative evaluation of patients with valvular stenosis. *Am J Cardiol* 1997;80:1464–1468.
4. Bruce CJ, Nishimura RA. Clinical assessment and management of mitral stenosis, valvular heart disease. *Cardiol Clin* 1998;16:375–403.
5. Ranganathan N, Lam JH, Wigle ED, et al. Morphology of the human mitral valve: the valve leaflets. *Circulation* 1970;41:459–467.
6. Roberts WC, Perloff JK. Mitral valvular disease: a clinicopathologic survey of the conditions causing the mitral valve to function abnormally. *Ann Intern Med* 1972;77:939–974.
7. Kennedy JW, Yarnall SR, Murray JA, et al. Quantitative angiocardiography: IV. Relationships of left atrial and ventricular pressure and volume in mitral valve disease. *Circulation* 1970;41:817–824.
8. Schlant RC, Alexander RW, O'Rourke RA, et al., eds. Mitral valve disease. In: *Hurst's the heart,* 8th ed. New York: McGraw-Hill, 1483–1518.
9. Selzer A, Cohn K. Natural history of mitral stenosis: a review. *Circulation* 1972;45:878–890.
10. Olson LJ, Subramanian R, Ackermann DM, et al. Surgical pathology of the mitral valve: a study of 712 cases spanning 21 years. *Mayo Clin Proc* 1987;62:22–34.
11. Wilkins G, Weyman A, Abascal V, et al. Percutaneous balloon dilatation of the mitral valve: an analysis of echocardiographic variables related to outcome and the mechanism of dilatation. *Br Heart J* 1988;60:299–308
12. Otto C, ed. Valvular stenosis: diagnosis, quantitation, and clinical approach. In: *Textbook of clinical echocardiography,* 2nd ed. Philadelphia: WB Saunders, 2000:229–264.
13. Nichol PM, Gilbert BW, Kisslo JA. Two-dimensional echocardiographic assessment of mitral stenosis. *Circulation* 1977;55:120–128.
14. Daniel W, Nellessen U, Schroder E, et al. Left atrial spontaneous echo contrast in mitral valve disease: an indicator for an increased thromboembolic risk. *J Am Coll Cardiol* 1988;11:1204–1211.
15. Chen YT, Kan MN, Chen JS, et al. Contributing factors to the formation of left atrial spontaneous echo contrast in mitral valvular disease. *J Ultrasound Med* 1990;9:151–155.
16. Liu CP, Ting CT, Yang TM, et al. Reduced left ventricular compliance in human mitral stenosis: role of reversible internal constraint. *Circulation* 1992;85:1447–1456.
17. Hatle L, Brubakk A, Tromsdal A, et al. Noninvasive assessment of pressure drop in mitral stenosis by Doppler ultrasound. *Br Heart J* 1978;40:131–140.
18. Oh JK, Seward JB, Tajik AJ. Hemodynamic assessment. In: *The echo manual,* 2nd ed. Philadelphia: Lippincott Williams & Wilkins, 1999:59–71.
19. Weyman AE, ed. Left ventricular inflow tract I: the mitral valve. In: *Principles and practice of echocardiography,* 2nd ed. Philadelphia: Lea & Febiger, 1994:391–497.
20. Oh JK, Seward JB, Tajik AJ. Valvular heart disease. In: *The echo manual,* 2nd ed. Philadelphia: Lippincott Williams & Wilkins, 1999:103–132.
21. Henry WL, Griffith JM, Michaelis LL, et al. Measurement of mitral orifice area in patients with mitral valve disease by real-time, two-dimensional echocardiography. *Circulation* 1975;51:827–831.
22. Wann LS, Weyman AE, Feigenbaum H, et al. Determination of mitral valve area by cross-sectional echocardiography. *Ann Intern Med* 1978;88:337–341.
23. Martin RP, Rakowski H, Kleiman JH, et al. Reliability and reproducibility of two-dimensional echocardiographic measurement of the stenotic mitral valve orifice area. *Am J Cardiol* 1979;43:560–568.

24. Libanoff AJ, Rodbard S. Atrioventricular pressure half-time: measure of mitral valve orifice area. *Circulation* 1968;38:144–150.
25. Hatle L, Angelsen B, Tromsdal A. Noninvasive assessment of atrioventricular pressure half-time by Doppler ultrasound. *Circulation* 1979;60:1096–1104.
26. Bruce C, Nishimura R. Newer advances in the diagnosis and treatment of mitral stenosis. *Curr Probl Cardiol* 1998;23:127–184.
27. Hatle L, Angelsen B, eds. Pulsed and continuous wave Doppler in the diagnosis and assessment of various heart lesions. In: *Doppler ultrasound in cardiology: physical principles and clinical applications.* Philadelphia: Lea & Febiger, 1982:76–89.
28. Braverman AC, Thomas JD, Lee R. Doppler echocardiographic estimation of mitral valve area during changing hemodynamic conditions. *Am J Cardiol* 1991;68:1485–1490.
29. Nakatani S, Masuyama T, Kodama K, et al. Value and limitations of Doppler echocardiography in the quantification of stenotic mitral valve area: comparison of the pressure half-time and the continuity equation methods. *Circulation* 1988;77:78–85.
30. Thomas JD, Wilkins G, Choong CYP, et al. Inaccuracy of mitral pressure half-time immediately after percutaneous mitral valvotomy: dependence on transmitral gradient and left atrial and ventricular compliance. *Circulation* 1988;78:980–993.
31. Thomas JD, Weyman AE. Doppler mitral pressure half-time: a clinical tool in search of theoretical justification. *J Am Coll Cardiol* 1987;10:923–929.
32. Wranne B, Msee PA, Loyd D. Analysis of different methods of assessing the stenotic mitral valve area with emphasis on the pressure gradient half-time concept. *Am J Cardiol* 1990;66:614–620.
33. Karp K, Teien D, Eriksson P. Doppler echocardiographic assessment on the valve area in patients with atrioventricular valve stenosis by application of the continuity equation. *J Intern Med* 1989;225:261–266.
34. Rodriguez L, Thomas JD, Monterroso V, et al. Validation of the proximal flow convergence method: calculation of orifice area in patients with mitral stenosis. *Circulation* 1993;88:1157–1165.
35. Deng Y, Matsumoto M, Wang X, et al. Estimation of mitral valve area in patients with mitral stenosis by the flow convergence region method: selection of aliasing velocity. *J Am Coll Cardiol* 1994;24:683–689.
36. Rifkin R, Harper K, Tighe D. Comparison of proximal isovelocity surface area method with pressure half-time and planimetry in the evaluation of mitral stenosis. *J Am Coll Cardiol* 1995;26:458–465.
37. Vandervoort PM, Rivera M, Mele D, et al. Application of color Doppler flow mapping to calculate effective regurgitant orifice area: an in vitro study and initial clinical observations. *Circulation* 1993;88:1150–1156.
38. Degertekin M, Basaran Y, Gencbay M, et al. Validation of flow convergence region method in assessing mitral valve area in the course of transthoracic and transesophageal echocardiographic studies. *Am Heart J* 1998;135:207–214.
39. Faletra F, Pezzano A, Fusco R, et al. Measurement of mitral valve area in mitral stenosis: four echocardiographic methods compared with direct measurement of anatomic orifices. *J Am Coll Cardiol* 1996;28:1190–1197.

QUESTIONS

1. What is the most common cause of MS in the adult patient?
   a. LA myxoma
   b. Severe mitral annular calcification
   c. Rheumatic heart disease
   d. Thrombus formation
2. Which definition of the modified Bernoulli equation is correct?
   a. It is a method to calculate mitral valve area.
   b. It converts peak pressure gradients to mean pressure gradients.
   c. It converts instantaneous velocities to instantaneous pressures.
   d. None of the above.

3. Which of the following statements about planimetry imaging "pitfalls" is/are correct?
    a. Inadequate imaging plane orientation can introduce measurement error.
    b. Gain settings that are too high can result in image saturation and a falsely narrow measurement of area.
    c. Gain settings that are too low can result in image dropout and introduce error into the valve area measurement.
    d. All of the above
4. The use of the continuity equation to calculate valve area in patients with MS is invalidated in which of the following clinical circumstances?
    a. After mitral valvuloplasty
    b. LV hypertrophy
    c. Mitral regurgitation
    d. None of the above
5. Which of the following valve areas is closest to normal?
    a. Less than 1 cm^2
    b. 4 to 6 cm^2
    c. More than 7 cm^2
    d. None of the above
6. Which of the following pressure half-time measurements corresponds to severe MV stenosis?
    a. More than 220 ms
    b. 60 to 80 ms
    c. Less than 60 ms
    d. 100 ms
7. Which of the following is not a component of the echocardiographic scoring system?
    a. Leaflet mobility
    b. Subvalvular involvement
    c. Chamber enlargement
    d. Calcium deposition
8. Which of the following is the best description of diastolic doming in patients with rheumatic MS?
    a. Bowing of the interatrial septum toward the right atrium in diastole
    b. The movement of the subvalvular apparatus in diastole
    c. The movement of the anterior mitral leaflet in diastole in which it becomes arched, with convexity toward the LV outflow tract
    d. None of the above
9. In which of the following clinical circumstances is error introduced into the pressure half-time method?
    a. Severe aortic regurgitation
    b. Decreased LV compliance
    c. Immediately after mitral balloon valvuloplasty
    d. All the above
10. Which of the following statements is correct with regard to the benefits of using the flow convergence method in calculating MV area?
    a. The flow convergence method can be used accurately when mitral regurgitation is present.
    b. Maximal flow rate is calculated from the product of the aliasing velocity and the area of a hemisphere.
    c. An angle correction factor is introduced to account for the inflow angle created by the mitral leaflets.
    d. All the above.

10

Mitral Valve Repair

Kristine J. Hirsch and Gregory M. Hirsch

History of Mitral Valve Repair

Mitral stenosis. The first successful mitral valvotomies were performed in the 1920s by Cutler and Levine in Boston (1) and Souttar in England (2). Subsequent attempts by both groups were disappointing, likely in part owing to the lack of such basic resources as blood transfusion, antibiotics, and safe anesthesia. After 25 years had elapsed, Charles P. Bailey, Dwight Harken, and Russell Brock had each devised successful methods of closed mitral valvotomy. Despite the development of safe cardiopulmonary bypass techniques, pioneered by Gibbon at Thomas Jefferson and refined by Kirklin at the Mayo Clinic, continued success with closed approaches delayed the widespread acceptance of "open heart" approaches to mitral commissurotomy until the 1970s.

Mitral regurgitation. Early attempts were made to repair regurgitant mitral valves (MVs) with ingenious closed approaches, such as circumferential annular sutures. With the advent of reasonably safe cardiopulmonary bypass, Lillehei and colleagues (3) first carried out direct repair in 1957. In 1961, Starr and Edwards (4) reported the first successful MV replacement, and after this, enthusiasm for mitral repair waned. In Europe, Carpentier, Duran, and others developed effective and reproducible methods to repair regurgitant MVs and were ultimately able to demonstrate the superiority of these methods over mitral replacement, stimulating renewed interest in mitral repair worldwide.

Indications for Mitral Valve Repair and Timing of Intervention

Mitral regurgitation. Historically, MV replacement was delayed until nearly intractable heart failure and often marked deterioration of left ventricular (LV) function developed. This strategy was based on the morbidity and mortality of the operation in addition to further loss of LV function postoperatively as a consequence of detachment of the chordal apparatus from the papillary muscles. *The advantages of mitral repair over mitral replacement include the preservation of LV function through preservation of the chordal attachments, low rates of thromboembolism, the lack of a requirement for anticoagulants (beyond aspirin), and excellent durability.* Given the excellent long-term results of modern mitral repair techniques, the threshold for surgical intervention has been appreciably lowered. The American College of Cardiology/American Heart Association Task Force on Practice Guidelines in Valvular Heart Disease recommends that patients with functional class II symptoms or higher and severe mitral regurgitation (MR) and asymptomatic patients with severe MR and echocardiographic evidence of LV dysfunction (LV end-systolic dimension ≥ 45 mm, ejection fraction ≤ 0.60) undergo repair. When a successful repair is probable, the weight of evidence favors surgical intervention in asymptomatic patients with severe MR and normal LV function (5).

Mitral stenosis. Similarly, the indications for the surgical repair of mitral stenosis (MS) have evolved to include patients in functional class III or higher with a valve area of 1.5 cm^2 or less. In patients who have favorable anatomy, catheter-based balloon mitral valvuloplasty is a competing recommendation (5).

Results of Mitral Valve Repair

With the development of standardized techniques for MV reconstruction, Deloche et al. (6) demonstrated that MV repair was feasible in 95% of patients with degenerative valve disease, 70% with rheumatic valve disease, and 75% with ischemic valve disease. The long-term results after MV repair were excellent, with very low rates of thromboembolism, reoperation,

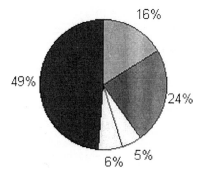

16%

49%

24%

6% 5%

FIG. 10.1. Pathologic anatomy of degenerative mitral valve disease (n = 1,072). Dilated annulus, 16% slice; elongated chordae, 24% slice; anterior and posterior chordal rupture, 5% slice; anterior chordal rupture, 6% slice; posterior chordal rupture, 49% slice. (From Gillinov AM, Cosgrove DM, Blackstone EH, et al. Durability of mitral valve repair for degenerative disease. *J Thorac Cardiovasc Surg* 1998;116:734–743, with permission.)

and valve-related mortality. Echocardiographic follow-up analysis revealed no or mild MR in 92% of patients. Gillinov et al. (7) analyzed 1,072 patients undergoing mitral repair for degenerative disease at the Cleveland Clinic. Although this study corroborated the excellent long-term results of Deloche et al. (92.9% freedom from reoperation at 10 years), the results varied when analyzed by anatomic subgroup (Fig. 10.1). Optimal results (97% freedom from reoperation at 10 years) were observed in patients with isolated posterior leaflet prolapse for which the surgical repair included posterior resection and ring annuloplasty. An isolated anterior leaflet repair, chordal-shortening techniques, posterior leaflet resection without annuloplasty, and annuloplasty alone all significantly decreased durability (7) (Fig. 10.2). In addition, residual MR of grade 2+ or higher at the termination of the procedure was shown to decrease the durability of repair (8).

Patients with rheumatic disease had significantly worse repair results (76% freedom from reoperation at 15 years) (6). Yau et al. (9) demonstrated improved risk-adjusted, long-term survival in patients with rheumatic disease undergoing mitral repair in comparison with mitral replacement.

ASSESSMENT OF THE PATIENT FOR MITRAL VALVE REPAIR

Preoperative Clinical Assessment

The cardiology referral for MV repair is based on clinical signs and symptoms and on echocardiographic and cardiac catheterization findings. Preoperative transthoracic echocardiographic (TTE) imaging often provides satisfactory information regarding the degree of MR or MS, annular size, involvement of anterior or posterior leaflets, chordal and papillary muscle structural integrity, and overall LV size and LV systolic function. In the absence of satisfactory TTE images, transesophageal echocardiography (TEE) provides improved visualization of MV pathology.

FIG. 10.2. Influence of valve pathology and operative technique on freedom from reoperation. **A:** Anterior leaflet prolapse versus posterior leaflet prolapse. The presentation is a risk-adjusted comparison with use of the multivariable equation for a patient undergoing resection and annuloplasty without chordal shortening and with intraoperative echocardiography. **B:** Chordal shortening versus no chordal shortening. The presentation is not risk-adjusted, showing both nonparametric and parametric estimates. **C:** Posterior leaflet resection with annuloplasty (with or without sliding repair) versus all other repair techniques. **D:** Use of intraoperative echocardiography versus no intraoperative echocardiography. (From Gillinov AM, Cosgrove DM, Blackstone EH, et al. Durability of mitral valve repair for degenerative disease. *J Thorac Cardiovasc Surg* 1998;116:734–743, with permission.)

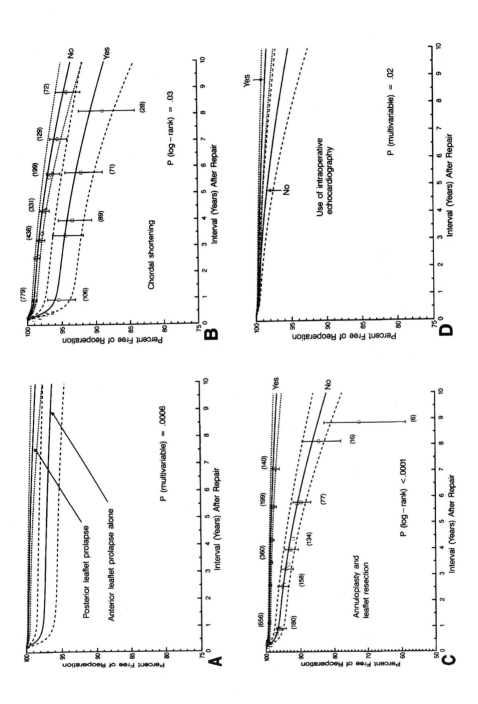

Intraoperative Transesophageal Echocardiographic Evaluation

Rationale. A detailed intraoperative TEE evaluation of the mitral apparatus is critical for planning surgery, assessing results, and predicting the long-term durability of the MV repair (7,10). A comprehensive and systematic approach to evaluating the mitral anatomy is described in Chapter 8. There are currently no widely accepted criteria for establishing which patients should undergo MV repair. The feasibility of repair depends on the anatomic lesions of the valve and the skill of the surgeon. A complete evaluation of the heart and great vessels by intraoperative TEE is critical because incidental findings (severe atherosclerotic aortic disease, undiagnosed aortic insufficiency, regional wall motion abnormalities suggestive of ischemia, left atrial [LA] thrombus, intracardiac masses) often significantly affect surgical planning.

Functional classification of mitral regurgitation. Carpentier (11) introduced a functional rather than a pathologic model of the regurgitant MV in which the focus is on the opening and closing motions of the leaflets.

Type I: normal leaflet motion: Leaflet motion in MR can be normal (type I), in which case the MR is caused by annular dilation that leads to failed coaptation or leaflet perforation (e.g., from endocarditis) (Fig. 10.3A,B).

Type II: excessive leaflet motion: When leaflet motion is excessive (type II), prolapse of the leaflet edge in systole beyond the plane of the annulus results in an eccentric regurgitant jet directed away from the prolapsing leaflet (Fig. 10.3C,D). Common causes of prolapse are chordal rupture or elongation, papillary muscle rupture, and papillary muscle elongation/dysfunction. It should be noted that papillary muscle dysfunction related to ischemic heart disease is associated with adjacent segmental wall motion abnormalities.

Type III: restricted leaflet motion: Restrictive leaflet motion may involve both inadequate opening in diastole (MS) secondary to commissural fusion (rheumatic disease) and inadequate closure in systole (MR) secondary to chordal thickening/fusion (rheumatic disease) or LV dilation. Inadequate closure keeps the valve edge below the plane of the annulus, resulting in a relative prolapse of the adjacent normal leaflet above the line of coaptation (Fig. 10.3E). The resultant regurgitant jet is directed toward the restricted leaflet. Various lesions can coexist, and the goal of repair is to address the component lesions systematically (Fig. 10.3F).

Nomenclature. The Carpentier nomenclature designates the posterior leaflet segments as P1, P2, and P3. P1 is adjacent to the anterolateral commissure, P2 is the middle scallop, and P3 is adjacent to the posteromedial commissure. The anterior leaflet has less clearly defined segments designated as A1, A2, and A3, corresponding to the adjacent posterior leaflet segments. The TEE short-axis view of the LV with some anteflexion provides the "fish mouth" view of the MV, in which the A3 and P3 segments are at the top of the screen and the A1 and P1 segments are at the bottom (anterior leaflet to the left) (Fig. 10.4A). In the surgeon's view, A3 and P3 are to the right, and A1 and P1 are to the left (anterior leaflet superior) (Fig. 10.4B). A simple way of demonstrating the surgical view is to tilt one's head to the left while viewing the echo image, thereby visualizing P1, P2, and P3 from left to right inferiorly and A1, A2, and A3 from left to right superiorly. At least three nomenclature systems are commonly used by surgical teams in repair of the MV (see Chapter 8). *Concordance in the use of nomenclature by the surgical team is important to avoid confusion and misdiagnosis.*

→

FIG. 10.3. Carpentier classification of leaflet motion. **A:** Type I, normal leaflet motion, depicted here with annular dilation and central mitral regurgitant (MR) jet. **B:** Type I, normal leaflet motion with leaflet perforation. Note normal degree of coaptation between anterior and posterior leaflets. **C:** Type II, flail of posterior leaflet, depicted here secondary to ruptured marginal chordae. The MR jet is directed anteriorly. **D:** Type II, flail of anterior leaflet, depicted here secondary to ruptured marginal chordae. The MR jet is directed posteriorly. **E:** Type III, restricted leaflet motion. The posterior leaflet is depicted here as tethered, causing a "relative prolapse" of the anterior leaflet. The MR jet is directed posteriorly. **F:** Types I and III, restricted leaflet motion, depicted here in a dilated failing heart. Annular dilation (type I) and leaflet restriction secondary to downward displacement of the papillary muscle heads (type III) commonly coexist in this condition.

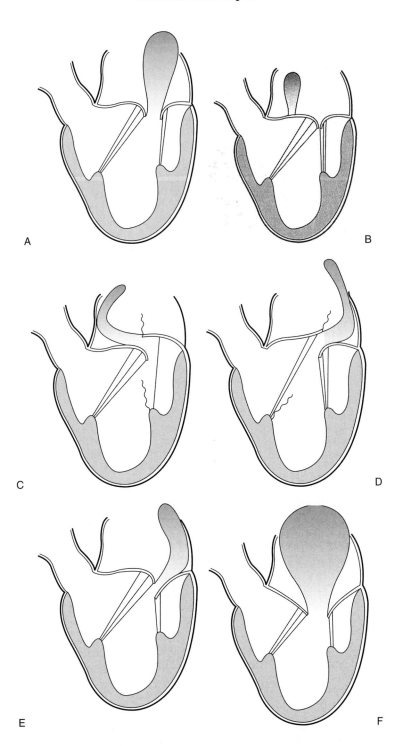

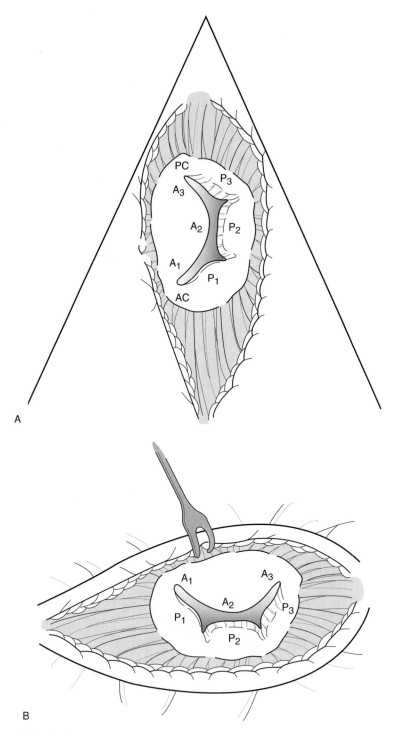

A

B

FIG. 10.4. Mitral valve leaflet segments. **A:** Echocardiographic short-axis or "fish mouth" view. **B:** Surgeon's view through open left atrium from the patient's right side. The echocardiographic view is rotated 90 degrees counterclockwise relative to the surgeon.

Reporting the transesophageal echocardiographic findings before mitral repair. The report of the findings before mitral repair must include the degree of MR or MS, the specific location of prolapsing or flail leaflet segments, areas of tethering and restriction, and areas of normal leaflet function. Leaflets should also be assessed for perforations, calcifications, excessive length, thickened appearance, and mobility. Annular calcification (most common posteriorly) should be noted. The subvalvular apparatus is assessed for chordal thickening, and for papillary muscle and ventricular wall function. Robust secondary chordae, which may be suitable for transposition to prolapsed leaflets, can often be identified by TEE. *Because the goal of the intraoperative TEE examination before repair is to evaluate the function of the MV, it is critical to evaluate the valve in a hemodynamic state comparable to that of the awake, ambulatory patient.* The use of inotropes or vasopressors may be necessary to achieve this end. The secondary effects of the valvular disease, including LA enlargement with or without thrombus, and the size and function of the left and right ventricles should be discussed with the surgeon.

Assessing the risk for systolic anterior motion. Systolic anterior motion (SAM) of the MV with resultant left ventricular outflow tract obstruction (LVOTO) develops in more than 16% of patients following MV repair (12–14). A complete TEE examination after repair will identify this complication. However, intraoperative TEE analysis of the mitral apparatus before bypass can identify the patients in whom this complication is likely to develop. The data allow the surgeon to perform a "sliding leaflet" procedure or modifications of this repair technique and thereby significantly reduce the occurrence of SAM (14–16).

The mechanism of SAM/LVOTO is multifactorial, the major cause being excess mitral leaflet tissue (as in the "floppy mitral valve" of myxomatous disease). Anteriorly displaced papillary muscles, a nondilated LV, and a narrow mitral-aortic angle have also been proposed as contributing factors (14). The incidence of SAM/LVOTO after MV repair has been shown to increase in patients with a more anterior position of the leaflet coaptation point. This may be the consequence of a relatively large posterior leaflet, shifting coaptation closer to the base of the anterior leaflet and causing both anterior displacement of the coaptation line and an increase in the amount of slack leaflet tissue in the outflow tract. An elongated anterior leaflet may cause a similar increase in the amount of slack leaflet available to obstruct LV outflow.

Maslow et al. (13) investigated various pre-repair TEE variables to determine the most useful measurements with which to assess the preoperative risk for SAM/LVOTO. These included the anterior leaflet (AL) and posterior leaflet (PL) lengths, used to determine the *AL/PL ratio,* and the distance from the coaptation point to the septum (*C-sept*) (Fig 10.5). The incidence of post-repair SAM/LVOTO was greater in patients with an AL/PL ratio below 1.0 than in patients with an AL/PL ratio above 3.0. SAM/LVOTO was more likely to develop in patients with a C-sept of 2.5 cm or less than in patients with a C-sept of 3.0 cm or more (13). The identification of patients at high risk for SAM/LVOTO affects the pharmacologic management of hemodynamics after bypass, which is aimed at reducing this complication (discussed later), and alters the surgical techniques described above.

Direct surgical inspection of the mitral apparatus. Before the use of intraoperative TEE became widespread, pre-repair valve analysis depended entirely on direct surgical inspection with the heart and mitral apparatus in the "tensed" state. This was accomplished by exposing the valve during ventricular fibrillation, either before application of the aortic cross-clamp or after cross-clamping with infusion of cold blood in the aortic root at physiologic pressure to reduce the risk for air embolization (17). In the current era, the surgeon plans most of the operation based on the intraoperative TEE findings, so that it is not necessary to evaluate the valve before the administration of cardioplegia. Although in the empty, flaccid heart nearly all leaflet edges can be shown to prolapse above the annular plane, direct inspection after cardioplegia remains a vital step in confirming the location of pathology and the suitability of the various valve structures for the planned repair (18). Leaflet prolapse or restriction is identified by the application of nerve hooks to the leaflet edge and comparison with "normal" leaflet segments, usually the P1 segment. Direct inspection allows the identification of ruptured or elongated chordae and of robust secondary chordae that can be transposed to prolapsing segments. Inspection of the papillary muscles determines the suitability of chordal-shortening approaches or the placement of artificial chords. Leaflet perforations and annular calcification are identified.

In MS, the degree of commissural fusion, leaflet calcification, and subchordal disease and the suitability of commissurotomy are determined by visual inspection.

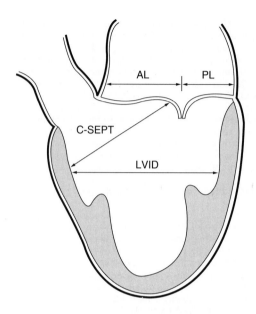

FIG. 10.5. Schematic demonstrating the transesophageal echocardiographic measurements used before repair to assess the risk for systolic anterior motion. *AL,* anterior leaflet length; *PL,* posterior leaflet length; *C sept,* distance from the coaptation point to the septum; *LVID,* left ventricular internal diameter in systole. (Adapted from Maslow AD, Regan MM, Haering JM, et al. Echocardiographic predictors of left ventricular outflow tract obstruction and systolic anterior motion of the mitral valve after mitral valve reconstruction for myxomatous valve disease. *J Am Coll Cardiol* 1999;34:2096–2104.)

SURGICAL REPAIR OF MITRAL REGURGITATION

Exposing the Mitral Valve

Good exposure of the MV is a prerequisite to adequate repair. Incision in the interatrial groove with bicaval cannulation is a widely used approach, with exposure improved by dissecting the left and right atria to allow a more medial incision (19). A transseptal approach with bicaval cannulation via a right atriotomy, with or without extension into the roof of the LA, also provides excellent exposure. If exposure is still difficult, the placement of annuloplasty ring sutures and the application of tension will "deliver" the valve into the surgical field. Left-sided pericardial traction sutures should be relaxed. Meticulous attention to myocardial protection, either by intermittent antegrade or a combination of antegrade and retrograde cardioplegia, is an absolute necessity to allow for the safe clamp time necessary to perform a complex repair. TEE can assist in the successful placement of a coronary sinus catheter, particularly in redo surgery in which the palpation of posterior structures is limited.

Repair Techniques

This section is intended to give the echocardiographer an appreciation of the common surgical procedures used in MV repair. A better understanding of the common repair techniques can guide the post-repair TEE evaluation.

Repair of leaflet prolapse

Isolated P2 prolapse: When resection and ring annuloplasty are performed, a prolapsed P2 segment is the most reliably repaired regurgitant lesion (7) (Fig. 10.6). Briefly, the P2 segment is resected from scallop to scallop in a quadrangular fashion. Intact chordae are detached from the papillary muscles (a robust, intact chord may be preserved to repair another prolapsing segment). The annulus is plicated with a horizontal mattress suture, and direct approximation of the leaflet edges is undertaken.

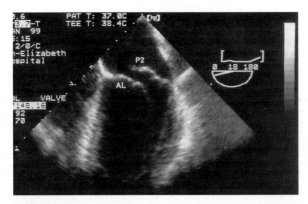

FIG. 10.6. Transesophageal four-chamber view of the mitral valve depicting prolapse/flail of the P2 segment of the posterior leaflet.

In the case of excessive leaflet length or other factors predisposing to SAM, or in all cases (author preference), a sliding plasty can be carried out (Fig. 10.7). In sliding leaflet plasty, after P2 resection, the P1 and P3 segments are partially detached from their hinge line, starting at the P2-facing edge. Horizontal mattress sutures are then placed through the annulus to reduce the gap left by the resection of P2. The leaflets are reattached to the annulus and their edges reapproximated. After leaflet repair, a ring annuloplasty is performed, with the ring sized to the anterior leaflet area and intercommissural distance.

Isolated anterior leaflet prolapse: Resection is not a reliable approach for the larger anterior leaflet, except for repair of a very small, focal prolapsing area by triangular resection (11). The prolapsing anterior leaflet (Fig. 10.8) can be repaired by means of chordal transfer, artificial chordal replacement, or chordal-shortening techniques. Chordal transfer involves transferring robust chords either from a secondary position on the anterior leaflet or from an adjacent posterior leaflet edge (the latter requiring a quadrangular resection, as described earlier). Artifical chords (Gore-Tex) can be placed from the papillary muscle head to the leaflet edge. A major challenge is adjusting the length of the chords, often by judging adjacent, nonprolapsing leaflet segments. Nevertheless, excellent long-term results have been demonstrated with chordal replacement (8). Finally, elongated chords can be shortened. The trenching technique, in which elongated chords are buried in a trench cut in the papillary muscle and sutured in place, was previously popular, but long-term durability was unsatisfactory (7,20). Papillary muscle shortening, especially for billowing valves in which multiple chords are elongated, has become popular. The method is efficient because multiple chords are shortened at once; however, exposure can be challenging, and long-term results are not yet available.

Bileaflet prolapse: In cases of prolapse of both the anterior and posterior leaflets (Fig. 10.9), a systematic approach combining quadrangular resection with chordal transposition, shortening, or replacement is required. If there is dominant posterior prolapse with a myxomatous, prolapsing anterior leaflet, isolated quadrangular resection with ring annuloplasty can be satisfactory (21).

Papillary muscle rupture: Rupture of a papillary muscle complicating an acute myocardial infarction can affect the entire papillary muscle (one third of cases), resulting in bileaflet flail, or only one head (two third of cases), resulting in flail of either the anterior or posterior leaflets. *The posteromedial papillary muscle is most often affected (75% of cases) because the coronary circulation to the inferior wall is not redundant.* A single ruptured papillary head can be reimplanted in adjacent endocardium. In cases with extensive necrosis of the papillary muscle and adjacent myocardium, an MV replacement with preservation of the remaining intact chords should be carried out (22).

Repair of ischemic mitral regurgitation: Patients with ischemic MR are a diverse group in regard to acuteness of presentation, LV function, and causes of MR (papillary muscle dysfunction, segmental LV wall dysfunction, leaflet restriction, annular dilation, chordal

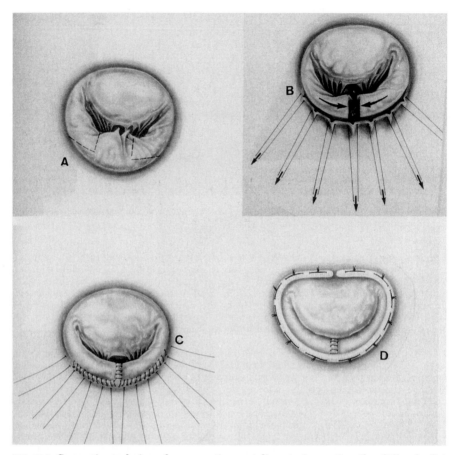

FIG. 10.7. Carpentier technique for preventing systolic anterior motion–the sliding leaflet technique. **A:** In cases of excess tissue of the mural leaflet, the quadrangular resection is completed by two triangular resections of the posterior leaflet remnants to correct excess leaflet tissue. **B:** Remnants are translated medially to close the gap. **C,D:** Repair is completed, and the ring is inserted to reinforce the repair. (From Jebara VA, Mihaileanu S, Acar C, et al. Left ventricular outflow tract obstruction after mitral valve repair: results of the sliding leaflet technique. *Circulation* 1992;88:30–34, with permission.)

rupture, papillary muscle rupture). A variety of procedures have been used to manage these problems, including the leaflet/chordal repair techniques described earlier, ring and suture annuloplasty for annular dilation/leaflet restriction, and valve replacement with or without chordal preservation. Although mitral repair is demonstrably superior to replacement for nonischemic MR, the issue remains unresolved for ischemic MR because of the heterogeneity of this patient population. For example, Duarte and colleagues (23) reported very good 10-year survival in patients with 3+ MR treated with coronary artery bypass grafting (CABG) alone. Rankin et al. (24) and Akins et al. (25) demonstrated improved results when the regurgitant MV was repaired rather than replaced, whereas Cohn et al. (26) reported better survival with replacement (with chordal preservation) than with repair. Of note, in the analysis of Cohn et al., repair of functional MR (secondary to annular dilatation or leaflet restriction) resulted in a 5-year survival of 43%, whereas replacement in this group resulted in a 5-year survival of 92%.

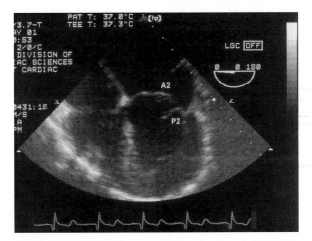

FIG. 10.8. Transesophageal four-chamber view of the mitral valve depicting prolapsing A2 segment of the anterior leaflet.

In summary, the issue of replacement versus repair remains uncertain in patients with mild-moderate ischemic MR undergoing CABG. In patients with severe MR, either mitral repair or mitral replacement with chordal preservation can yield acceptable results.

Mitral ring annuloplasty in cardiomyopathy. One of the most exciting developments has been mitral ring annuloplasty for patients with congestive heart failure (CHF) and moderate to severe MR. Functional MR in CHF is caused by failed leaflet coaptation resulting from a combination of annular enlargement and ventricular dilation, the latter leading to leaflet restriction (27,28). Mitral ring annuloplasty in patients with New York Heart Association class IV CHF and MR results in a 2-year survival of 70% (29). Hence, mitral ring annuloplasty offers another therapeutic option besides transplantation in a subset of patients with CHF, severe functional limitation, and an otherwise dismal prognosis.

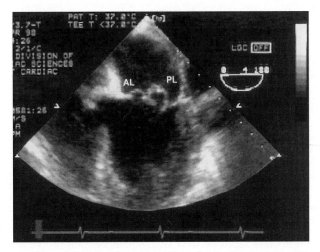

FIG. 10.9. Transesophageal five-chamber view of the mitral valve depicting bileaflet prolapse.

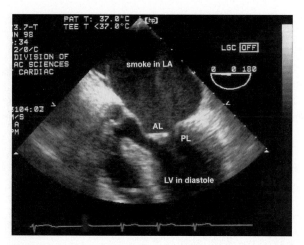

FIG. 10.10. Transesophageal five-chamber view of the mitral valve depicting mitral stenosis with "smoke" (spontaneous contrast) in an enlarged left atrium (*LA*). Note the hockey stick deformity of the anterior leaflet (*AL*) and marked narrowing of the mitral orifice in diastole.

Mitral repair in rheumatic disease

Mitral stenosis: The symptoms of patients with some degree of leaflet pliability can be relieved by open commissurotomy and chordal fenestration in lieu of replacement (Fig. 10.10). The anterolateral commissure is often fused to a greater degree than the posteromedial commissure. With a nerve hook distracting either leaflet edge, the fused portions of the leaflets/commissures are divided; great care must be taken to respect the chordal attachments to the papillary muscle heads. This incision can be carried down from the leaflet through the fused chords. In minimally calcified valves with good pliability on echocardiography, comparable results can be achieved with percutaneous balloon valvuloplasty (30).

Mitral regurgitation: Repair of rheumatic MR is a very challenging endeavor. Leaflet restriction can be relieved through aggressive chordal fenestration with fanning of the involved papillary muscle heads. Leaflet decalcification and the transposition of chords from a secondary position back to the leaflet edge can give good results. Ring annuloplasty may be necessary, but care must be taken in mixed lesions that relief of MS is maintained.

Special Surgical Considerations

Calcified mitral annulus. The presence of annular calcification considerably complicates mitral repair or replacement, increasing the risk for ventricular rupture, damage to the circumflex coronary artery, and postoperative paravalvular MR, and it must be identified in the TEE examination (31). Calcification is most commonly seen in the posterior annulus but can extend into the leaflet tissue or the ventricular myocardium, and rarely to the anterior annulus. It is distinguished from the calcification of rheumatic disease, in which primary leaflet calcification may extend to the annulus with concomitant calcification of subchordal structures. Annular calcification in association with MR occurs most frequently in the elderly and in patients with Marfan syndrome or Barlow disease. Carpentier et al. (32) reported successful en bloc resection of the entire calcium deposit with subsequent repair in 98% of cases, with a 3.3% mortality (Fig 10.11). Once the calcium is resected, the atrioventricular groove is repaired with vertical mattress sutures. The posterior leaflet (or its remnants in the case of a P2 resection) is then reattached.

Cases at high risk for systolic anterior motion. The surgical approach to MV repair may be modified in cases identified to be at high risk for SAM. In the case of dominant

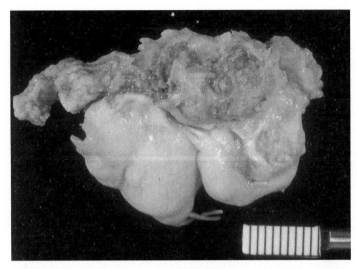

FIG. 10.11. P2 segment with adjacent annular calcium. The patient was a 72-year-old woman with marked calcium deposition in the posterior annulus and P2 prolapse with severe mitral regurgitation. En bloc resection was carried out with repair, as described in the text.

posterior leaflet prolapse, sliding leaflet plasty can be carried out after P2 resection and the excessive height of the remnants of the posterior leaflet reduced by the resection of leaflet tissue from the annulus-facing edge (33). If an anteriorly displaced line of coaptation is identified after leaflet resection has been performed, some modification can be achieved by bending a rigid ring so that the anteroposterior diameter is increased, which reduces the volume of anterior leaflet tissue available to obstruct the LVOT. Accurate ring sizing and avoidance of undersizing the annuloplasty ring also reduce the risk for LVOTO secondary to SAM. Finally, post-repair hemodynamic management should be attempted, as outlined later.

ASSESSMENT OF THE MITRAL VALVE AFTER REPAIR

Surgical Valve Assessment

After packs and retraction sutures have been removed to prevent distortion of the valve and ventricle, the passive leak test is performed by forcefully injecting saline solution into the LV. This test remains useful in determining gross inadequacies of repair; a large leak by this test is generally confirmed as severe MR by TEE. *Patients with a competent valve following the leak test may still have significant valvular insufficiency by TEE secondary to ischemic wall dysfunction or SAM in the beating, volume-loaded heart* (34).

Transesophageal Echocardiographic Assessment of Adequacy of Repair

Post-repair assessment by TEE in the physiologically optimized heart has become the gold standard in determining the adequacy of MV repair. "Immediate failures" are detected in approximately 6% to 8% of patients, who then may undergo further reparative techniques or replacement during the same procedure (35,36). Post-repair MR of grade 1+ or 2+ increases the incidence of late reoperation threefold in comparison with trace or no MR after

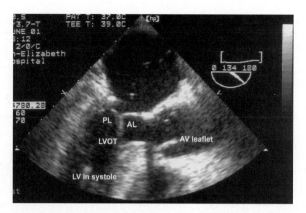

FIG. 10.12. Transesophageal longitudinal view depicting obstruction of the left ventricular outflow tract (LVOT) by leaflet tips during systole (systolic anterior motion with left ventricular outflow tract obstruction). Color Doppler in this situation would show turbulence in the left ventricular outflow tract and a posteriorly directed mitral regurgitant jet.

repair (37). *Thus, post-repair TEE information is essential in determining whether immediate reintervention during the same surgery is warranted.*

Transesophageal Echocardiographic Assessment of Complications of Mitral Valve Repair

Systolic anterior motion/left ventricular outlet tract obstruction. SAM of the MV leaflets with resultant dynamic LV outflow tract obstruction is a known complication of MV repair, as discussed earlier. The echocardiographic findings demonstrate a characteristic systolic bending of the leaflet tips into the outflow tract, turbulent flow in the LVOT, and commonly MR (usually as a posteriorly directed jet) (Fig 10.12). Gradients across the LVOT are increased from baseline as a result of dynamic outflow obstruction. *When SAM/LVOTO occurs after MV repair, hemodynamic maneuvers must be attempted before the results are declared inadequate. Inotropic agents, vasodilators, and low-volume states all exacerbate this condition and perhaps provoke it in susceptible patients.* With the discontinuation of these agents and manipulation of the cardiovascular status by volume loading with or without the administration of alpha agents, SAM/LVOTO often resolves. In some patients with a significant LVOT gradient, beta-blockers may be useful in resolving the LVOTO (38). With persistent SAM/LVOTO, surgical reintervention may be necessary.

Coronary artery injury. Injury to the circumflex coronary artery is a rare but frequently fatal complication of either mitral repair or mitral replacement (39). *Intraoperative TEE findings of new segmental wall motion abnormalities in the lateral wall or inferoposterior regions may suggest circumflex injury, and grafting of the distal coronary artery may be indicated* (40).

Ventricular rupture. Disruption of the atrioventricular groove or rupture of the LV between the papillary muscle insertions and the atrioventricular groove is a feared and devastating complication of MV surgery. Factors predisposing to rupture include female sex, advanced age, annular calcification, and high-profile valve replacement devices in patients with a small LV cavity. *Recognition of LV rupture can be aided by TEE, which often demonstrates continuous entrainment of intracardiac air.* Repair by placement of an endocardial patch has been shown to be superior to attempts to stem the bleeding by placing external sutures or patches (41).

Aortic valve leaflet injury. Deep suture placement in the anterior annulus can inadvertently injure the left or noncoronary leaflets of the aortic valve. Massive aortic insufficiency noted either clinically or by TEE alerts the surgeon to this possibility. Simple leaflet tethering may be relieved by suture removal and replacement, whereas tears in the aortic leaflets may require aortic valve replacement or more complex repair (42).

Pitfalls of Transesophageal Echocardiographic Examination after Mitral Valve Repair

Unreliability of pressure half-time results after repair of mitral stenosis. A major assumption of the pressure half-time technique in valve area calculations is that LA and LV compliance does not significantly affect the rate of pressure decline across the stenotic orifice. In clinically stable MS, this assumption appears valid, but immediately following MV repair, LA and LV compliance is markedly altered and does not reach equilibrium for 24 to 72 hours. *Thus, the pressure half-time method of calculating the MV area after MS repair may not be accurate in the immediate postoperative period.*

Inadequacy of hemodynamic state inadequate to expose mitral regurgitation. General anesthesia can effectively mask MR by lowering preload, decreasing afterload, and decreasing the inotropic state of the heart. Before TEE assessment of the MV, manipulation (volume loading, administration of an inotrope or alpha agonist) should be attempted to attain hemodynamics that approximate those of the ambulatory state. This detail is critical in both pre-repair and post-repair TEE evaluations to assess the degree of mitral insufficiency accurately.

DECISION TO REINTERVENE

The decision to reintervene because of an imperfect result is a difficult one, in part because of a conflicting literature concerning the significance of mild-moderate residual MR. Fix et al. (36) found no increase in long-term mortality in patients with grade 1 to 2+ MR after repair, although a trend to increased late reoperation was noted. In contrast, Sheikh et al. (43) noted an increase in postoperative morbidity and mortality in patients with grade 2+ or higher residual MR. Interpretation of the post-repair TEE data may reveal the cause of residual MR, and cooperation between the echocardiographer and surgeon will allow a determination of the likelihood of a more successful repair. *The decision to reintervene must also take into account the condition of the heart, the potential for injury during a second cross-clamp period, and the potential need for valve replacement with its attendant costs.* These decisions must be made in the "heat of battle" and require echocardiographers with a firm and confident grasp of TEE interpretation, surgeons with an awareness of their capabilities, and a clear understanding by the entire team of the short-term implications of reintervention and the long-term implications of residual MR.

SUMMARY

The establishment of intraoperative TEE as the standard of care in MV repair places the intraoperative echocardiographer and the surgeon in a close working relationship in which real-time decisions with tremendous implications for the patient are made on a daily basis.

REFERENCES

1. Cutler EC, Levine SA. Cardiotomy and valvulotomy for mitral stenosis: experimental observations and clinical notes concerning an operated case with recovery. *Boston Med Surg J* 1923;188:1023–1027.
2. Souttar H. The surgical treatment of mitral stenosis. *Br Med J* 1925;2:603–606.
3. Lillehei CW, Got VL, Dewfall RA, et al. Surgical correction of pure mitral insufficiency by annuloplasty under direct vision. *Lancet* 1957;1:446.
4. Starr A, Edwards ML. Mitral replacement: clinical experience with a ball valve prosthesis. *Ann Surg* 1961;154:726.

5. Bonow RO, Carabello B, De Leon AC, et al. ACC/AHA guidelines for the management of patients with valvular heart disease: executive summary. A report of the American College of Cardiology/American Heart Association Task Force on Practice Guidelines (Committee on Management of Patients with Valvular Heart Disease). *J Heart Valve Dis* 1998;7:672–707.
6. Deloche A, Jebara VA, Relland JY, et al. Valve repair with Carpentier techniques. *J Thorac Cardiovasc Surg* 1990;99:990–1002.
7. Gillinov AM, Cosgrove DM, Blackstone EH, et al. Durability of mitral valve repair for degenerative disease. *J Thorac Cardiovasc Surg* 1998;116:734–743.
8. David TE, Omran A, Armstrong S, et al. Long-term results of mitral valve repair for myxomatous disease with and without chordal replacement with expanded polytetrafluoroethylene sutures. *J Thorac Cardiovasc Surg* 1998;115:1279–1286.
9. Yau TM, El-Ghoneimi YA, Armstrong S, et al. Mitral valve repair and replacement for rheumatic disease. *J Thorac Cardiovasc Surg* 2000;119:53–61.
10. Foster GP, Isselbacher EM, Rose GA, et al. Accurate localization of mitral regurgitant defects using multiplane transesophageal echocardiography. *Ann Thorac Surg* 1998;65:1025–1031.
11. Carpentier A. Honored guest's address: Cardiac valves surgery—the "French correction." *J Thorac Cardiovasc Surg* 1983;86:323–337.
12. Lee KS, Stewart WJ, Lever HM, et al. Mechanism of outflow tract obstruction causing failed mitral valve repair: anterior displacement of leaflet coaptation. *Circulation* 1994;88:24–29.
13. Maslow AD, Regan MM, Haering JM, et al. Echocardiographic predictors of left ventricular outflow tract obstruction and systolic anterior motion of the mitral valve after mitral valve reconstruction for myxomatous valve disease. *J Am Coll Cardiol* 1999;34:2096–2104.
14. Jebara VA, Mihaileanu S, Acar C, et al. Left ventricular outflow tract obstruction after mitral valve repair: results of the sliding leaflet technique. *Circulation* 1993;88:30–34.
15. Perier P, Claunizer B, Mistarz K. Carpentier "sliding leaflet" technique for repair of the mitral valve: early results. *Ann Thorac Surg* 1994;57:383–386.
16. Gillinov AM, Cosgrove DM. Modified sliding leaflet technique for repair of the mitral valve. *Ann Thorac Surg* 1999;68:2356–2357.
17. DeVarennes B. Personal communication.
18. Shah PM, Raney AA, Duran CMF, et al. Multiplane transesophageal echocardiography: a roadmap for mitral valve repair. *J Heart Valve Dis* 1998;8:625–629.
19. Larbalastier RI, Chard RB, Cohn LH. Optimal approach to the mitral valve: dissection of the interatrial groove. *Ann Thorac Surg* 1992;54:1186–1188.
20. Phillips MR, Daly RC, Schaff HV, et al. Repair of anterior leaflet mitral valve prolapse: chordal replacement versus chordal shortening. *Ann Thorac Surg* 2000;69:25–29.
21. Gillinov MA, Cosgrove DM, Wahli S, et al. Is anterior leaflet repair always necessary in repair of bileaflet mitral valve prolapse? *Ann Thorac Surg* 1999;68:820–824.
22. David TE. Techniques and results of mitral valve repair for ischemic mitral regurgitation. *J Card Surg* 1994;9:274–277.
23. Duarte IG, Shen Y, MacDonald MJ, et al. Treatment of moderate mitral regurgitation and coronary disease by coronary bypass alone: late results. *Ann Thorac Surg* 1999;68:426–430.
24. Rankin JS, Fenely MP, Hickey MS, et al. A clinical comparison of mitral valve repair versus valve replacement in ischemic mitral regurgitation. *J Thorac Cardiovasc Surg* 1988;95:165–175.
25. Akins CW, Hilgenberg AD, Buckley MJ, et al. Mitral valve reconstruction versus replacement for degenerative or ischemic mitral regurgitation. *Ann Thorac Surg* 1994;58:668–676.
26. Cohn LH, Rizzo RJ, Adams DH, et al. The effect of pathophysiology on the surgical treatment of ischemic mitral regurgitation: operative and late risks of repair versus replacement. *Eur J Cardiothorac Surg* 1995;9:568–574.
27. Kono T, Sabbah HN, Stein PD, et al. Left ventricular shape as a determinant of functional mitral regurgitation in patients with severe heart failure secondary to either coronary artery disease or idiopathic dilated cardiomyopathy. *Am J Cardiol* 1991;68:355–359.

28. Kiyoshige K, Oki T, Fukuda N, et al. Changes in left ventricular inflow and pulmonary venous flow velocities during preload alteration in dilated heart. *Clin Cardiol* 1996;19:38–44.
29. Smolens IA, Pagani FD, Bolling SF. Mitral valve repair in heart failure. *Eur J Heart Failure* 2000;2:365–371.
30. Reyes VP, Raju BS, Wynne J, et al. Percutaneous balloon valvuloplasty compared with open surgical commissurotomy for mitral stenosis. *N Engl J Med* 1994;331:961–967.
31. Cammack PL, Edie RN, Edmunds LH. Bar calcification of the mitral annulus: a risk factor in mitral valve operations. *J Thorac Cardiovasc Surg* 1987;94:399–404.
32. Carpentier AF, Pellerin M, Fuzellier JF, et al. Extensive calcification of the mitral valve annulus: pathology and surgical management. *J Thorac Cardiovasc Surg* 1996;111:718–730.
33. Jebara VA, Mihaileanu S, Acar C, et al. Left ventricular outflow tract obstruction after mitral valve repair: results of the sliding leaflet technique. *Circulation* 1993;88:II-30–II-34.
34. Chitwood WR Jr. Mitral valve repair: an odyssey to save the valves! *J Heart Valve Dis* 1998;7:255–261.
35. Saiki Y, Kasegawa H, Kawase M, et al. Intraoperative TEE during mitral valve repair: does it predict early and late postoperative mitral valve dysfunction? *Ann Thorac Surg* 1998;66:1277–1281.
36. Fix J, Isada L, Cosgrove D, et al. Do patients with less than "echo-perfect" results from mitral valve repair by intraoperative echocardiography have a different outcome? *Circulation* 1993;88:II-39–II-48.
37. Gillinov AM, Cosgrove DM, Lytle BW, et al. Reoperation for failure of mitral valve repair. *J Thorac Cardiovasc Surg* 1997;113:467–475.
38. Grossi EA, Galloway AC, Parish MA, et al. Experience with twenty-eight cases of systolic anterior motion after mitral valve reconstruction by the Carpentier technique. *J Thorac Cardiovasc Surg* 1992;103:466–470.
39. Danielson GK, Cooper E, Tweedale DN. Circumflex coronary artery injury during mitral valve replacement. *Ann Thorac Surg* 1967;4:53–59.
40. Travilla G, Pacini D. Damage to the circumflex coronary artery during mitral valve repair with sliding leaflet technique. *Ann Thorac Surg* 1998;66:2091–2093.
41. Karlson KJ, Ashraf MM, Berger RL. Rupture of left ventricle following mitral valve replacement. *Ann Thorac Surg* 1988;46:590–597.
42. Hill AC, Bansal RC, Razzouk AJ, et al. Echocardiographic recognition of iatrogenic aortic valve leaflet perforation. *Ann Thorac Surg* 1997;64:684–689.
43. Sheikh K, DeBruijn N, Rankin J, et al. The utility of transesophageal echocardiography and Doppler color flow imaging in patients undergoing cardiac valve surgery. *J Am Coll Cardiol* 1990;15:363–372.

QUESTIONS

1. Which of the following is true about ischemic papillary muscle rupture?
   a. Rupture is caused by fewer chordal attachments to the posteromedial papillary muscle.
   b. Rupture most commonly involves the anterior papillary muscle.
   c. A lack of dual blood supply to the myocardium subtending the posterior papillary muscle makes it the one most commonly involved in ischemic papillary rupture.
   d. Rupture most commonly involves the entire papillary muscle.
   e. Rupture usually results in bileaflet flail.
2. Mitral ring annuloplasty
   a. Can increase the risk for SAM if the ring is oversized
   b. Improves the durability of repair techniques
   c. Decreases the risk for atrioventricular groove disruption
   d. Improves visualization of the mitral apparatus by TEE after MV repair
   e. Increases the risk for MS after MV repair

3. After MV repair, SAM/LVOTO
   a. Can be identified before surgery
   b. Can be successfully treated by increasing the afterload
   c. Should be treated with dopaminergic agents
   d. Can be treated by undersizing the mitral annuloplasty ring
   e. Is more likely in patients with a preoperative AL/PL ratio greater than 3
4. Anterior leaflet prolapse repair
   a. May involve resection of P2
   b. Is the most durable of all leaflet repairs
   c. Requires at least a small triangular resection of a large anterior leaflet
   d. Results are improved with chordal-shortening procedures
   e. Long-term results are poor after chordal replacement with Gore-Tex
5. Intraoperative TEE evaluation for mitral repair
   a. Fails to depict localized leaflet prolapse accurately
   b. Accurately measures postrepair stenosis by the pressure half-time technique after open commissurotomy
   c. Allows inexperienced observers to identify normal and abnormal leaflet segments accurately
   d. Does not correlate well with postoperative TTE findings
   e. Improves the long-term durability of mitral repair
6. In type III leaflet abnormality
   a. Of both leaflets, one would expect an eccentric jet of MR
   b. Of the posterior leaflet, one would expect a posteriorly directed MR jet
   c. Of the anterior leaflet, one would expect a posteriorly directed MR jet
   d. Effective resolution of MR by mitral repair does not alter the long-term outcome of patients with severe CHF before surgery
   e. MR cannot be treated with a mitral annuloplasty ring alone
7. In MS of rheumatic origin
   a. Adequate repair is achieved in more than 90% of cases with good long-term results
   b. Repair is commonly complicated by annular calcification
   c. Balloon mitral commissurotomy may provide adequate treatment
   d. TEE is unable to predict the degree of stenosis accurately before surgery with the pressure half-time method
   e. Chordal fenestration has been shown to improve long-term durability.
8. The surgical view of the MV
   a. Places the P3 and A3 segments to the surgeon's right
   b. Allows accurate assessment of leaflet prolapse after the administration of cardioplegia
   c. Is most easily replicated with the echocardiographer's head tilted to the right and the TEE image in the fish mouth view
   d. Easily demonstrates the continuity of the posterior leaflet with the LVOT and aortic valve apparatus
   e. Reliably demonstrates a competent valve if the passive leak test result is negative
9. Late MV repair failure
   a. Is rarely caused by the progression of valvular disease
   b. Is rarely a consequence of procedure-related failures
   c. Is most often caused by endocarditis
   d. Is more likely with the use of an annuloplasty ring
   e. And reoperation are more likely when the trenching technique of chordal shortening is used
10. The American College of Cardiology/American Heart Association practice guidelines recommend MV repair
   a. For patients with severe MR and marked LV dysfunction only
   b. For asymptomatic patients with severe MR and LV dilation
   c. Over percutaneous balloon valvuloplasty for patients with severe MS and pliable leaflets
   d. For patients with MS, functional class II symptoms, and an MV area of 2 cm^2
   e. For patients with severe MR so long as atrial fibrillation is absent

Aortic Regurgitation

Ira S. Cohen

The exquisite sensitivity of transesophageal echocardiography (TEE) in identifying regurgitation is manifested by its ability to detect the minute regurgitant jets engineered into the design of the St. Jude prosthetic valve to flush platelet aggregates off the valve surface. Early efforts at quantification of the severity of aortic regurgitation (AR) were based on the distribution of flow of the regurgitant jet into the left ventricular (LV) cavity. The assessment of the severity of valvular insufficiency is complicated by the dramatic effects of even transient changes in loading conditions on Doppler indices of AR severity. Acute increases in peripheral vascular resistance (e.g., during isometric exercise or the administration of vasopressors) can increase the apparent degree of valvular insufficiency by increasing systemic vascular resistance and the impedance to peripheral runoff. Conversely, vasodilators (e.g., volatile anesthetics, angiotensin-converting enzyme inhibitors, calcium channel blockers) reduce peripheral vascular resistance and decrease the apparent degree of insufficiency, both clinically and by Doppler interrogation. The physical properties (e.g., distensibility, elasticity, compliance) of the source (aorta) and recipient (LV) of regurgitant flow, in addition to the size of the regurgitant orifice and the physical properties of the involved valve, are other variables that further complicate assessment. Because the operating room environment is one in which a multitude of factors affect both the preload and afterload of the ventricle, the potential impact of these changes must be borne in mind when the apparent severity of a valvular lesion is evaluated. In fact, some clinicians feel it is not possible to assess regurgitant lesions accurately in the operating room environment.

As a result of the multitude of factors influencing any assessment of the severity of AR, the estimate should be based on an integration of the results of all Doppler approaches providing technically adequate data in any given patient. TEE estimates the grade of AR tend to be overestimates. Methods for assessing the severity of AR with Doppler have evolved along with advances in Doppler technology since Ward et al. (1) first described the use of pulsed Doppler in conjunction with M-mode echocardiography and auscultation to detect aortic insufficiency. The general approaches to assessing the severity of AR with TEE are presented in the order of their relative clinical applicability, and approaches adapted from transthoracic echocardiography (TTE) are included. Color mapping of the LV outflow tract (LVOT) has traditionally been regarded as the most accurate echocardiographic assessment (2–7). Currently under investigation are methods that appear to be less dependent on loading conditions, and their efficacy is not as thoroughly documented (4,6). Measurement of the width of the vena contracta, the narrowest cross-sectional area of the regurgitant jet as it traverses the valve plane, is emerging as an attractive approach (8). The proximity of the TEE probe to the aortic root and LVOT and the ability to interrogate these structures with the higher-frequency TEE signal make it possible to delineate the size of the regurgitant jet relative to adjacent structures more accurately than can be done with TTE techniques. Such data are often mutually reinforcing despite the problems that have been outlined.

In the operating room, TEE can help delineate potential problems before the patient leaves. The mechanism of AR in cases of aortic dissection can be assessed and used to guide surgery (9–14). For example, the efficacy of resuspension, as opposed to replacement, of a prolapsed aortic valve to correct AR resulting from a Stanford type A dissection is proportional to the percentage of the annulus dissected and, to a lesser extent, the initial diameter of the aortic root (13). The superior resolution of TEE is particularly helpful in defining the anatomic location of regurgitant lesions related to prosthetic heart valves and the suture line of insertion of the valve. The anatomic continuity of the anterior mitral leaflet with the posterior aortic root creates potential problems in the mitral and aortic valves associated with the debridement of calcification in either annulus or the placement of "overbiting" sutures when a prosthesis is inserted. The potential for poor seating of the valve and paravalvular leaks as well as other complications of surgery can be analyzed with TEE and resolved while the patient is still in the operating room.

RECOMMENDED VIEWS

In AR, but not in stenotic lesions, useful information can be obtained from interrogation both parallel and perpendicular to the regurgitant jet because its area of distribution is one of the major variables used in the assessment of severity. The most useful views are generally obtained from the mid esophagus (ME) when the angle of interrogation from a standard ME four-chamber view is changed to approximately 120 degrees to visualize the LVOT and proximal aorta in a long-axis view (ME aortic valve long-axis view). The ME aortic valve short-axis view at approximately 45 degrees allows excellent resolution of the individual cusps of the aortic valve.

Alternatively, but less frequently, good views can be obtained from a transgastric (TG) position at an angle of either 0 degree (deep TG long-axis view) or approximately 120 degrees (TG long-axis view), and these approaches have the advantage of being more nearly parallel to the direction of blood flow, which is essential for quantitative Doppler analysis. In general, these views are not optimal for visualizing the height or cross-sectional area of an AR jet immediately below the valve plane. However, they may be the only means of assessing the outflow tract in the presence of a prosthetic mitral valve (MV), which frequently causes acoustic shadowing of the aortic annulus in more standard views.

The pressure gradient between the regurgitant and recipient chambers in regurgitant valvular lesions is always high. By the simplified Bernoulli equation, the gradient equals four times the square of the peak jet velocity. Again, aligning a Doppler beam parallel to the flow is best accomplished in the TG views. Whereas in stenotic lesions absolute gradient information is critical, in regurgitant lesions, it is the rate of change in pressure gradients that provides clinically useful information. Fortunately, color Doppler techniques for the assessment of AR lesions provide useful information that is, to a significant degree, independent of the angle of the beam to the regurgitant flow.

When color flow Doppler is used, the appropriate gain setting for mapping is obtained by first setting the gain high enough that random color pixels appear within or outside the blood pool. Gain is then decreased until these random color pixels disappear. Failure to standardize the color examination in this manner leads to invalid data and is the source of the so-called "dial-a-jet" phenomenon, in which overgaining the Doppler signal can expand the apparent size of the jet.

APPROACHES TO THE QUANTITATIVE ASSESSMENT OF AORTIC REGURGITATION

Color Flow Mapping

In the initial efforts at quantifying AR, pulsed wave Doppler was used to map the depth of penetration of the regurgitant jet into the LV cavity. This approach entailed several problems related to the effects of a high-pressure gradient crossing a narrow regurgitant orifice (see later discussion). A better approach was developed in which jet mapping from the then newly introduced color flow Doppler technique was used (3,15). Two techniques for color flow mapping are recommended.

Ratio of jet height to left ventricular outflow diameter. Long-axis imaging of the LVOT is used to measure the height of the regurgitant jet immediately below the aortic valve plane, which is then compared with the diameter of the outflow tract at that same point (16). The optimal views are the 120-degree ME aortic valve long-axis view and the ME five-chamber view (Fig. 11.1; see Color Plate 16 following page 212). The long-axis view that shows the maximal height of the color jet is selected for analysis. The maximal height during diastole is identified during slow motion freeze-frame review. The analysis is performed with the "on-board" package of the ultrasound machine. Alternatively, an M-mode cursor can be placed perpendicular to the outflow tract. If color flow mapping is then activated, the regurgitant jet will appear in color in the M-mode view of the outflow tract, and the relative dimensions can be measured from this display by using the caliper function of the ultrasound machine (Fig. 11.2; see Color Plate 17 following page 212). This is generally the easier of the two methods of analysis to perform (Table 11.1).

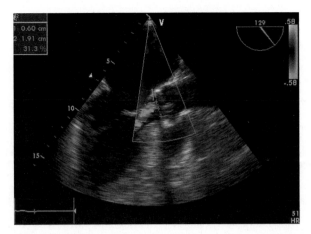

FIG. 11.1. Midesophageal aortic valve long-axis view demonstrating calculation of the ratio of aortic insufficiency height to left ventricular outflow tract diameter. The internal caliper on the echocardiography system is used to make these measurements. In this example, the ratio is 31%, indicating mild aortic insufficiency. (See Color Plate 16 following page 212.)

Ratio of jet area to left ventricular outflow tract area. In the second color flow mapping technique, the area of the regurgitant jet is compared with the area of the LVOT (Fig. 11.3; see Color Plate 18 following page 212). The preferred view for this approach is the ME aortic valve short-axis view, but with the probe advanced to immediately below the valve plane. Again, diastole is evaluated by slow motion freeze-frame review, and the maximal jet area is traced and compared with the area of the LVOT. The process is simplified by using the software analysis package of the machine. This method is slightly more accurate than the height-diameter ratio method but is technically more difficult to perform.

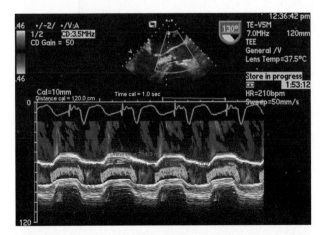

FIG. 11.2. Color M-mode assessment of aortic regurgitation. From the midesophageal aortic valve long-axis view the M-mode cursor is positioned perpindicular to the aortic root as close to the origin of the regurgitant jet as possible. The jet and the outflow tract are well delineated in the color M-mode display. Caliper measurement of the jet height (75 mm) is compared to that of the root (214.3 mm) and the resulting ratio of 35% corresponds to 2+ aortic regurgitation (see Table 11.1). (See Color Plate 17 following page 212.)

TABLE 11.1. SCORING OF SEVERITY OF AORTIC REGURGITATION

Method of evaluation (view)	Trivial (0–1+)	Mild (1+–2+)	Moderate (2+–3+)	Severe (3+–4+)
AI jet height/LVOT diameter (ME AV LAX)	1%–24%	25%–46%	47%–64%	>65%
AI areal/LVOT area (ME AV SAX)	<4%	4%–24%	25%–59%	>60%
Jet depth mapping (ME LAX)	LVOT	Mid anterior mitral leaflet	Tip anterior mitral leaflet	Papillary muscle head
Vena contracta mapping (ME LAX, ME AV SAX)				Width >6 mm Area >7.5 mm²
Aortic diastolic flow reversal (UE aortic arch LAX)				Holodiastolic retrograde flow in the descending aorta
Slope of AR jet decay (TG LAX, deep TG LAX)			≥2 m/s	≥3 m/s
Pressure half-time (TG LAX, deep TG LAX)		>500 ms	200–500 ms	<200 ms

AI, aortic insufficiency; LVOT, left ventricular outflow tract; ME, midesophageal; AV, aortic valve; LAX, long axis; SAX, short axis; UE, upper esophageal; AR, aortic regurgitation; TG, transgastric.

Caveats. In practice, these approaches provide reliable estimates of severity and consequently have become widely regarded as among the best and most easily applied methods of Doppler assessment (16). They do, however, require technically adequate views and color flow images that cannot always be obtained and may be affected by changes in loading conditions (Table 11.1).

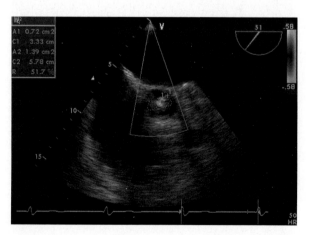

FIG. 11.3. Midesophageal aortic valve short-axis view in the same patient as in Figure 11.1 demonstrating the jet area/left ventricular outflow tract area method. The ratio of the areas is 51%, indicating moderate mitral regurgitation. The patient therefore has mild-moderate aortic insufficiency. (See Color Plate 18 following page 212.)

Color Flow Mapping of the Depth of the Regurgitant Jet

Technique. In the first Doppler approach to quantification of the severity of AR, pulsed wave Doppler was used to map the depth to which the regurgitant jet extended into the LV cavity (17–19) (Table 11.1). Color Doppler has supplanted that approach. The maximal depth below the two-dimensional aortic valve plane at which the jet can be detected by color Doppler imaging determines the equivalent angiographic grade of insufficiency. The size of the heart varies with body surface area, so the scale is based on anatomic landmarks instead of depth below the valve plane. Depth is recorded in relation to MV structures because more than 90% of regurgitant jets are oriented toward the anterior mitral leaflet as a result of the Coanda effect. In the less common situation in which the jet is oriented along the interventricular septum, the depth at which it can be detected along the septum is compared with a corresponding depth in relation to MV structures to estimate angiographic severity.

Limitations. As in any form of valvular insufficiency, a large pressure gradient exists between the two chambers where the leak is occurring. Depending on the location, a pressure head of 60 to 110 mm Hg or greater drives the regurgitant jet through a small orifice. Accordingly, a small regurgitant jet frequently extends far into the recipient chamber despite a leak that is hemodynamically insignificant. In vitro analysis of models of AR suggests that the depth is more an index of the gradient between the aorta and LV than of the angiographic grade of severity (15,20).

Use of the color flow map of regurgitant flow as an index of severity is further complicated by the entrainment of blood from a high-velocity jet entering a low-pressure chamber. This leads to color Doppler overestimation of the apparent depth of the regurgitant jet. *Measurements of the apparent depth are more likely to be affected by this phenomenon than are measurements of jet height, which are made close to the aortic valve plane.*

Mapping the Vena Contracta

The *vena contracta* is the narrowest portion of the jet crossing the valve plane and can be identified by visualizing the convergence zone of color flow as it approaches the valve plane. The width of the vena contracta can be measured as it passes through the regurgitant orifice to exit the valve plane (6,21). To optimize visualization, the echo sector is narrowed and the depth decreased to maximize the valve size and frame rate. Long- and short-axis views are then obtained from the ME, as outlined earlier. The largest diameter of the vena contracta during any portion of diastole is measured in the long-axis plane of the jet, or planimetry of its area is performed in the short-axis view at the valve plane. In a small series of patients undergoing TEE, a vena contracta width of more than 6 mm or an area of more than 7.5 mm² predicted severe AR (6). More importantly, and in contrast to observations made during assessments of the severity of mitral regurgitation with this technique (22), changes in afterload obtained with phenylephrine or volume loading did not change the size of the vena contracta, findings suggesting that this measurement may be load-independent (6,23,24). If additional clinical studies validate the accuracy and reproducibility of this method, it will likely become the method of choice for intraoperative assessment because of its relative ease of acquisition and apparent load independence.

Aortic Diastolic Flow Reversal

Another early index of the severity of aortic insufficiency was based on the demonstration of retrograde diastolic flow in the ascending or descending aorta or the aortic arch (17), which can be assessed by interrogating the aorta in a plane near the arch (upper esophageal aortic arch long-axis view), as demonstrated in Figure 11.4 (see Color Plate 19 following page 212). This view is obtained by withdrawing the probe from the ME position and rotating it posteriorly to visualize the descending aorta at 0 degree in circular cross section. In patients with a tortuous aorta, the angle necessary for a short-axis view may vary considerably. As the probe is withdrawn into the upper esophagus, the plane elongates as the arch is cut tangentially at a point slightly deeper than 20 cm from the incisors. Angulation with firm retroflexion from this position generally allows

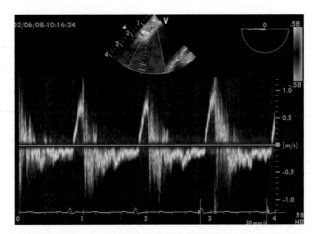

FIG. 11.4. Upper esophageal aortic arch long-axis view demonstrating severe aortic regurgitation, evidenced by flow reversal within the distal aortic arch during diastole. Note flow away from the probe, below the baseline, throughout diastole (holodiastolic flow). (See Color Plate 19 following page 212.)

interrogation of the high arch. Images of the ascending and descending portions of the aorta are typically acquired only with significant obliquity and thus are not generally used in clinical spectral Doppler examinations. However, because the flow abnormality is assessed by comparing the areas under the curves of systolic and diastolic flow independently of the absolute flow velocities, the inability to assess true flow velocities is not a contraindication. The areas under the systolic and diastolic flow curves are measured and the ratio calculated.

Normally, a minor retrograde flow pattern can be detected in the ascending aorta and proximal descending aorta related to runoff into the great vessels and coronary bed. In AR, holodiastolic retrograde flow can be observed. As aortic insufficiency becomes more severe, the degree of apparent retrograde aortic flow relative to antegrade aortic flow increases (17). In general, the further distally in the aorta (e.g., descending or abdominal aorta) holodiastolic retrograde flow is detected, the more severe the AR.

This assessment remains a useful adjunct for confirming the severity of AR but is less accurate in the presence of significant aortic stenosis (7,25,26). *Importantly, the usefulness of the descending aortic diastolic reversal of flow as an index of severe AR intraoperatively has been confirmed in patients in whom the LVOT cannot be adequately imaged on TEE for technical reasons (e.g., interposed MV prosthesis creating an acoustic shadow that obscures the LV outflow). In these patients, color flow mapping of the regurgitant jet is not possible (5).*

Slope of Aortic Regurgitant Jet Decay

Analysis of a continuous wave Doppler wave form of aortic insufficiency from the TG long-axis or deep TG long-axis view is used because the Doppler beam is aligned parallel to the regurgitant jet flow. Basal esophageal views of the LVOT are generally obtained at too great an angle to the flow for an accurate jet to be acquired. It is essential that a smooth waveform with an intact envelope be recorded for analysis to be meaningful.

The principle of this analysis is that the velocity of the regurgitant jet is directly related to the pressure gradient between the central aorta and the LV in diastole, in accordance with the Bernoulli equation. When a large defect is in the valve, the pressures will equalize more rapidly because more blood leaks through the valve per unit of time. Therefore, the pressure gradient between the aorta and the LV decreases more rapidly in severe regurgitation, and as a result, the velocity of the jet also diminishes more rapidly. The slope of the rate of decay of the velocity is therefore a measure of the severity of regurgitation. A slope of AR velocity decay of 2 to 3 m/s suggests moderately severe or severe (grades 3+ to 4+) AR. Rapid equalization of the pressure gradient can result in premature closure of the MV before the onset of ventricular systole, indicative of severe AR, or in extreme cases, premature opening of the aortic valve in diastole. For an analysis of the slope of the AR jet on continuous wave Doppler, two technical criteria must be met:

1. A smooth velocity envelope must be defined by continuous wave Doppler.
2. It must be confirmed that the core of the regurgitant jet has been interrogated. With appropriate interrogation, the peak regurgitant jet velocity measurement should approximate the value calculated with the Bernoulli equation from the gradient between the arterial diastolic pressure and the LV diastolic pressure (velocity equals the square root of the pressure gradient divided by 4). Typically, jet velocities are high (>4 m/s) because the initial diastolic pressure gradient between the aorta and LV is generally 60 to 80 mm Hg. The exception is in severe AR, in which the aortic and LV diastolic pressures may be similar. Otherwise, lower velocities on the spectral display suggest that the true regurgitant jet is not being interrogated directly.

Pressure Half-Time Measurement

Alternatively, a pressure half-time can be calculated. This is defined as the interval between the time when the transvalvular AR pressure gradient is maximal and the time when the pressure gradient is half the maximum. The computer analysis package determines the pressure half-time from the slope of the AR jet decay (Fig. 11.5; see Color Plate 20 following page 212). A pressure half-time of less than 200 ms suggests severe AR (27). *Factors related to LV and aortic compliance and the presence of high LV diastolic pressures (heart failure, restrictive physiology, diastolic dysfunction) all potentially cause the gradient to dissipate more rapidly and artifactually worsen the apparent severity of the lesion.* Accordingly, these two methods of analysis of the decay curve should be used mainly to confirm the color flow findings.

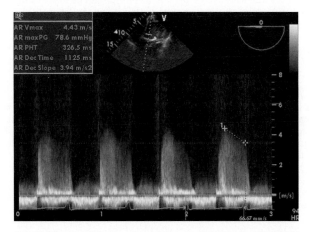

FIG. 11.5. Transgastric long-axis view with nearly parallel Doppler beam alignment demonstrating the aortic regurgitant jet velocity profile. The pressure half-time is 218 m/s, with a slope of 3.94 m/s indicating moderate to severe aortic regurgitation. (See Color Plate 20 following page 212.)

Calculation of Regurgitant Volume

The AR volume can be calculated from the difference between the LV stroke volume and the right ventricular (RV) stroke volume. The LV stroke volume is calculated by multiplying the cross-sectional area of the LVOT by the time-velocity integral of LVOT flow. The RV stroke volume is then estimated from the pulmonary outflow tract diameter and time velocity integral calculated in a similar fashion. However, obtaining accurate measurements of the necessary parameters in an intraoperative situation is time-consuming and technically challenging, so that this approach is impractical.

Role of the Doppler Signal Characteristics in the Assessment of Aortic Regurgitation

Because the blood flow velocity is directly related to the pressure differential, the *diastolic* velocity is always high (4.0–5.0 m/s) in comparison with the *systolic* velocities of 1.0 to 1.7 m/s across normal valves. The to-and-fro systolic and diastolic Doppler signal is easily detected as abnormal by even an untrained ear when heard through the audio system of the ultrasound machine. The sound becomes louder and its tone purer as the alignment of the probe becomes more closely parallel to the core of the jet. High-velocity jets do not *necessarily* mean severe regurgitation is present. If the gain settings are constant, the *intensity* of the spectral Doppler signal is directly related to the severity of the leak. This is because the larger the regurgitant flow, the greater the number of red blood cells contained therein to reflect the ultrasound beam. Consequently, more severe regurgitant lesions tend to produce more intense Doppler signals.

In more severe lesions, the velocity of the antegrade flow through the regurgitant valve may be increased in comparison with that in normal subjects. This is a consequence of the increased stroke volume that develops because the heart must eject both the regurgitant and the normal stroke volume through the aortic annulus, which is a fairly rigid structure. The velocity of systolic flow in the LVOT increases with significant insufficiency, and outflow tract velocities above 1.5 m/s suggest stenosis of the outflow tract relative to the volume of blood flowing through it and support a diagnosis of significant regurgitation. The clinical corollary of this phenomenon is the development of a functional systolic ejection murmur of *relative* aortic stenosis, heard during auscultation of the heart in addition to the diastolic murmur of aortic insufficiency. However, this technique can be misleading in patients with a hyperdynamic state, who also can present with outflow tract flow velocities between 1.5 and 2.0 m/s.

SUMMARY

The intraoperative assessment of AR with TEE is generally best accomplished by measuring the jet height in the LVOT just below the aortic valve plane. More recent studies suggest that it is practical to measure the width of the vena contracta because this measurement is less load-dependent than others. The assessment of diastolic flow reversal in the aorta itself remains an important and useful approach that has been reconfirmed. The other approaches discussed in this chapter are useful and can play an ancillary role, reinforcing the practitioner's confidence in making a definitive assessment.

REFERENCES

1. Ward JM, Baker DW, Rubenstein SA, et al. Detection of aortic insufficiency by pulse Doppler echocardiography. *J Clin Ultrasound* 1977;5:5–10.
2. Meyerowitz CB, Jacobs LE, Kotler MN, et al. Assessment of aortic regurgitation by transesophageal echocardiography: correlation with angiographic determination. *Echocardiography* 1993;10:269–278.

3. Rafferty T, Durkin MA, Sittig D, et al. Transesophageal color flow Doppler imaging for aortic insufficiency in patients having cardiac operations. *J Thorac Cardiovasc Surg* 1992;104:521–525.
4. Sato Y, Kawazoe K, Kamata J, et al. Clinical usefulness of the effective regurgitant orifice area determined by transesophageal echocardiography in patients with eccentric aortic regurgitation. *J Heart Valve Dis* 1997;6:580–586.
5. Sutton DC, Kluger R, Ahmed SU, et al. Flow reversal in the descending aorta: a guide to intraoperative assessment of aortic regurgitation with transesophageal echocardiography. *J Thorac Cardiovasc Surg* 1994;108:576–582.
6. Willett DL, Hall SA, Jessen ME, et al. Assessment of aortic regurgitation by transesophageal color Doppler imaging of the vena contracta: validation against an intraoperative aortic flow probe. *J Am Coll Cardiol* 2001;37:1450–1455.
7. Zarauza J, Ares M, Vilchez FG, et al. An integrated approach to the quantification of aortic regurgitation by Doppler echocardiography. *Am Heart J* 1998;136:1030–1041.
8. Yoganathan A, Cape E, Sung H, et al. Review of hydrodynamic principles for the cardiologist: applications to the study of blood flow and jets by imaging techniques. *J Am Coll Cardiol* 1988;12:1344–1353.
9. Adam MC, Tribouilloy C, Mirode A, et al. Contribution of transesophageal and transthoracic echography in the evaluation of the mechanism and quantification of regurgitation in mitral and aortic bioprosthetic valves [in French]. *Arch Mal Coeur Vaiss* 1993;86: 1345–1350.
10. Hioki J, Shibutani T, Naito T, et al. Aortic valve insufficiency caused by nonpenetrating chest trauma difficult to distinguish from infective endocarditis with transesophageal echocardiography: a case report [in Japanese]. *J Cardiol* 1997;29:143–149.
11. Oda H, Tanaka T, Yamazaki Y, et al. A case of nonpenetrating traumatic aortic regurgitation detected by transesophageal echocardiography. *Tohoku J Exp Med* 1997;182: 93–101.
12. Brandstatt P, Carlioz R, Fontaine B, et al. Acute post-traumatic aortic insufficiency: transesophageal echocardiography in the diagnosis and therapy of the lesions [in French]. *Ann Cardiol Angeiol (Paris)* 1998;47:563–567.
13. Keane MG, Wiegers SE, Yang E, et al. Structural determinants of aortic regurgitation in type A dissection and the role of valvular resuspension as determined by intraoperative transesophageal echocardiography. *Am J Cardiol* 2000;85:604–610.
14. Movsowitz HD, Levine RA, Hilgenberg AD, et al. Transesophageal echocardiographic description of the mechanisms of aortic regurgitation in acute type A aortic dissection: implications for aortic valve repair. *J Am Coll Cardiol* 2000;36:884–890.
15. Switzer DF, Yoganathan AP, Nanda NC, et al. Calibration of color Doppler flow mapping during extreme hemodynamic conditions in vitro: a foundation for a reliable quantitative grading system for aortic incompetence. *Circulation* 1987;75:837–846.
16. Perry J, Helmcke F, Nanda N, et al. Evaluation of aortic insufficiency by Doppler color flow mapping. *J Am Coll Cardiol* 1987;9:952–959.
17. Quinones MA, Young JB, Waggoner AD, et al. Assessment of pulsed Doppler echocardiography in detection and quantification of aortic and mitral regurgitation. *Br Heart J* 1980;44:612–620.
18. Toguchi M, Ichimiya S, Yokoi K, et al. Clinical investigation of aortic insufficiency by means of pulsed Doppler echocardiography. *Jpn Heart J* 1981;22:537–550.
19. Ciobanu M, Abbasi AS, Allen M, et al. Pulsed Doppler echocardiography in the diagnosis and estimation of severity of aortic insufficiency. *Am J Cardiol* 1982;49:339–343.
20. Taylor AL, Eichhorn EJ, Brickner ME, et al. Aortic valve morphology: an important in vitro determinant of proximal regurgitant jet width by Doppler color flow mapping. *J Am Coll Cardiol* 1990;16:405–412.
21. Tribouilloy CM, Enriquez-Sarano M, Bailey KR, et al. Assessment of severity of aortic regurgitation using the width of the vena contracta: a clinical color Doppler imaging study. *Circulation* 2000;102:558–564.
22. Kizilbash AM, Willett DL, Brickner ME, et al. Effects of afterload reduction on vena contracta width in mitral regurgitation. *J Am Coll Cardiol* 1998;32:427–431.
23. Ishii M, Jones M, Shiota T, et al. Evaluation of eccentric aortic regurgitation by color Doppler jet and color Doppler–imaged vena contracta measurements: an animal study of quantified aortic regurgitation. *Am Heart J* 1996;132:796–804.

24. Ishii M, Jones M, Shiota T, et al. Quantifying aortic regurgitation by using the color Doppler–imaged vena contracta: a chronic animal model study. *Circulation* 1997;96:2009–2015.
25. Diebold B, Peronneau P, Blanchard D, et al. Non-invasive quantification of aortic regurgitation by Doppler echocardiography. *Br Heart J* 1983;49:167–173.
26. Reimold SC, Maier SE, Aggarwal K, et al. Aortic flow velocity patterns in chronic aortic regurgitation: implications for Doppler echocardiography. *J Am Soc Echocardiogr* 1996;9:675–683.
27. Labovitz AJ, Ferrara RP, Kern MJ, et al. Quantitative evaluation of aortic insufficiency by continuous wave Doppler echocardiography. *J Am Coll Cardiol* 1986;8:1341–1347.

QUESTIONS

1. Which of the following factors can affect the degree of AR during an operative examination?
   a. Administration of vasopressors
   b. Presence of volatile anesthetics
   c. Patient's volume status
   d. All of the above
2. Which TEE view is most helpful in evaluating the aortic valve in a patient with a St. Jude mitral valve?
   a. ME four-chamber view
   b. ME aortic valve long-axis view
   c. ME aortic valve short-axis view
   d. TG long-axis view
3. Which view allows for optimal Doppler beam alignment in a patient with AR?
   a. ME four-chamber view
   b. ME aortic valve long-axis view
   c. ME aortic valve short-axis view
   d. TG short-axis view
   e. Deep TG long-axis view
4. When the ratio of the AR jet height to the LVOT diameter is used to quantify the degree of AR, the following is true
   a. One must optimize the color gain setting
   b. The ME aortic valve long-axis view is preferred
   c. The ratio for AR with a grade of 4+ is more than 65%
   d. All of the above
5. When the pressure half-time method is used to quantify the severity of AR, which of the following will NOT artificially worsen the apparent severity of the AR?
   a. Congestive heart failure
   b. Restrictive physiology
   c. Diastolic dysfunction
   d. Acute myocardial infarction
   e. Acute hemorrhage
6. Obtaining diastolic aortic flow reversal in a patient with AR with TEE is difficult. The following statements regarding techniques are true **except**
   a. The upper esophageal aortic arch long-axis view is useful.
   b. Obtaining accurate flow velocities is essential.
   c. Holodiastolic flow in the distal aorta indicates severe AR.
   d. AR end-diastolic velocity profiles in the descending aorta correlate better with AR severity than those in the ascending aorta.
7. Which statement about continuous wave Doppler analysis of AR is true?
   a. Parallel alignment with the regurgitant jet is essential.
   b. The deep TG long-axis and TG long-axis views are preferred.
   c. ME views are seldom adequate because of poor beam alignment.
   d. A smooth wave form with an intact envelope is necessary.
   e. All of the above.

8. Which principle is not important in an evaluation of the slope of AR jet decay with Doppler?
   a. Pulsed wave Doppler is preferred because of "cleaner" envelopes.
   b. The velocity of the regurgitant jet is directly proportional to the pressure gradient between the aorta and the LV in diastole.
   c. A large regurgitant lesion will equalize the pressure gradient between the aorta and the LV more quickly.
   d. The velocity of the AR jet diminishes more quickly as the severity of AR increases.
9. Which of the following observations is useful to remember in an attempt to optimize the Doppler beam alignment in a patient with AR?
   a. The velocity should be high (4–5 m/s).
   b. AR has a loud and pure audio tone as the jet is entered.
   c. The intensity (darkness) of the spectral Doppler signal is proportional to the severity of the leak.
   d. Patients with significant AR frequently have LVOT velocities greater than 1.5 m/s.
   e. All of the above.
10. All of the following indicate severe AR **except**
   a. Pressure half-time of less than 500 ms
   b. Ratio of height of the AR jet in the LVOT to the diameter of the LVOT above 65%
   c. Ratio of area of AR jet in LVOT to area of LVOT above 60%
   d. Diastolic flow reversal in the descending aorta

Aortic Stenosis

Ira S. Cohen

With the exception of coronary artery bypass grafting procedures, aortic valve replacement for critical aortic stenosis (AS) is probably the most common indication for cardiac surgery in patients past the age of 65 years. The overwhelming majority of patients in this age group have atherosclerotic degenerative changes of a tricuspid valve as the pathophysiologic substrate. In contrast, most patients undergoing aortic valve replacement for AS in the 35- to 55-year-old age group have a bicuspid aortic valve, which typically calcifies early. Aortic valve involvement by rheumatic disease occurs much less frequently than in the pre-antibiotic era, typically causes commissural fusion, and is almost invariably associated with mitral valve (MV) disease.

Generally, critical AS is diagnosed preoperatively. Symptoms of hemodynamically significant AS indicating a clinical need for valve replacement are congestive heart failure (often starting as exertional dyspnea), syncope, and angina. Provided other potential causes of these symptoms have been excluded, their presence is of paramount clinical significance because they are associated with a poor prognosis. This is so even if the estimated valve areas fall only within the "severe" range because the calculated areas are just estimates based on both measurements and theoretic assumptions. AS can cause angina in the absence of coronary artery disease because the tissue turgor of the hypertrophic wall compromises coronary flow reserve by restricting the dilation of penetrating vessels. Cardiac catheterization is therefore required to exclude critical coronary artery disease (which coexists in approximately 50% of cases) in the subset of patients with angina.

The rate of progression of stenosis can be fairly rapid and tends to be linear for a given individual, but it is not predictable based on the initial echocardiographic findings (1,2). The issue of whether to replace a noncritically stenotic valve prophylactically is increasingly important. This is a highly controversial issue, and intraoperative data may be required to reach a decision. Accordingly, the intraoperative echocardiographer must be adept with the techniques used to assess the severity of AS (Table 12.1).

EVALUATION OF THE AORTIC VALVE

Two-Dimensional Planimetry of the Orifice

The area of the normal aortic valve is between 2.6 and 3.5 cm^2 (Fig. 12.1). AS is considered severe when the aortic valve area is less than 0.8 to 0.9 cm^2 or less than 0.5 to 0.6 cm^2/m^2. Early echocardiographers looked at the characteristics of aortic leaflet motion in an attempt to determine the severity of aortic obstruction. Separation of the aortic leaflets by less than 8 mm in a two-dimensional long-axis view suggested critical disease, whereas separation by more than 12 mm suggested noncritical disease (3) (Fig. 12.1). In addition, fluttering of an aortic leaflet on M-mode echocardiography was felt to be better than two-dimensional separation as a discriminator of noncritical disease (4). These findings have been superseded by later techniques.

Two-dimensional echocardiography in the midesophageal (ME) aortic valve short-axis view images the short-axis plane of the aortic valve and allows planimetry of the aortic valve orifice. Accurate planimetry requires that the imaging plane and machine settings be optimized as follows:

1. Obtain a true short-axis view of the aortic valve with all three leaflets in view.
2. Optimize the image by adjusting the gain settings. *Excessive gain leads to an underestimation of valve area because of a "blooming artifact" from the bright echoes of the thickened valve leaflets.*

TABLE 12.1. SEVERITY OF AORTIC STENOSIS

Method of evaluation	Normal	Mild	Moderate	Severe
Peak velocity (m/sc)	1.0–1.7			>4.5
Mean gradient (mm Hg)		<20	20–50	>50
Maximal pressure gradient (mm Hg)		<36	>50	>80
TVI$_{LVOT}$ TVI$_{AV}$ ratio				<0.25
AVA (cm^2)	2.6–3.5	1.0–1.5	0.80–1.0	<0.80

TVI, time-velocity integral; LVOT, left ventricular outflow tract; AVA, aortic valve area.

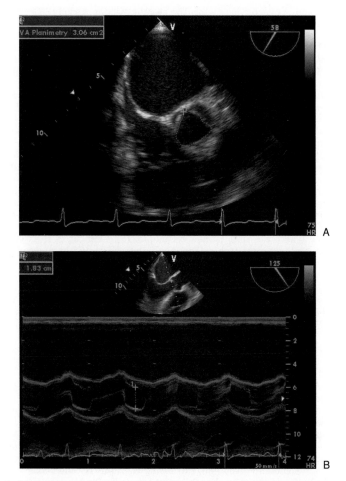

FIG. 12.1. A: Midesophageal aortic valve short-axis view of a normal aortic valve with a planimetric area of 3.06 cm^2. **B:** Two-dimensional M-mode (motion mode) midesophageal aortic valve long-axis view demonstrating cusp separation of 18 mm in the same patient.

3. Use color flow Doppler imaging to aid in adjusting the probe depth and angle of the imaging plane so as to interrogate the *narrowest orifice*.
4. Use the electronic tracing caliper of the ultrasound machine to trace the orifice and so obtain its area (Fig. 12.1).

This technique is limited by an inability to determine whether the actual minimal orifice is being imaged or whether the plane chosen for measurement is at an angle to the true minimal orifice.

The accuracy of planimetry has been assessed by comparing it with the "gold standard" reference technique used in the catheterization laboratory to calculate aortic valve area, the Gorlin equation:

$$AVA = \frac{cardiac\ output}{44.3(SEP)(HR)\sqrt{mean\ gradient}}$$

where 44.3 is an empiric correction factor. The systolic ejection period (SEP) is factored in because we are assessing flow through the valve only in systole.

Because the Gorlin equation–derived aortic valve area is *directly* dependent on the cardiac output (CO) and inversely dependent on the *square root* of the gradient, an accurate measurement of the CO is critical. Multiple beats must be averaged when thermodilution estimates of CO are used, especially if the patient is not in normal sinus rhythm. *It also follows that if the CO increases, the mean gradient must increase if the area is to remain constant.* In fact, the Gorlin equation–derived area may increase with output, and its accuracy in these situations is the subject of active debate in the catheterization community.

Although successful measurement by transthoracic echocardiographic (TTE) planimetry has been reported, transesophageal echocardiography (TEE), with its superior resolution, would be expected to be more effective in making this measurement accurately (5). Stoddard et al. (6), using a single-plane TEE probe, reported a high degree of correlation between TEE planimetric aortic valve area and aortic valve area determined by TTE and the continuity equation in both normal and impaired ventricles, and a superior correlation with aortic valve area determined by catheterization and the standard Gorlin formula. Hoffman et al. (7) showed excellent correlation of the planimetric result and the Gorlin formula–determined area. The use of multiplane rather than single-plane probes facilitates obtaining adequate studies and is more accurate than biplane techniques (8). Changes in the CO should not cause changes in a planimetric area, so that the technique should be as good in patients with a low *or* normal CO (9), and it has been suggested to be more accurate than the Gorlin equation at low or high output.

TEE is not as accurate in the presence of significant valvular calcification (10), and not all observers have reported uniformly good correlations of TEE planimetric valve areas with Gorlin formula valve areas (11). Consequently, the results of both two-dimensional and Doppler assessment should be used to assess the severity of AS reliably.

Quantitative Doppler Assessment of Aortic Stenosis

The severity of AS is assessed quantitatively with Doppler echocardiography in two ways: measuring the gradient across the valve with the modified Bernoulli equation or estimating the aortic valve area with the continuity equation (12–14). Both techniques require that the ultrasound beam be parallel to the transvalvular blood flow.

Transesophageal echocardiographic Doppler views for assessing aortic stenosis. In AS, aligning the transesophageal transducer parallel to the left ventricular outflow tract (LVOT) and aortic valve can be challenging. The deep transgastric (TG) long-axis and TG long-axis views are commonly used (15). Advancing from the TG short-axis view and anteroflexion of the probe head to visualize the heart from near the LV apex allow acquisition of the deep TG long-axis view. Counterclockwise rotation of the probe as it is advanced may facilitate this. The TG long-axis view is obtained with the probe at the midpapillary level and the imaging plane rotated to 120 to 140 degrees. Both techniques offer an excellent approach to aortic valve flow dynamics; however, the patient's anatomy will dictate which view provides the best interrogation of transvalvular blood flow.

A note of caution is necessary in a discussion of Doppler imaging and the angle of incidence. It is tempting to correct for nonparallel orientation of the Doppler beam to the flow of blood. Many echocardiographic systems provide a means to correct the angle of interrogation visually. The correction is obtained by multiplying the Doppler shift velocity by the cosine of the incident angle of the beam to the aortic flow. *It is generally accepted that this is not a reliable method to use in quantitative Doppler analysis. Because the interaction of beam and blood flow occurs in three dimensions, two-dimensional imaging is unable to determine the true angle of incidence to the jet accurately.* With turbulent jets, as in AS, judging the alignment with flow is particularly difficult (16). Such jets may be very eccentrically directed to the two-dimensional plane visualized, so that apparent "correction" by looking at a color flow map of the jet can be very imprecise. Obtaining the highest-velocity smooth envelope is a better way to confirm accuracy.

Doppler determination of the aortic valve gradient: modified Bernoulli equation. The Bernoulli equation is used to calculate transaortic valve pressure gradients (Table 12.2). The modified Bernoulli equation states that the maximal pressure gradient equals four times the square of the peak jet velocity and allows calculation of the peak instantaneous gradient across any orifice. Thus, if the peak blood flow velocity across the aortic valve is 4 m/s, the calculated peak gradient $= 4 \times 4^2 = 64$ mm Hg. The mean gradient is calculated by averaging the instantaneous gradients over time. This function is accomplished by tracing the aortic flow velocity profile and using the analysis program of the ultrasound machine (Fig. 12.2). Alternatively, the mean velocity can be estimated from the peak velocity and the mean gradient calculated as $2.4(v_{max})^2$. The mean gradient, in particular, correlates well with invasively determined gradients and is most often used in evaluating the severity of AS (16). It is imperative that a true peak velocity be obtained for this estimate to be valid. A well-defined velocity curve with a smooth envelope is generally a valid one.

Discrepancies often occur between catheterization and echocardiographic pressure gradients in AS. The peak echocardiographic gradient measures the peak *instantaneous* gradient between the LV and aorta. This is often higher than the peak-to-peak gradient (between the peak LV pressure and the generally *later* peak aortic pressure) routinely entered on cardiac catheterization reports (Fig. 12.3). Also, a rapid recovery of pressure distal to the stenosis reduces or abolishes the gradient within several centimeters of the valve orifice as the flow becomes more laminar (the phenomenon of "pressure recovery") (17). The peak gradient can be influenced by the flow volume on the ventricular side of the valve plane. Remember that the simplified Bernoulli equation ignores the impact of the LVOT blood flow velocity. *However, the Bernoulli equation must factor in the LVOT blood flow velocity when it exceeds 1.5 m/s, as commonly occurs in associated aortic insufficiency or other high-output states, to avoid overestimation of the pressure gradient* (Table 12.2). For example, if the outflow tract velocity is 1.7 m/s and the peak transvalvular velocity is 4 m/s, the actual gradient is $4 \times (4^2 - 1.7^2) = 4 \times (16 - 2.89) = 4 \times 13.1 = 52.4$ mm Hg, instead of the 64 mm Hg predicted by the simplified Bernoulli equation.

Hemodynamically significant AS is generally associated with a mean gradient of 50 mm Hg or more or a maximal velocity of 4.5 m/s or more (Table 12.1). The exception is in patients with a low ejection fraction, who may not be able to generate a high gradient. In these patients, gradients as low as 20 to 30 mm Hg may be associated with critical stenosis, and

TABLE 12.2. EQUATIONS FOR AORTIC TRANSVALVULAR GRADIENTS

Peak Gradient (Simplified Bernoulli Equation)
Peak Gradient (mm Hg) $= 4$ (Aortic Peak Velocity)^2
Mean Gradient
Mean Gradient (mm Hg) $= 4$ (Mean Velocity)^2
$= 2.4$ $(v_{max})^2$
Peak Gradient with Significant Aortic Regurgitation (Modified Bernoulli Equation)
Gradient $= 4$ [(Peak Aortic Velocity)^2 $-$ (LVOT Velocity)^2]

LVOT, left ventricular outflow tract.

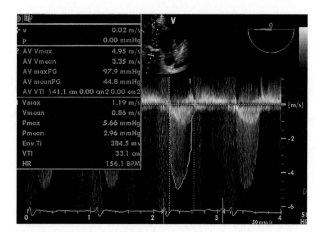

FIG. 12.2. Deep transgastric view with parallel continuous wave Doppler beam alignment in a patient with severe aortic stenosis. Aortic stenosis tracing is labeled *2 (outer envelope),* with a maximal aortic valve velocity of 4.95 m/s and a Bernoulli equation–derived peak aortic valve gradient of 97.9 mm Hg. Aortic valve time-velocity integral *(TVI)* is 141.1 cm. Tracing *1* is of the left ventricular outflow tract *(LVOT)* velocity. LVOT maximal velocity is 1.19 m/s, and LVOT TVI is 33.1 cm.

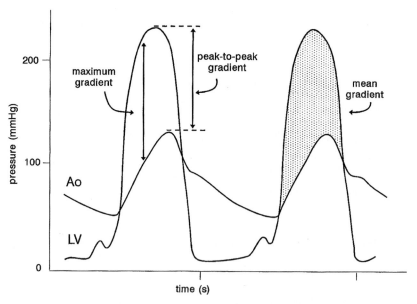

FIG. 12.3. Example of left ventricular (LV) and aortic (Ao) pressures measured with fluid-filled catheters in a patient with severe aortic stenosis. The maximal instantaneous gradient is greater than the peak-to-peak gradient. The *shaded area* indicates the mean gradient. (From Otto CM. *Textbook of clinical echocardiography,* 2nd ed. Philadelphia: WB Saunders, 2000:238, with permission.)

TABLE 12.3. CALCULATION OF AORTIC VALVE AREA WITH THE CONTINUITY EQUATION

Continuity Equation ("What goes in must come out.")
LVOT Stroke Volume = AV Stroke Volume
Stroke Volume = CSA × TVI
Therefore,
$$TVI_{LVOT} \times Area_{LVOT} = TVI_{AV} \times Area_{AV}$$
$$Area_{AV} = \frac{TVI_{LVOT} \times Area_{LVOT}}{TVI_{AV}}$$
Aortic Valve Area
LVOT Velocity (m/s, maximal)
LVOT Diameter (cm, inner to inner, mid systole)
LVOT Area (cm^2) = πr^2
AV Area (cm^2, continuity equation)

LVOT, left ventricular outflow tract; AV, aortic valve; CSA, cross-sectional area; TVI, time-velocity integral.

the continuity equation *and* planimetry should be used to exclude significant AS (see later discussion).

Doppler Estimation of the Aortic Valve Area: The Continuity Equation

The continuity equation states that the volume of blood that enters the stenotic aortic orifice is equal to the volume of blood that exits it. If we can calculate the volume of flow entering a stenotic aortic valve through the LVOT and measure the velocity at which it exits the stenotic valve, then the equation can be rearranged to solve for the area of the stenotic valve (18) (Table 12.3).

One first must calculate the cross-sectional area of the LVOT. In the ME aortic valve long-axis view (120 degrees), the LVOT annular diameter is obtained by measuring the *inner* dimension (endocardium to endocardium) of the LVOT at the insertion point of the aortic valve leaflets in mid systole with the electronic calipers (Fig. 12.4). The diameter of the LVOT is generally approximately 2.0 ± 0.2 cm and varies somewhat with body surface area. Inaccuracies in measurement of the outflow tract can account for much of the error in this technique because the radius is squared in the continuity equation. The most common discrepancies occur during the imaging of elderly women, who often have a smaller outflow tract (and body surface area) than average, and large men, who often have a larger outflow tract (and body surface area). If we assume that the LVOT is a circle, one calculates its area as πr^2.

The LVOT time-velocity integral (TVI) is then determined by either of two methods. Pulsed wave Doppler can be used, with the sample volume just proximal to the aortic valve cusps within the LVOT (Fig. 12.5). The sample volume is gradually moved toward the aortic valve until a smooth LVOT velocity profile is obtained *at the level of the outflow tract where the annular dimension was obtained*. The internal calculation package available on all echocardiographic machines traces the LVOT velocity, allowing calculation of the LVOT TVI. Pulsed wave Doppler is essential for this flow measurement because it must be made at the level at which the outflow tract was measured to calculate the stroke volume through that area. An alternative method, which is less well validated, uses continuous wave Doppler interrogation through the aortic valve. If the alignment is correct, a more intense lower-velocity inner envelope representing the lower-velocity LVOT flow is imaged within the higher-velocity aortic jet envelope and can be traced as previously described to calculate the LVOT TVI (19) (Fig. 12.2).

Finally, the aortic valve TVI is traced from the larger envelope of the continuous wave Doppler profile (Fig. 12.2). These measurements require that the Doppler probe be as close to parallel as possible to the direction of flow (usually from the deep TG long-axis view). The resulting values for the LVOT diameter, LVOT TVI, and aortic valve TVI are entered

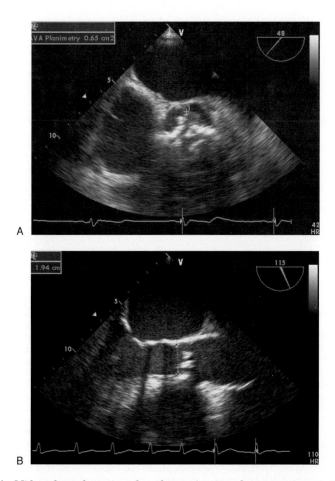

FIG. 12.4. A: Midesophageal aortic valve short-axis view demonstrating aortic stenosis and a tricuspid aortic valve with heavy calcification. Aortic valve area by planimetry is 0.65 cm^2. **B:** Midesophageal aortic valve long-axis view in mid systole with measurement of the left ventricular outflow tract (LVOT) diameter (1.94 cm). The diameter is measured from the inner surfaces (endocardium to endocardium) of the LVOT at the insertion points of the aortic cusps. The continuity equation–derived aortic valve area is 0.70 cm^2. Continuous wave Doppler values are from Figure 12.2.

into the continuity equation to solve for the aortic valve area. Some clinicians use the peak velocity instead of the TVI in these analyses, although the TVI should correlate better from a theoretic standpoint.

Technical Considerations

AS is a technically challenging valvular lesion to assess by Doppler TTE, and the limitations imposed by the angle of incidence of the Doppler beam in TEE are even more of a challenge. Often, the orientation of the jet is such that the transducer cannot be aligned parallel to it.

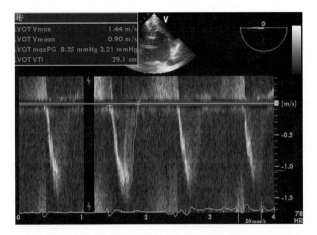

FIG. 12.5. Deep transgastric view of the aortic valve with pulsed wave Doppler assessment of the left ventricular outflow tract (LVOT) flow velocity. The LVOT time-velocity integral is assessed to be 39.1 cm. Note correlation with inner envelope technique valve area of 33.1 cm (same patient as in Fig. 12.2).

Acceptance of an inadequate jet as representative of the true jet is a significant source of error in estimating the severity of stenosis. Unless a clearly defined velocity envelope can be seen, no quantitative estimate of severity should be made.

The jet of mitral insufficiency can easily be mistaken for that of AS. Both jets have several features in common: they are negative, high-velocity jets when interrogated from the mid to low esophagus, tend to peak in mid systole, and may lie in the same path of interrogation because the Doppler beam often traverses both the anterior left atrium and the adjacent posterior aortic root. In the latter situation, anteriorly oriented mitral regurgitant (MR) jets and stenotic aortic jets can be interrogated. It is important to document visually that an MR jet is not traversed when color Doppler imaging is used. In cases in which this is difficult, it is useful to look at the time of onset of an MR jet during pulsed Doppler recording to determine the relationship of the onset of flow velocity to the electrocardiographic QRS complex for reference. MR jets start early (during isovolumic systole) because the LV pressure exceeds the LA pressure (normal, 0–12 mm Hg) almost as soon as LV contraction begins. AS jets start later in systole because flow begins when the LV pressure exceeds the central aortic diastolic pressure (60–90 mm Hg). This is generally in the mid or latter portion of the QRS complex. It may be helpful to look at the aortic valve morphology to assess whether significant obstruction is suggested by the mobility of the valve on two-dimensional imaging. It should be borne in mind, however, that in a low-output state, aortic valve motion may be decreased by reduced CO rather than by significant stenosis.

SPECIAL CONSIDERATIONS

Assessment of Low Cardiac Output: The "Dimensionless" Index

From a hemodynamic standpoint, it is critically important to understand that *the gradient across a stenosis varies with the flow across the stenosis* (20,21). The gradient will increase during exercise or in a hyperadrenergic state (e.g., in the operating room), but the valve area remains constant because it is directly proportional to the CO. This relationship is reflected in the Gorlin formula used to calculate valve areas, in which the gradient is in the denominator and the CO is in the numerator. In patients with a normal CO, significant and possibly critical stenosis usually results in a peak pressure gradient of 50 mm Hg or higher (often >100 mm Hg). However, in patients with a low CO, a peak gradient in potentially critical stenosis may be in the range of 20 to 30 mm Hg. Gradients this low with a normal CO are generally minor and not hemodynamically important. Therefore, the CO is an important determinant of the significance of a given valve gradient.

Patients with poor LV performance are unable to mount sufficient CO to produce mean and peak pressure gradients in the range of 50 mm Hg or higher. In patients with a low LV ejection fraction, the echocardiographer must use the aortic valve area and LVOT TVI / aortic valve TVI ratio calculations, which are less dependent on cardiac performance, to quantify the degree of AS (Table 12.1). When this so-called *dimensionless index* is used, a ratio of 0.25 or less generally denotes critical disease. In general, but not always, the surgical outcome of these patients is poorer than that of patients with high gradients and normal baseline function (22). In addition, the use of dobutamine has been suggested to determine whether a low gradient is caused by intrinsic myocardial disease or valvular disease. A significant increase in gradient and output with a constant valve area suggests severe valvular disease, but the significance of other changes is debated.

Assessment of Aortic Stenosis in Aortic Regurgitation

In aortic insufficiency, because of the leak in the aortic valve, the volume of blood that must be ejected from the ventricle during systole increases. The reason is that the forward stroke volume now equals the volume of blood returning from the lungs plus the volume leaking back from the aorta. The latter can exceed 50% of the forward stroke volume. This increased volume must be ejected through the LVOT, which has only a limited ability to dilate to accommodate it. Therefore, velocity in the LVOT increases because the area is relatively stenotic for the volume of blood traversing it. The increased velocity in the outflow tract is exaggerated in the aorta by the acceleration resulting from the narrowing caused by the valvular stenosis. If the LVOT velocity is 1.5 m/s or more, it must be corrected for with the modified Bernoulli equation to calculate the true valve gradient accurately. The outflow tract velocity should be sampled just below the aortic valve plane from the TEE approach.

This method for gradient determination entails several potential problems, and a full clinical and standard echocardiographic assessment of the patient should always be performed before a more aggressive diagnostic or therapeutic approach is entertained. A two-dimensional echocardiographic assessment of LV function should routinely be performed before "small" gradients are reported as insignificant, as is discussed previously.

Postoperative Subaortic Obstruction

The anterior MV leaflet and the intraventricular septum are relatively close to each other. In a small percentage of patients in whom the septum is hypertrophic as an adaptive response to AS, the septum bulges into the outflow tract and may appear to underlie most of the right coronary cusp in the ME 120-degree TEE long-axis view (mirrored in the parasternal long-axis TTE view preoperatively). The so-called sigmoid septum, seen in some older patients with or without hypertrophy, has a similar appearance (23). Valvular AS can also coexist with idiopathic hypertrophic subaortic stenosis and systolic anterior motion (SAM) of the MV (24). When the afterload imposed on the LV chamber is removed by replacement of the stenotic aortic valve, the anterior mitral leaflet is more closely juxtaposed to the septum, and SAM may develop, causing a secondary subaortic stenosis physiologically identical to that of idiopathic hypertrophic subaortic stenosis (see Fig. 3.14). The classic finding is the so-called dagger-shaped jet seen in dynamic subaortic obstruction, caused by an increase in the gradient late in systole as the MV moves closer to the septum when the ventricle becomes smaller. A similar phenomenon can occur with redundant, elongated mitral leaflets after a "floppy" MV is repaired (25,26), particularly when a circumferential annuloplasty has been performed as a part of the repair. This is less common with use of an incomplete ring. Occasionally, postoperative intracavitary gradients or midcavity obliteration occurs in ventricles that are markedly hypertrophic in response to the stenotic valve.

The result of all of these phenomena is that weaning from bypass may be difficult as a consequence of hypotension. In this situation, interrogation of the LVOT in the long-axis view demonstrates SAM of the MV. Color flow Doppler shows the mosaic appearance of high-velocity aliasing flow caused by the resultant gradient across the LVOT. Interrogation by continuous wave Doppler demonstrates a high velocity proportional to the gradient caused by the obstruction that can be quantified with the modified Bernoulli equation. *The treatment for the resultant hypotension is counterintuitive; the patient requires volume loading to increase the LV volume and the negative inotropic effect of beta blockers to decrease contractility and prolong the diastolic filling period by slowing the heart.* On rare occasions, the obstruction may be intractable, and septal myomectomy (27) or MV replacement with a low-profile prosthetic valve is required.

SUMMARY

Assessment of the stenotic aortic valve remains a challenge. Echocardiography provided valuable insights into the rate of progression by permitting serial noninvasive measurements for the first time. As is generally the case in echocardiography, the application of a variety of techniques allows a more reliable estimate of the severity of disease, particularly if the results support each other. In clinical practice, however, the integration of patient data is essential, and a good correlation of the clinical and echocardiographic findings remains essential. Accordingly, echocardiographers must be thoroughly familiar with the application of all these techniques for an optimal assessment of AS in the operating room.

REFERENCES

1. Roger VL, Tajik AJ. Progression of aortic stenosis in adults: new insights provided by Doppler echocardiography. *J Heart Valve Dis* 1993;2:114–118.
2. Rosenhek R, Binder T, Porenta G, et al. Predictors of outcome in severe, asymptomatic aortic stenosis. *N Engl J Med* 2000;343:611–617.
3. Godley RW, Green D, Dillion JC, et al. Reliability of two-dimensional echocardiography in assessing the severity of valvular aortic stenosis. *Chest* 1981;79:657–662.
4. Chin ML, Bernstein RF, Child JS, et al. Aortic valve systolic flutter as a screening test for severe aortic stenosis. *Am J Cardiol* 1983;51:981–985.
5. Okura H, Yoshida K, Hozumi T, et al. Planimetry and transthoracic two-dimensional echocardiography in noninvasive assessment of aortic valve area in patients with valvular aortic stenosis. *J Am Coll Cardiol* 1997;30:753–759.
6. Stoddard MF, Arce J, Liddell NE, et al. Two-dimensional transesophageal echocardiographic determination of aortic valve area in adults with aortic stenosis. *Am Heart J* 1991;122:1415–1422.
7. Hoffmann R, Flachskampf FA, Hanrath P. Planimetry of orifice area in aortic stenosis using multiplane transesophageal echocardiography. *J Am Coll Cardiol* 1993;22:529–534.
8. Kim KS, Maxted W, Nanda NC, et al. Comparison of multiplane and biplane transesophageal echocardiography in the assessment of aortic stenosis. *Am J Cardiol* 1997;79:436–441.
9. Tardif JC, Miller DS, Pandian NG, et al. Effects of variations in flow on aortic valve area in aortic stenosis based on in vivo planimetry of aortic valve area by multiplane transesophageal echocardiography. *Am J Cardiol* 1995;76:193–198.
10. De la Fuente Galan L, San Roman Calvar JA, Munoz San Jose JC, et al. Influence of the degree of aortic valve calcification on the estimate of valvular area using planimetry with transesophageal echocardiography [in Spanish]. *Rev Esp Cardiol* 1996;49:663–668.
11. Bernard Y, Meneveau N, Vuillemenot A, et al. Planimetry of aortic valve area using multiplane transoesophageal echocardiography is not a reliable method for assessing severity of aortic stenosis. *Heart* 1997;78:68–73.
12. Owen AN, Simon P, Moidl R, et al. Measurement of aortic flow velocity during transesophageal echocardiography in the transgastric five-chamber view. *J Am Soc Echocardiogr* 1995;8:874–878.

13. Skjaerpe T, Hegrenaes L, Hatle L. Noninvasive estimation of valve area in patients with aortic stenosis by Doppler ultrasound and two-dimensional echocardiography. *Circulation* 1985;72:810–818.
14. Hatle L, Angelsen BA, Tromsdal A. Non-invasive assessment of aortic stenosis by Doppler ultrasound. *Br Heart J* 1980;43:284–292.
15. Harris SN, Luther MA, Perrino AC. Multiplane transesophageal echocardiography acquisition of ascending aortic flow velocities: a comparison with established techniques. *J Am Soc Echocardiogr* 1999,12:754–760.
16. Cooper J, Pinheiro L, Fan P, et al. A practical approach to cardiovascular Doppler ultrasound. In: Nanda V, ed. *Doppler echocardiography*. Baltimore: Williams & Wilkins, 1993: 59–68.
17. Laskey WK, Kussmaul WG. Pressure recovery in aortic valve stenosis. *Circulation* 1994;89:116–121.
18. Richards KL. Assessment of aortic and pulmonic stenosis by echocardiography. *Circulation* 1991;84:I182–I187.
19. Maslow AD, Mashikian J, Haering JM, et al. TEE evaluation of native aortic valve area: utility of the double envelope technique. *J Cardiothorac Vasc Anesth* 2001;15:293–299.
20. Burwash IG, Pearlman AS, Kraft CD, et al. Flow dependence of measures of aortic stenosis severity during exercise. *J Am Coll Cardiol* 1994;24:1342–1350.
21. Burwash IG, Thomas DD, Sadahiro M, et al. Dependence of Gorlin formula and continuity equation valve areas on transvalvular volume flow rate in valvular aortic stenosis. *Circulation* 1994;89:827–835.
22. Brogan WC 3rd, Grayburn PA, Lange RA, et al. Prognosis after valve replacement in patients with severe aortic stenosis and a low transvalvular pressure gradient. *J Am Coll Cardiol* 1993;21:1657–1660.
23. Maron BJ, Gottdiener JS, Roberts WC, et al. Nongenetically transmitted disproportionate ventricular septal thickening associated with left ventricular outflow obstruction. *Br Heart J* 1979;41:345–349.
24. Chung KJ, Manning JA, Gramiak R. Echocardiography in coexisting hypertrophic subaortic stenosis and fixed left ventricular outflow obstruction. *Circulation* 1974; 49:673–677.
25. Kronzon I, Cohen ML, Winer HE, et al. Left ventricular outflow obstruction: a complication of mitral valvuloplasty. *J Am Coll Cardiol* 1984;4:825–828.
26. Mihaileanu S, Marino JP, Chauvaud S, et al. Left ventricular outflow obstruction after mitral valve repair (Carpentier's technique). Proposed mechanisms of disease. *Circulation* 1988;78:I78–I84.
27. Turina M. Asymmetric septal hypertrophy should be resected during aortic valve replacement. *Z Kardiol* 1986;75:198–200.

QUESTIONS

1. Use of the Gorlin equation in the catheterization suite has all of the following limitations **except**
   a. In patients with aortic insufficiency, the aortic valve area may be falsely elevated.
   b. The CO of multiple beats must be averaged for patients in atrial fibrillation.
   c. The peak-to-peak gradient is required.
   d. The systolic ejection period must be calculated.
2. The following statements regarding the usefulness of planimetry in the evaluation of AS are true **except**
   a. The ME aortic valve short-axis view is preferred.
   b. The results of planimetry correlate extremely well with catheterization-derived determinations of the aortic valve area.
   c. An adequate planimetry-derived determination of the aortic valve area depends on an adequate CO.
   d. Significant valvular calcification decreases the accuracy of planimetry-derived determinations of area.

3. All of the following statements regarding continuous wave Doppler evaluation of the aortic valve are true **except**
   a. The preferred view is the deep TG long-axis view because of the parallel alignment of the Doppler beam with flow.
   b. The deep TG long-axis view offers a correlation of more than 0.9 with TTE-derived aortic valve flow velocities.
   c. If a mitral prosthetic valve is present, the TG long-axis view at 120 degrees can be used to obtain aortic valve flow velocities.
   d. Accurate flow velocities can be obtained with the ME views by electronically steering (angle correction) the resulting signal.
4. A patient is determined to have the following Doppler parameters: LVOT velocity, 1.7 m/s; aortic valve velocity, 4.6 m/s. The pressure gradient across the aortic valve is
   a. 84.64 mm Hg
   b. 73.00 mm Hg
   c. 33.64 mm Hg
   d. 11.56 mm Hg
5. In regard to pressure gradients in the LV and aortic valve, the following is/are true:
   a. The Doppler-derived maximal instantaneous gradient approximates the catheterization-derived maximal instantaneous gradient.
   b. The peak-to-peak gradient is usually the highest gradient recorded.
   c. The Doppler-derived maximal instantaneous gradient is comparable with the peak-to-peak catheterization gradient.
   d. All of the above.
6. A patient has an LV ejection fraction of 10%. Which measurements are preferred in determining the severity of the AS?
   a. Peak aortic valve flow velocity
   b. Aortic valve mean gradient
   c. Planimetric aortic valve area
   d. LVOT TVI/aortic valve TVI ratio
   e. **a** and **b**
   f. **c** and **d**
   g. All of the above
7. When the continuity equation is used, which of the following statements regarding measurement of the LVOT diameter is true?
   a. The diameter is measured 1 cm proximal to the aortic valve.
   b. The diameter is measured at the insertion point of the aortic valve leaflets.
   c. The diameter is measured at the leaflet tips.
   d. The chance of introducing error into this measurement is small.
8. A patient is found to have aortic sclerosis. What maneuvers will increase the gradient across the aortic valve?
   a. Exercise
   b. Aortic insufficiency
   c. Acute myocardial ischemia
   d. **a** and **b**
   e. All of the above
9. All of the following statements regarding SAM of the MV are true **except**
   a. It commonly occurs following a noncircumferential ring annuloplasty.
   b. It occurs in patients with redundant anterior MV leaflets.
   c. The pathophysiology is similar to that of idiopathic hypertrophic subaortic stenosis.
   d. It can develop after aortic valve replacement because of changes in LV geometry.
10. Treatment for SAM can include which of the following
   a. MV replacement
   b. Volume expansion
   c. Reduction in inotropes
   d. All of the above

13

Prosthetic Valves

Albert T. Cheung

The first successful artificial heart valves were implanted in 1960. Starr implanted a Starr-Edwards caged-ball valve in a patient with rheumatic mitral stenosis, and Harken implanted the Harken caged-ball prosthesis in the subcoronary aortic position in a patient with rheumatic aortic stenosis and regurgitation. During the next 30 years, prosthetic valves of various designs made by different manufacturers became available for clinical use. As a consequence of these developments, a large number of patients have many different kinds of prosthetic valves. This effort is ongoing, and new types of prosthetic valves are continually being developed and are in various stages of clinical testing.

ROLE OF TRANSESOPHAGEAL ECHOCARDIOGRAPHY IN THE EVALUATION OF PROSTHETIC CARDIAC VALVES

Multiplane transesophageal echocardiography (TEE) is considered the diagnostic technique of choice for identifying the type of prosthesis, assessing its function, and diagnosing dysfunction (1–5). With the combination of two-dimensional imaging, color flow and spectral Doppler, the ability of TEE to integrate structural information and hemodynamic function is unparalleled. However, the evaluation of prosthetic heart valves poses special problems because mechanical valves and the components of bioprosthetic valves have poor acoustic properties, so that it is difficult to image valves and surrounding soft tissues in detail with ultrasound. In addition, the small size of the valves and their mechanical components makes detailed examination of the motion of the stent and occluder mechanisms difficult.

Typically, the imaging resolution that can be achieved with transthoracic echocardiography does not permit a detailed assessment of prosthetic valve function. The increased imaging resolution provided by TEE is a major advantage in determining the cause of prosthetic valve dysfunction. The clinical role of TEE includes evaluation of the native valve before valve replacement, evaluation of prosthetic valve function immediately after implantation, and the diagnosis of prosthetic valve dysfunction (Table 13.1).

High-resolution two-dimensional imaging can distinguish between normal and abnormal motion of the valve leaflets and occluder mechanisms. Abnormal motion of the valve stent or dehiscence of the prosthetic valve annulus can be also detected. In addition, vegetations, calcifications, pannus, and thrombus on the prosthetic valve can be identified by two-dimensional imaging.

Color Doppler flow imaging can distinguish normal closure and leakage regurgitant jets from pathologic transvalvular or paravalvular regurgitant jets. Quantification of blood flow velocity with spectral Doppler techniques often permits an estimation of transvalvular pressure gradients and the effective orifice area of a prosthetic valve (6–8).

TECHNICAL CONSIDERATIONS IN THE TRANSESOPHAGEAL ECHOCARDIOGRAPHIC EXAMINATION OF PATIENTS WITH PROSTHETIC VALVES

Many of the approaches used to evaluate native valve function can be applied to the evaluation of prosthetic heart valves, but certain special considerations are necessary. The metallic and polymeric components of mechanical and biologic valves do not transmit ultrasound. These material components produce highly specular echoes, and the images of distal structures are impaired by shadowing. Decreasing the transmit gain helps to minimize imaging artifacts and resolve detail in the vicinity of nonbiologic materials. To compensate for ultrasound shadowing, it is necessary to select multiple imaging planes from both above and below the prosthetic valve. For example, the midesophageal (ME) aortic valve long-axis imaging

TABLE 13.1. CLINICAL ROLE OF TRANSESOPHAGEAL ECHOCARDIOGRAPHY IN ASSESSING PROSTHETIC HEART VALVES

TEE evaluation before valve replacement
1. Verify disease of native valve.
2. Assess the extent of annular calcification.
3. Estimate the annular diameter of the native valve. In aortic valve disease, a small annulus may dictate the type of valve to be implanted.
4. Evaluate the feasibility of valve repair. Because of the limitations of prosthetic valves, it is almost always preferable to repair a valve rather than replace it.

TEE evaluation immediately after valve replacement
1. Verify that all leaflets or occluders move normally.
2. Verify the absence of paravalvular regurgitation.
3. Verify that no air remains in the cardiac chambers.
4. Verify that there is no left ventricular outflow tract obstruction by struts or subvalvular apparatus.

TEE diagnosis of prosthetic valve dysfunction
1. Identification of prosthetic valve type.
2. Detection and quantification of transvalvular or paravalvular regurgitation.
3. Detection of annular dehiscence.
4. Detection of vegetations consistent with endocarditis.
5. Detection of thrombosis or pannus formation on the valve.
6. Detection and quantification of valve stenosis.
7. Detection of tissue degeneration or calcification.

plane will not reliably display the motion of a mechanical aortic prosthesis because of shadowing from the valve sewing ring. If the probe is advanced to the transgastric (TG) position, prosthetic aortic leaflet motion can be observed without interference from the sewing ring. Similarly, imaging the ventricular side of a mitral prosthetic valve may require TG midventricular or deep TG long-axis imaging planes.

Doppler echocardiography can be used to estimate the transvalvular pressure gradient across bileaflet, tilting-disc, and biologic valves that have a centrally directed, linear transvalvular flow. In contrast, for caged-ball or caged-disc valves, in which the occluder alters the direction of blood flow through the valve, the Bernoulli equation does not accurately estimate the transvalvular pressure gradient.

ECHOCARDIOGRAPHIC CHARACTERISTICS OF THE VARIOUS TYPES OF PROSTHETIC CARDIAC VALVES

Each type of prosthetic valve has distinct echocardiographic features and hemodynamic characteristics. The type of prosthetic valve is determined by the shape and motion of the structural components. By providing comparisons with the manufacturer's specifications for the normal range of motion of the valve components, Doppler assessment of the average transvalvular pressure gradient and average effective orifice area verifies normal functioning of the prosthesis. In general, prosthetic valves are classified as mechanical or biologic (Table 13.2).

Mechanical Heart Valves

Mechanical heart valves are more durable than biologic valves but are thrombogenic, so that the patient requires systemic anticoagulation. For this reason, mechanical valves are typically preferred for younger patients. The Silastic, metal, and pyrolytic carbon components of mechanical valves are poor conductors of ultrasound and cause acoustic shadowing, reverberations, and strong specular signals.

TABLE 13.2. PROSTHETIC VALVE TYPES

Valve	Description
Bioprosthetic	
Allograft	Indistinguishable from the native valve, used only in the aortic position (Cryolife aortic allograft).
Porcine bioprostheses	Porcine aortic valve on polypropylene mount with three support struts (e. g., Hancock, Carpentier-Edwards, St. Jude BioImplant.)
Bovine pericardial	Trileaflet valve fashioned from bovine pericardium in Dacron-covered support frame with three struts (e. g., Ionescu-Shiley, Carpentier-Edwards Pericardial, Sorin Pericarbon, Mitroflow).
Stentless	Reinforced porcine aortic root (Medtronic Freestyle, Toronto Stentless Porcine Valve).
Mechanical	**Description**
Ball-in-cage	Circular sewing ring with two U-shaped arches containing a Silastic ball (e. g., Starr-Edwards, Harken, Braunwald-Cutter).
Caged-disc	Circular sewing ring with short cage containing a lightweight Silastic centrally occluding disc (e. g., Beall, Kay-Shiley, Kay-Suzuki, Starr-Edwards model 6520).
Tilting-disc	Eccentrically hinged single tilting disc in circular ring opening to form two orifices (e. g., Bjork-Shiley, Medtronic Hall, Sorin Allcarbon monoleaflet, Lillehei-Kastor, Omniscience, Wada-Cutter).
Bileaflet	Two semicircular hinged leaflets in a circular ring opening almost perpendicularly to form three orifices (e. g., St. Jude, Carbomedics, Edwards MIRA, Sorin Bicarbon, ATS).

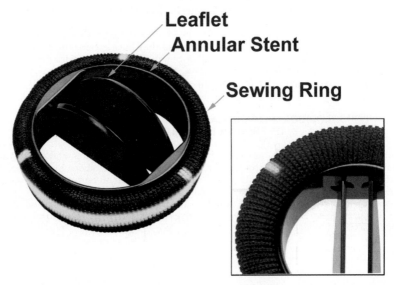

Leaflet

Annular Stent

Sewing Ring

FIG. 13.1. Carbomedic R-series mechanical bileaflet prosthetic aortic valve. The valve consists of two semicircular pyrolytic carbon leaflets supported within a pyrolytic carbon annular stent surrounded by the sewing ring. The *insert* shows a close-up view of the hinge points of the leaflets. The valve is designed to permit a small amount of leakage backflow at the hinge points.

Bileaflet Valves (St. Jude, Carbomedic)

The bileaflet mechanical valve prostheses are the most commonly implanted mechanical valves because of their outstanding record of durability and large valve orifice area in relation to stent diameter. They can be implanted in the aortic, mitral, or tricuspid position. The valves are constructed of two semicircular leaflets suspended from four hinge points in a circular annulus surrounded by a sewing ring (Fig. 13.1). When the leaflets open, three separate orifices are formed within the valve annulus.

A systematic TEE examination of the prosthetic valve includes verification of normal leaflet motion, proper seating of the prosthesis within the native valve annulus, and normal blood flow pattern through the valve. In addition, the TEE examination should verify the absence of paravalvular regurgitation and abnormal transvalvular regurgitation. Finally, TEE can estimate the transvalvular pressure gradient or calculate the effective orifice area of the valve.

Recommended examination sequence

1. *Confirm leaflet motion.* Two-dimensional imaging confirms the opening and closure of the two mechanical leaflets. In the short-axis imaging plane, the two leaflets in the open position produce two linear shadows within a circular annulus. For valves implanted in the mitral position, leaflet motion is best examined in the ME long-axis views (Fig. 13.2; see Color Plate 21 following page 212). Multiplane rotation through the valve to generate a cross-sectional imaging plane that is perpendicular to the two leaflets permits

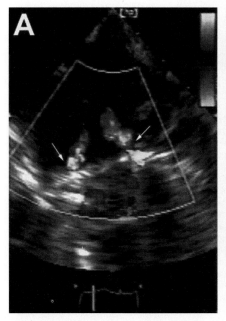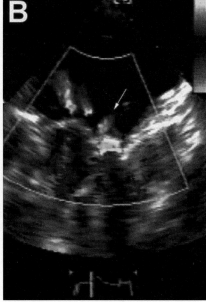

FIG. 13.2. Bileaflet mechanical prosthesis, mitral position. Color Doppler flow transesophageal echocardiographic midesophageal mitral valve commissural view at a multiplane angle of 60 degrees (**A**) and long-axis view at a multiplane angle of 150 degrees (**B**) show the normal appearance of leakage regurgitant jets that are characteristic of bileaflet valves. **A:** Individual leakage jets originate from the hinge points of the leaflets (*arrows*) and are directed toward the center of the valve. **B:** A third normal leakage regurgitant jet (*arrow*) can be visualized originating at the point of contact between the leaflet and the valve stent. (See Color Plate 21 following page 212.)

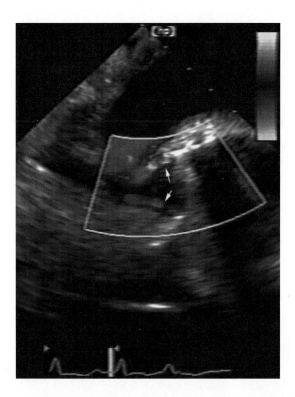

FIG. 13.3. Bileaflet mechanical prosthesis in the aortic position. Transesophageal echocardiographic midesophageal aortic valve long-axis view at a multiplane angle of 135 degrees in a patient with a bileaflet mechanical prosthesis in the aortic position. Color Doppler flow imaging in diastole shows the normal appearance of the two leakage regurgitant jets that originate at the leaflet hinge points (arrows). Note that ultrasound shadowing caused by the valve stent makes it difficult to assess the motion of the leaflets from this imaging angle. The transgastric long-axis or the deep transgastric long-axis view through the aortic valve (not shown) is necessary to evaluate the motion of the individual leaflets. (See Color Plate 22 following page 212.)

the motion of both leaflets to be observed simultaneously (Fig. 13.2B; see Color Plate 21 following page 212). The two leaflets tilt open symmetrically to an angle of 85 to 90 degrees and close at an angle of 30 degrees in relation to the plane of the annulus. Leaflet motion of a valve implanted in the aortic position is more difficult to evaluate (Fig. 13.3; see Color Plate 22 following page 212). Acoustic shadowing from the sewing ring and leaflets typically obscures leaflet motion in the ME aortic valve long-axis view. Individual leaflet motion is better visualized in the TG long-axis and deep TG long-axis views, which provide unobstructed views of the aortic valve in the far field through the left ventricle and left ventricular outflow tract (LVOT).

2. *Confirm proper valve seating.* Incomplete fixation of the prosthetic sewing ring to the native annulus or dehiscence of the sewing ring will cause paravalvular regurgitation. Paravalvular regurgitation is defined as regurgitation originating outside the prosthetic valve annulus or sewing ring. The most common cause of incomplete fixation immediately after prosthetic implantation is a severely calcified native valve annulus. Prosthetic endocarditis is the most common cause of late valve dehiscence and can produce a "rocking" motion of the entire valve apparatus on two-dimensional imaging. Proper seating of the prosthetic valve, paravalvular regurgitation, and dehiscence are best identified from the multiplane long-axis images of the valve.

3. *Confirm normal blood flow patterns and the absence of pathologic transvalvular and paravalvular regurgitation.* Color flow Doppler imaging will demonstrate central antegrade flow through the valve annulus when the leaflets open and small characteristic regurgitant jets during leaflet closure. A small amount of regurgitation is normal for bileaflet prosthetic valves and is caused by closure backflow and leakage backflow. Closure backflow is the reversal of flow required for closure of the leaflets. Leakage backflow occurs after the closure of mechanical valves, originates from the four hinge points of the leaflets, and produces four centrally directed regurgitant jets (Figs. 13.2 and 13.3; see Color Plates 21 and 22 following page 212). The leakage backflow jets originating from the hinge points are best visualized in the long-axis

image through the prosthetic valve at a multiplane angle aligned parallel to the leaflets (Fig. 13.2A; see Color Plate 21 following page 212). The bileaflet valves are designed to permit a small amount of regurgitation at the hinge points to prevent the formation of thrombus within the hinge mechanism. These small regurgitant jets are often referred to as *cleansing jets*. Sometimes, small leakage backflow jets originating along the edge of the leaflet where it meets the annulus during closure can also be imaged by color Doppler (Fig. 13.2B; see Color Plate 21 following page 212). Normal physiologic regurgitant jets are small and short in duration and can be distinguished from pathologic transvalvular regurgitation based on their size, location, and duration.

Pathologic regurgitation in which a jet originates within the sewing ring is called *transvalvular regurgitation*. Pathologic transvalvular regurgitation immediately after valve implantation indicates malfunctioning of the valve leaflets. Intraoperative causes of leaflet malfunction include retained tissue that prevents valve closure, a misplaced suture that interferes with leaflet motion, and debris within the hinges that traps the leaflet in a fixed position. Regurgitant jets originating outside the sewing ring are always pathologic; this situation is referred to as *paravalvular regurgitation*.

4. *Calculate valve gradient and effective orifice area.* Continuous wave Doppler and the simplified Bernoulli equation are used to quantify the hemodynamic performance of a prosthetic valve (see Fig. 13.12). Even though bileaflet valves when open form three separate orifices with slightly different flow characteristics through the central orifice, Bernoulli calculations of the peak and mean transvalvular pressure gradients are accurate. Additionally, the effective valve orifice area can be determined with the continuity equation (Table 13.3; see Fig. 13.13). Doppler verification that the transvalvular gradient and effective orifice area are appropriate for the valve size is particularly important for valves implanted in the aortic position, where it is difficult to verify normal leaflet motion with two-dimensional imaging.

Caged-Ball Valves (Starr-Edwards and Harken)

Caged-ball valves were the first prosthetic valves implanted in humans. They consist of a Silastic or metal ball occluder housed in a wire cage with three or four struts. The ball occluder casts a large acoustic shadow, and its motion within the cage is best imaged in the long-axis plane of the valve (Fig. 13.4A; see Color Plate 23 following page 212). In the short-axis imaging plane, the ball occluder can be imaged within the wire struts. Doppler color flow imaging in the short-axis plane of the valve demonstrates blood flow between the wire struts through the outside perimeter of the ball occluder (Fig. 13.4B; see Color Plate 23 following page 212).

Caged-Disc Valves (Beall and Kay-Shiley)

Caged-disc valves consist of a disc occluder housed within a wire cage. Motion of the disc occluder up and down within the wire cage is best imaged in the long-axis plane. Doppler color flow imaging should demonstrate flow through the central orifice in the plane of the stent, then out the side of the wire cage between the stent and the disc occluder. The multidirectional blood flow through the valve precludes reliable Doppler estimates of the valve orifice area and transvalvular gradient.

TABLE 13.3. DETERMINING THE EFFECTIVE ORIFICE AREA OF PROSTHETIC AORTIC VALVES

$$EOA = LVOT_{area}(TVI_{transvalvular}/TVI_{LVOT})$$

Where
EOA = effective orifice area of prosthetic valve
$LVOT_{area}$ = cross-sectional area of left ventricular outflow tract
= π(diameter of LVOT/2)^2
$TVI_{transvalvular}$ = time-velocity integral of blood flow across prosthetic aortic valve
TVI_{LVOT} = time-velocity integral of blood flow across LVOT

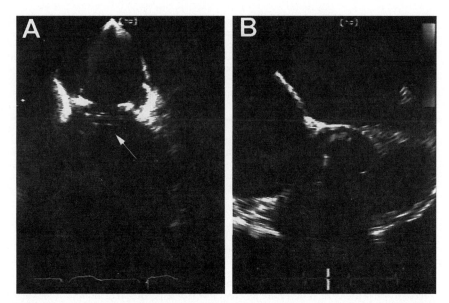

FIG. 13.4. Starr-Edwards caged-ball mechanical valve. **A:** Transesophageal echocardiographic midesophageal four-chamber view of a caged-ball valve prosthesis in the mitral position at end-diastole. The Silastic ball occluder (*arrow*) contained within the wire cage causes ultrasound shadowing and makes it difficult to image the distal side of the valve. **B:** Transesophageal echocardiographic midesophageal aortic valve short-axis view during systole in a patient with a caged-ball valve in the aortic position. Note the three metal struts of the cage. Color Doppler flow imaging demonstrates blood flow through the valve at the perimeter of the Silastic ball occluder. Again, the Silastic ball occluder causes ultrasound shadowing that obscures both two-dimensional and color flow Doppler views of the distal valve. (See Color Plate 23 following page 212.)

Tilting-Disc Valves (Bjork-Shiley and Medtronic Hall)

Tilting-disc valves are used in the aortic or mitral position. They consist of a disc occluder supported by struts. The single disc occluder pivots open 60 to 80 degrees to form two orifices of different size and shape. They have a low profile and offer the advantage of providing a large orifice size in relation to the stent size.

Recommended examination sequence

1. *Confirm proper tilting action* of the occluder in the long-axis imaging plane.
2. *Confirm that the disc occluder properly tilts open and closed* in the short-axis imaging plane by observing one edge of the disc occluder moving in and out of the imaging plane.
3. *Doppler color flow* images showing small leakage backflow jets at the hinge point of the disc occluder or along the site of contact between the disc and the stent are normal findings.
4. *Abnormal findings.* Strut fracture is a serious complication that can cause occluder malfunction and even disc embolization. Other complications, such as thrombus or pannus formation on the valve, can impair occluder motion, resulting in stenosis or transvalvular regurgitation (Fig. 13.5).

Biologic or Tissue Valves

Biologic valves do not require systemic anticoagulation, but their effective life span is only 12 to 15 years. They are typically reserved for elderly patients or patients who cannot tolerate

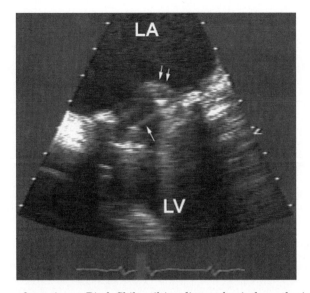

FIG. 13.5. Pannus formation on Bjork-Shiley tilting-disc mechanical prosthesis in the mitral position. Transesophageal echocardiographic midesophageal four-chamber view during systole in a patient with a tilting-disc mechanical prosthesis in the mitral position. The single disc occluder (*single arrow*) fails to close completely during systole and open completely during diastole (not shown). Pannus formation on the valve (*double arrows*) limits the motion of the disc occluder, causing both prosthetic mitral stenosis and transvalvular mitral regurgitation.

anticoagulation. The effective orifice area of a stented biologic valve is slightly less than that of a bileaflet mechanical valve of the same annular diameter. The biologic components have favorable acoustic properties and permit imaging by ultrasound. In general, the same principles used to examine native cardiac valves can be applied to the TEE examination of biologic valve prostheses.

Stented Porcine Heterografts (Carpentier-Edwards and Hancock)

Stented porcine heterografts are constructed from a glutaraldehyde-preserved porcine aortic xenograft mounted on a cloth-covered wire frame with an attached sewing ring (Fig. 13.6). They can be implanted in the aortic, mitral, or tricuspid position. In the short axis, the three leaflets supported by struts open to form a central orifice in the shape of a bulging triangle. In the long axis, the valve leaflets separate symmetrically when open and coapt at the center of the valve when closed. The struts that support the leaflets extend from the base of the annulus and point toward the downstream side of the valve. Doppler color flow imaging can sometimes detect a small closure or leakage backflow jet originating from the central coaptation point.

Stented Bovine Pericardial Valves

Stented bovine pericardial valves are constructed from bovine pericardium fashioned into three leaflets supported by a wire frame with three struts attached to a sewing ring (Fig. 13.7). Previously, the bovine pericardial valves were approved only for implantation

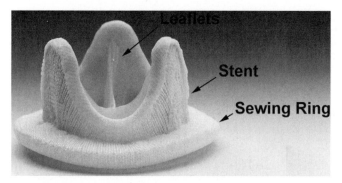

FIG. 13.6. Carpentier-Edwards model 6625 porcine bioprosthetic mitral valve. The valve is constructed from a porcine aortic xenograft mounted on a wire stent surrounded by a sewing ring.

in the aortic position, but they have been recently approved for use in the mitral position. The pericardial bioprosthetic valves have a lower profile than the stented porcine bioprosthetic valves, but the echocardiographic appearance of these valves is very similar to that of a stented porcine aortic heterograft. The pericardial bioprosthesis when implanted in the mitral position sometimes exhibits mild central transvalvular regurgitation immediately after implantation that diminishes over time.

Stentless Valves

Stentless bioprosthetic valves are fabric-reinforced, glutaraldehyde-preserved porcine aortic heterografts constructed without the wire frame, stents, and sewing ring. They are designed

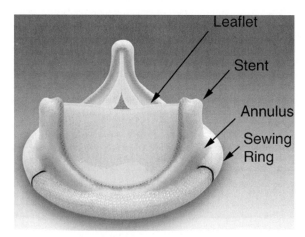

FIG. 13.7. Carpentier-Edwards model 6900 bovine pericardial bioprosthetic mitral valve. The valve leaflets are constructed from bovine pericardium mounted on a wire stent surrounded by a sewing ring.

for use in the aortic position or for replacement of the aortic root. Elimination of the stent and sewing ring increases the effective orifice area that can be achieved after valve replacement, so that these valves are particularly useful in patients with a native aortic valve annulus less than 20 mm in diameter. Elimination of the stent also permits greater freedom of movement of the valve leaflets and annulus and may increase the longevity of the valve. However, the competency of the stentless aortic valve is contingent on the geometry of the aortic root. Mismatching of the annular size, malalignment of the leaflets in the annular plane, or dilation of the aortic root will alter leaflet coaptation and cause regurgitation. For this reason, it is important for the intraoperative echocardiographic examination to size the native annulus accurately and verify that the ascending aorta is not dilated and that the diameter of the sinotubular junction matches or is within 10% of the diameter of the stentless valve (9) (Fig. 13.8). The echocardiographic appearance of the stentless valve is virtually indistinguishable from that of the native aortic valve. Implantation of the stentless valve within the native aortic root increases the thickness of the vessel wall at the region of overlap and makes paravalvular regurgitation possible. Trace or mild central aortic regurgitation is detectable up to 25% of the time immediately after implantation of the stentless bioprosthetic valve.

Allograft Valves

Cryopreserved human aortic root allografts are commercially available for implantation. They are sized according to the aortic valve annulus diameter in a range of 20 to 26 mm. Absence of a stent requires that the annular size of the allograft match the size of the native valve annulus to ensure valve competence. Implantation of an undersized allograft in patients with a native aortic valve annulus diameter larger than 27 mm may result in aortic regurgitation. Allograft aortic root replacement is commonly performed for endocarditis with aortic root abscess. The echocardiographic appearance of the aortic allograft is indistinguishable from that of the native aortic valve and aortic root.

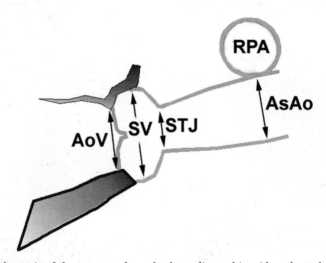

FIG. 13.8. Schematic of the transesophageal echocardiographic midesophageal aortic valve long-axis imaging plane demonstrating the anatomic landmarks used to measure the diameter of the native aortic valve annulus (*AoV*), sinus of Valsalva (*SV*), sinotubular junction (*STJ*), and ascending aorta (*AsAo*) at the level of the right pulmonary artery (*RPA*).

PROSTHETIC VALVE DYSFUNCTION: CLINICAL CAVEATS FOR ECHOCARDIOGRAPHIC DIAGNOSIS

Prosthetic valve dysfunction can result in regurgitation, stenosis, or hemolysis. TEE is recognized as the diagnostic examination of choice for the diagnosis and evaluation of suspected prosthetic valve dysfunction.

Prosthetic Valve Regurgitation

When the Doppler examination reveals regurgitation in a prosthetic valve, it is important to distinguish physiologic from pathologic regurgitation.

Normal backflow patterns. A small amount of regurgitation is normally observed in all mechanical prosthetic valves and in approximately 10% of bioprosthetic valves. **Closure backflow** is the reversal of flow required for closure of the valve. In contrast, **leakage backflow** occurs after closure of mechanical valves and originates from the hinges and the regions of coaptation between the occluders and the valve ring (Figs. 13.2 and 13.3; see Color Plates 21 and 22 following page 212). Physiologic regurgitation jets are small and short in duration. The leakage backflow patterns for each valve type are unique and distinct from pathologic regurgitation.

Pathologic transvalvular regurgitation. In bioprosthetic valves, pathologic transvalvular regurgitation is commonly associated with chronic degenerative changes, including leaflet calcification, perforation, tears, and prolapse (Fig. 13.9; see Color Plate 24 following page 212), and with leaflet destruction caused by endocarditis. In mechanical prosthetic valves,

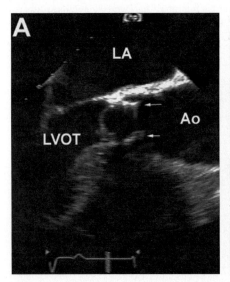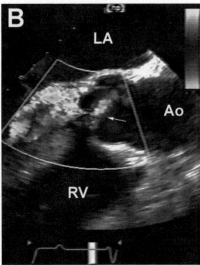

FIG. 13.9. Transvalvular regurgitation, porcine bioprosthetic valve in the aortic position. Transesophageal echocardiographic midesophageal aortic valve long-axis image at a multiplane angle of 150 degrees in a patient with a porcine bioprosthetic valve in the aortic position. Two-dimensional imaging (**A**) in diastole shows the valve struts (*arrows*) that support the leaflets. The leaflets prolapse into the left ventricular outflow tract. Color Doppler flow imaging during diastole (**B**) shows the aortic regurgitant jet (*arrow*) originating between the valve struts, indicating transvalvular regurgitation caused by structural degeneration of the bioprosthetic valve. (See Color Plate 24 following page 212.)

pathologic transvalvular regurgitation develops when the formation of pannus, thrombus, vegetations or the presence of foreign material on valve components prevents complete closure of the occluder. Two-dimensional imaging of leaflet or occluder motion in mechanical valves is useful for detecting transvalvular regurgitation caused by pannus, thrombus, or vegetations impinging on the occluder. Systems to grade the degree of valvular regurgitation (e.g., Doppler measurements of regurgitant fraction, regurgitant jet area, jet length, and vena contracta or jet width) also apply in assessing the clinical severity of prosthetic valve regurgitation.

Paravalvular regurgitation. Paravalvular regurgitation is caused by incomplete fixation of the prosthetic sewing ring to the native annulus or dehiscence of the sewing ring. Incomplete fixation is typically a consequence of native annular calcification, which increases the difficulty of prosthetic implantation. Dehiscence is often associated with endocarditis. Paravalvular regurgitant jets imaged with color Doppler flow originate outside the sewing ring, characteristically track along the walls of the receiving chamber, and usually produce zones of flow acceleration adjacent to the site of regurgitation in the chamber proximal to the prosthetic valve (Fig. 13.10; see Color Plate 25 following page 212). Dehiscence of part of the sewing ring may destabilize the prosthetic valve, producing a "rocking" motion of the entire prosthesis and a visible separation of the native and prosthetic valve annulus on two-dimensional imaging (Fig. 13.11).

Prosthetic Valve Stenosis

Compared with the native valve, all prosthetic valves are mildly stenotic, depending on the valve type and size and on the hemodynamic condition of the patient. The mean pressure gradient across prosthetic valves calculated with the simplified Bernoulli equation depends on the prosthetic valve type, position, and size. For this reason, the manufacturer's package insert, which lists the hemodynamic specifications for the particular valve type according

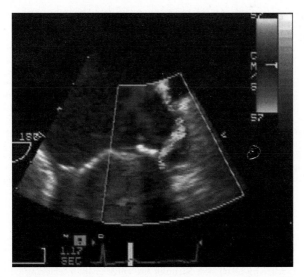

FIG. 13.10. Paravalvular regurgitation. Transesophageal echocardiographic midesophageal view at a multiplane angle of 22 degrees of a mechanical bileaflet prosthesis in the mitral position demonstrates an eccentric paravalvular regurgitant jet originating outside the prosthetic annulus. (See Color Plate 25 following page 212.)

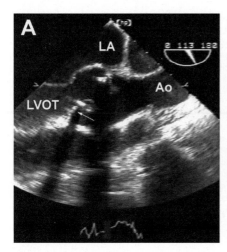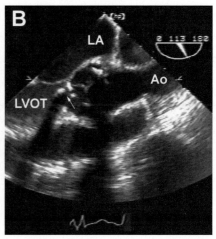

FIG. 13.11. Dehiscence, bovine pericardial bioprosthesis in the aortic position. Transesophageal echocardiographic midesophageal aortic valve long-axis image shows dehiscence of a pericardial bovine bioprosthesis in the aortic position. In systole (**A**), the anterior region of the prosthetic stent (*arrow*) is displaced toward the left ventricular side of the native aortic valve annulus. In diastole (**B**), the anterior region of the prosthetic stent is completely detached from the aortic valve annulus (*arrow*). Dehiscence with partial annular detachment produces a "rocking" motion of the prosthetic valve and paravalvular regurgitation in the region of separation. LVOT, left ventricular outflow tract; Ao, aorta.

to annular size, is often used as a reference when the hemodynamic performance of a prosthetic valve is examined. The peak transvalvular gradient for valves in the mitral position averages 4 mm Hg, and the peak transvalvular gradient for valves in the aortic position averages 20 to 30 mm Hg (Fig. 13.12). The continuity method can also be used to estimate the effective orifice area of prosthetic valves in the mitral or aortic position (Table 13.3). In this method, Doppler is used to measure the time-velocity integral (TVI) across the prosthetic valve in relation to the cross-sectional area and the TVI through the LVOT. Average values for the effective orifice area estimated by the continuity equation range from 2.5 to 3.0 cm^2 for valves in the mitral position and 1.5 to 2.0 cm^2 for valves in the aortic position (Fig. 13.13). Stenosis of bioprosthetic valves is caused by chronic degenerative changes that result in leaflet calcification, thickening, and rigidity, so that the leaflet cannot open completely. Degenerative changes and restricted leaflet mobility can be detected by the two-dimensional examination. In mechanical valves, stenosis can be caused by thrombus, pannus, vegetation, suture, or even retained subvalvular structures that trap the occluder mechanism in the closed position or restrict its ability to open completely (Figs. 13.5 and 13.14).

Thrombosis

Acute thrombosis, usually a result of inadequate anticoagulation, can cause stenosis or regurgitation by obstructing blood flow through the valve or by interfering with leaflet opening and closure. In this condition, two-dimensional imaging is used to detect thrombus on the valve apparatus that interferes with leaflet motion. Incomplete range of motion of the occluder device may be a sign of thrombus or pannus formation in patients with mechanical

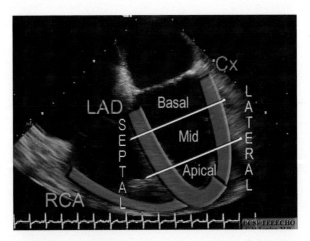

COLOR PLATE 1. Midesophageal four-chamber anatomic segments and perfusion. Segmental anatomy of the left ventricle in the midesophageal four-chamber view according to the American Society of Echocardiography classification system. Also depicted are the approximate perfusion zones of the left anterior descending (*LAD*), circumflex (*CX*), and right coronary (*RCA*) arteries. (Courtesy of M. London, M.D., http://www.ucsf.edu/teeecho) (See Figure 4.4.)

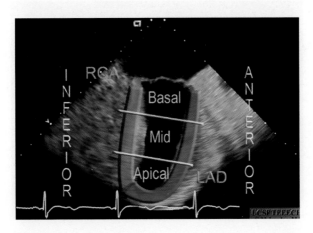

COLOR PLATE 2. Midesophageal two-chamber anatomic segments and perfusion. Segmental anatomy of the left ventricle in the midesophageal two-chamber view according to the American Society of Echocardiography classification system. Also depicted are the approximate perfusion zones of the left anterior descending (*LAD*) and right coronary (*RCA*) arteries. (Courtesy of M. London, M.D., http://www.ucsf.edu/teeecho) (See Figure 4.5.)

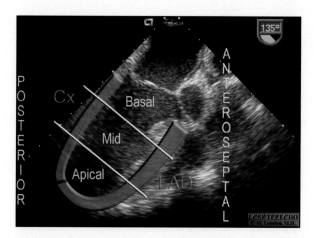

COLOR PLATE 3. Midesophageal long-axis anatomic segments and perfusion. Segmental anatomy of the left ventricle in the midesophageal long-axis view according to the American Society of Echocardiography classification system. Also depicted are the approximate perfusion zones of the major left anterior descending (*LAD*) and circumflex (*CX*) arteries. (Courtesy of M. London, M.D., http://www.ucsf.edu/teeecho) (See Figure 4.6.)

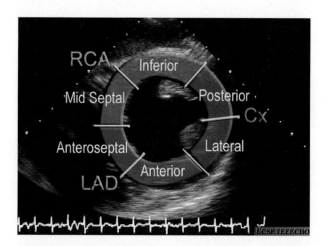

COLOR PLATE 4. Transgastric short-axis anatomic segments and perfusion. Segmental anatomy of the left ventricle in the transgastric short-axis view according to the American Society of Echocardiography classification system. Also depicted are the approximate perfusion zones of the major left anterior descending (*LAD*), circumflex (*CX*), and right coronary (*RCA*) arteries. (Courtesy of M. London, M.D., http://www.ucsf.edu/teeecho) (See Figure 4.7.)

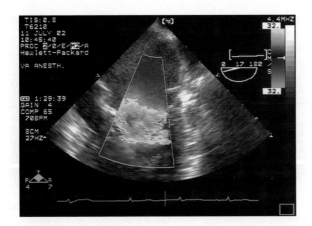

COLOR PLATE 5. Aliasing of color display. Blood flow through the mitral valve (midesophageal four-chamber view) during early diastole results in aliasing in the color flow mapper. Flow velocity accelerates in the left atrium as blood is funneled to the mitral valve orifice, shown as the color code of dark blue transitioning to light blue, and reaches 32 cm/s (the Nyquist limit), as seen on the color bar. As a result, aliasing signals are coded bright yellow, then red, as the velocity reaches a maximum at the level of the leaflet tips. Once in the left ventricle, the blood flow decelerates to fall below the Nyquist limit and is again appropriately coded blue by the echocardiographic system. (See Figure 5.14.)

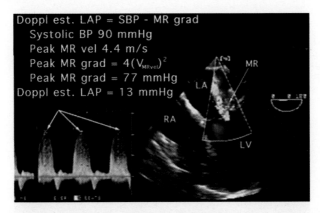

COLOR PLATE 6. The left atrial pressure can be estimated by using the mitral regurgitation velocity profile. The peak ventriculoatrial pressure gradient, measured by using the peak velocity of the mitral regurgitation profile (*arrow*) and the simplified Bernoulli equation, is subtracted from the known systolic blood pressure. In this case, the systolic blood pressure was 122 mm Hg, and the peak velocity was 5.18 m/s (107 mm Hg). The Doppler-estimated left atrial pressure was 15 mm Hg. The known pulmonary capillary wedge pressure was 14 mm Hg. LAP, left atrial pressure; MR, mitral regurgitation; RA, right atrial pressure; LV, left ventricle; vel, velocity; grad, gradient; SBP, systolic blood pressure; V_{Mrvel}, peak velocity of the mitral regurgitant flow profile. (See Figure 6.9.)

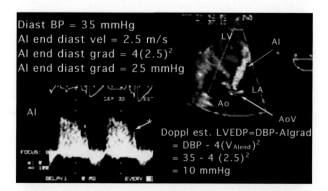

COLOR PLATE 7. The left ventricular end-diastolic pressure can be estimated by using the aortic valve insufficiency velocity profile. The aortic-ventricular gradient, measured from the end-diastolic velocity of the aortic insufficiency regurgitation profile (*arrow*) and the simplified Bernoulli equation, is subtracted from the systemic pressure. In this case, the diastolic pressure was 45 mm Hg, and the late peak velocity was 2.91 m/s (gradient = 34 mm Hg). The estimated left ventricular end-diastolic pressure is 11 mm Hg (45 − 35 mm Hg). Diast BP, systemic diastolic blood pressure; AI, aortic insufficiency; diast, diastolic; vel, velocity; grad, gradient; LVEDP, left ventricular end-diastolic pressure; V_{Aiend}, end-diastolic velocity of the aortic insufficiency jet; Ao, ascending aorta; LA, left atrium; LV, left ventricle. (See Figure 6.10.)

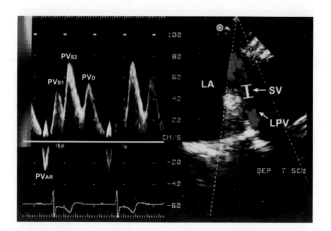

COLOR PLATE 8. Doppler pulmonary venous blood flow (*PVDF*) velocity profile. Left atrial (*LA*) filling can be assessed by placing a pulsed wave Doppler sample volume (2–4 mm) approximately 1.0 cm into a pulmonary vein (*PV*) orifice where it joins the LA. LAA, left atrial appendage; LUPV, left upper pulmonary vein; PV_{AR}, late diastolic retrograde velocity; PV_{S1}, first systolic component; PV_{S2}, second systolic component; PV_D, diastolic component; SV, sample volume; LPV, left pulmonary vein. (See Figure 7.5A.)

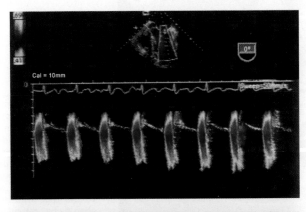

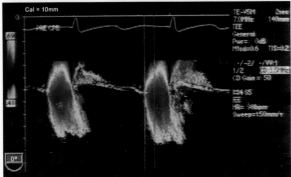

COLOR PLATE 9. Transmitral color M-mode Doppler flow propagation velocity (Vp) is obtained by placing the M-mode cursor through the center of the mitral inflow region in a transesophageal midesophageal four-chamber view and measuring the slope of the first aliasing velocity. (See Figure 7.8.)

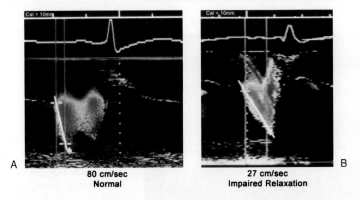

A   80 cm/sec   27 cm/sec   B
Normal   Impaired Relaxation

COLOR PLATE 10. In comparison with the transmitral color M-mode (motion mode) propagation velocity (Vp) in a normal subject (**A**), Vp is reduced in a patient with impaired left ventricular relaxation (**B**). (See Figure 7.9.)

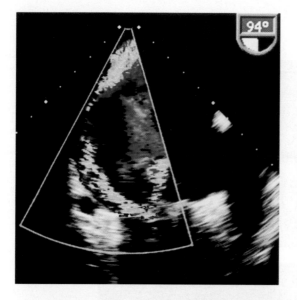

COLOR PLATE 11. Eccentric mitral regurgitant jet. This is a color Doppler scan of the mitral valve in the midesophageal four-chamber view. Note the severe mitral regurgitant jet, which "hugs" the posterior wall of the left atrium all the way to the top. Wall-hugging jets should be considered severe until proven otherwise. (See Figure 8.5.)

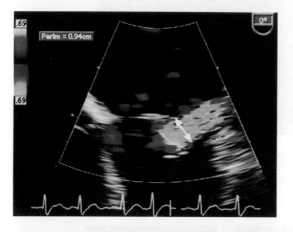

COLOR PLATE 12. Measurement of the vena contracta. This is a color Doppler scan of the mitral valve in the midesophageal four-chamber view. The diameter of the base of the mitral regurgitant jet correlates with the severity of regurgitation. (See Figure 8.6.)

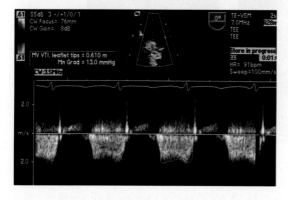

COLOR PLATE 13. A diastolic spectral profile of mitral inflow has been obtained with continuous wave Doppler in this patient with mitral stenosis. The profile has been traced out, and a mean pressure gradient of 13 mm Hg has been calculated with the software available within the machine. Note that the inflow velocities are close to 2 m/s. (See Figure 9.5.)

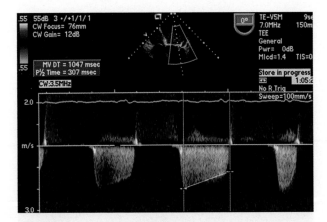

COLOR PLATE 14. A diastolic spectral profile of mitral inflow obtained with continuous wave Doppler. Severe mitral stenosis is confirmed by a pressure half-time measurement of 307 ms. (See Figure 9.7.)

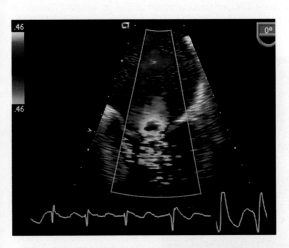

COLOR PLATE 15. Color Doppler imaging from this midesophageal four-chamber view of the mitral valve demonstrates proximal isovelocity surface area (PISA) or flow convergence on the left atrial side of the mitral valve. (See Figure 9.9.)

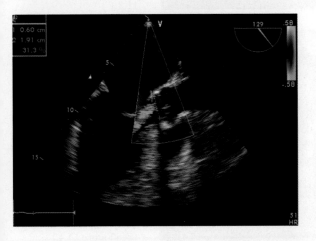

COLOR PLATE 16. Midesophageal aortic valve long-axis view demonstrating calculation of the ratio of aortic insufficiency height to left ventricular outflow tract diameter. The internal caliper on the echocardiography system is used to make these measurements. In this example, the ratio is 31%, indicating mild aortic insufficiency. (See Figure 11.1.)

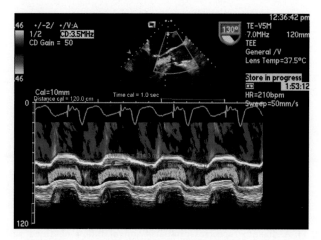

COLOR PLATE 17. Color M-mode assessment of aortic regurgitation. From the midesophageal aortic valve long-axis view the M-mode cursor is positioned perpindicular to the aortic root as close to the origin of the regurgitant jet as possible. The jet and the outflow tract are well delineated in the color M-mode display. Caliper measurement of the jet height (75 mm) is compared to that of the root (214.3 mm) and the resulting ratio of 35% corresponds to 2⁺ AR. (See Figure 11.2.)

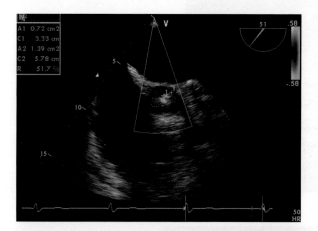

COLOR PLATE 18. Midesophageal aortic valve short-axis view in the same patient as in Figure 11.1 demonstrating the jet area/left ventricular outflow tract area method. The ratio of the areas is 51%, indicating moderate mitral regurgitation. The patient therefore has mild-moderate aortic insufficiency. (See Figure 11.3.)

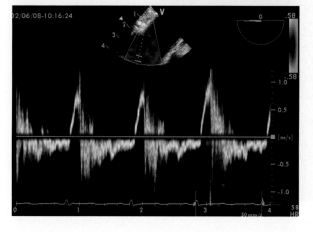

COLOR PLATE 19. Upper esophageal aortic arch long-axis view demonstrating severe aortic regurgitation, evidenced by flow reversal within the distal aortic arch during diastole. Note flow away from the probe, below the baseline, throughout diastole (holodiastolic flow). (See Figure 11.4.)

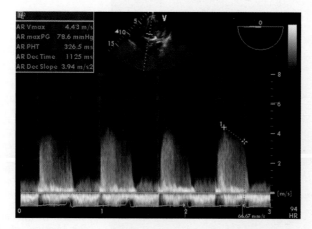

COLOR PLATE 20. Transgastric long-axis view with nearly parallel Doppler beam alignment demonstrating the aortic regurgitant jet velocity profile. The pressure half-time is 218 m/s, with a slope of 3.94 m/s indicating moderate to severe aortic regurgitation. (See Figure 11.5.)

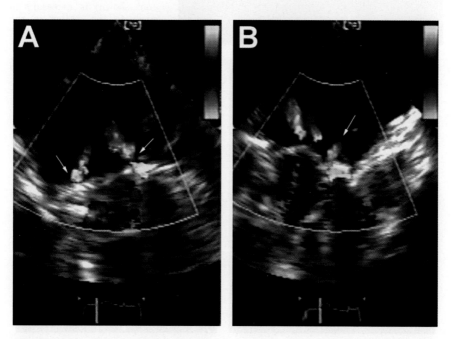

COLOR PLATE 21. Bileaflet mechanical prosthesis, mitral position. Color Doppler flow transesophageal echocardiographic midesophageal mitral valve commissural view at a multiplane angle of 60 degrees (**A**) and long-axis view at a multiplane angle of 150 degrees (**B**) show the normal appearance of leakage regurgitant jets that are characteristic of bileaflet valves. **A:** Individual leakage jets originate from the hinge points of the leaflets (*arrows*) and are directed toward the center of the valve. **B:** A third normal leakage regurgitant jet (*arrow*) can be visualized originating at the point of contact between the leaflet and the valve stent. (See Figure 13.2.)

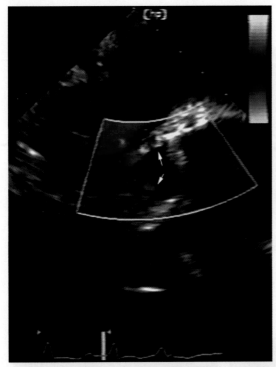

COLOR PLATE 22. Bileaflet mechanical prosthesis in the aortic position. Transesophageal echocardiographic midesophageal aortic valve long-axis view at a multiplane angle of 135 degrees in a patient with a bileaflet mechanical prosthesis in the aortic position. Color Doppler flow imaging in diastole shows the normal appearance of the two leakage regurgitant jets that originate at the leaflet hinge points (*arrows*). Note that ultrasound shadowing caused by the valve stent makes it difficult to assess the motion of the leaflets from this imaging angle. The transgastric long-axis or the deep transgastric long-axis view through the aortic valve (not shown) is necessary to evaluate the motion of the individual leaflets. (See Figure 13.3.)

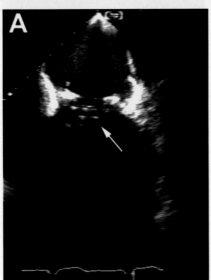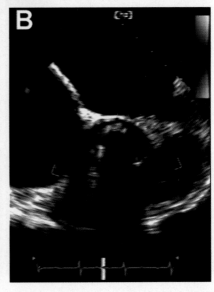

COLOR PLATE 23. Starr-Edwards caged-ball mechanical valve. **A:** Transesophageal echocardiographic midesophageal four-chamber view of a caged-ball valve prosthesis in the mitral position at end-diastole. The Silastic ball occluder (*arrow*) contained within the wire cage causes ultrasound shadowing and makes it difficult to image the distal side of the valve. **B:** Transesophageal echocardiographic midesophageal aortic valve short-axis view during systole in a patient with a caged-ball valve in the aortic position. Note the three metal struts of the cage. Color Doppler flow imaging demonstrates blood flow through the valve at the perimeter of the Silastic ball occluder. Again, the Silastic ball occluder causes ultrasound shadowing that obscures both two-dimensional and color flow Doppler views of the distal valve. (See Figure 13.4.)

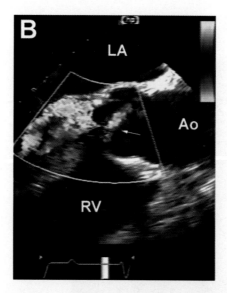

COLOR PLATE 24. Transvalvular regurgitation, porcine bioprosthetic valve in the aortic position. Transesophageal echocardiographic midesophageal aortic valve long-axis image at a multiplane angle of 150 degrees in a patient with a porcine bioprosthetic valve in the aortic position. Color Doppler flow imaging during diastole (**B**) shows the aortic regurgitant jet (*arrow*) originating between the valve struts, indicating transvalvular regurgitation caused by structural degeneration of the bioprosthetic valve. (See Figure 13.9B.)

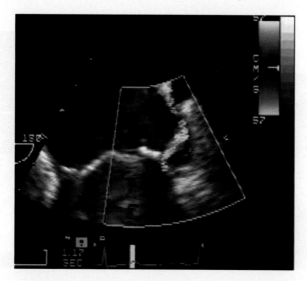

COLOR PLATE 25. Paravalvular regurgitation. Transesophageal echocardiographic midesophageal view at a multiplane angle of 22 degrees of a mechanical bileaflet prosthesis in the mitral position demonstrates an eccentric paravalvular regurgitant jet originating outside the prosthetic annulus. (See Figure 13.10.)

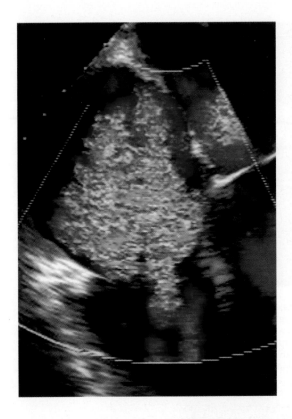

COLOR PLATE 26. Color flow Doppler image demonstrating severe tricuspid regurgitation. (See Figure 14.8.)

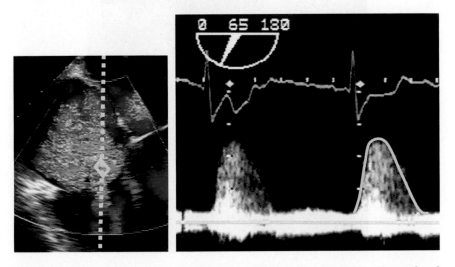

COLOR PLATE 27. Continuous wave Doppler image of tricuspid regurgitation. A sample calculation of the pulmonary artery systolic pressure follows: $\Delta P = 4(2.6)^2$; Systolic Pulmonary Artery Pressure = 27 + Right Atrial Pressure (15); Systolic Pulmonary Artery Pressure = 42 mm Hg. (See Figure 14.10.)

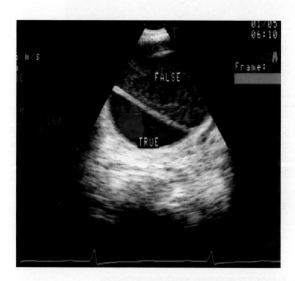

COLOR PLATE 28. A color Doppler image of Figure 16.6 demonstrating early systolic flow within the true lumen. (See Figure 16.7.)

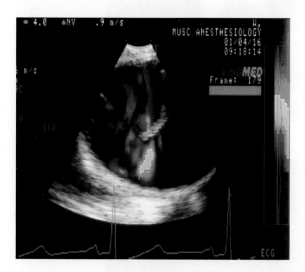

COLOR PLATE 29. A color flow image of Figure 16.8 demonstrating flow from the true lumen to the false lumen through the entry site. (See Figure 16.9.)

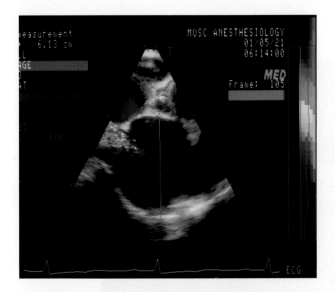

COLOR PLATE 30. Ascending aortic aneurysm with dilation in the proximal ascending aorta resulting in poor coaptation of the aorta valve leaflets and a central jet of aortic regurgitation. (See Figure 16.11.)

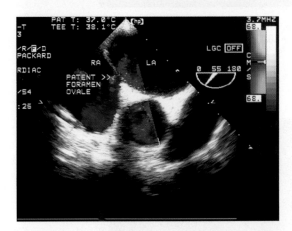

COLOR PLATE 31. Intracardiac shunt (patent foramen ovale) across the intraatrial septum. (See Figure 17.3.)

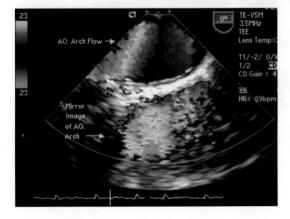

COLOR PLATE 32. A **mirror image** of the true aortic arch is seen in the far field. Note that the false arch is the same size as the true structure. The color flow Doppler signals are also duplicated. (See Figure 19.14.)

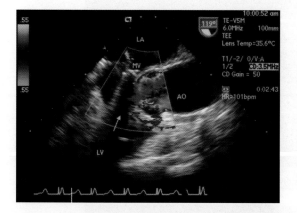

COLOR PLATE 33. Acoustic shadowing in color flow Doppler caused by a prosthetic mitral valve ring in the midesophageal aortic valve long-axis view. The *arrow* points to the long axial shadow. (See Figure 19.16.)

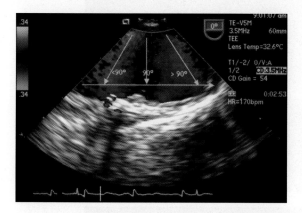

COLOR PLATE 34. Nonparallel beam angle color flow Doppler artifact in the aortic arch. The direction of blood flow is indicated by the *horizontal arrow*. The *angled arrows* indicate the direction of the Doppler ultrasound interrogating beam. (See Figure 19.17.)

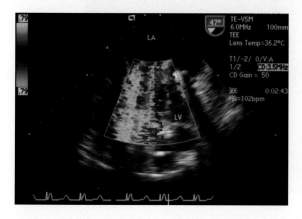

COLOR PLATE 35. Color flow Doppler **reverberations** are seen distal to a mechanical mitral valve in this midesophageal commissural view. (See Figure 19.19.)

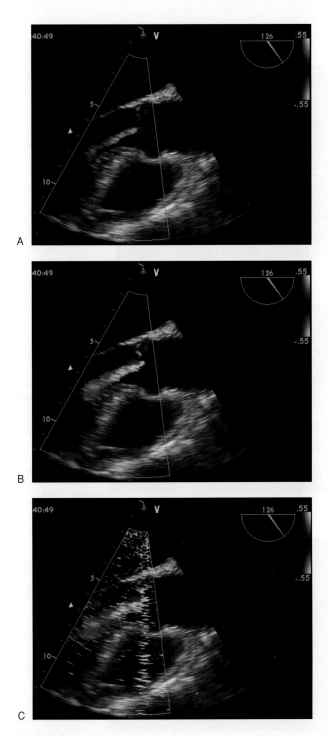

COLOR PLATE 36. Midesophageal aortic valve long-axis view in a patient with aortic insufficiency. **A:** The color gain is set too low, so that the width of the aortic insufficiency jet is underestimated. **B:** The color gain is correctly set. **C:** The color gain is too high. (See Figure 20.5.)

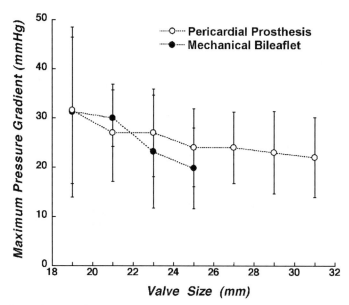

FIG. 13.12. Normal maximal transvalvular pressure gradients for aortic valve prostheses. The pressure gradients are determined with the simplified Bernoulli equation (see text). Values are the mean. *Error bars* indicate the standard deviation. (Data from Reisner SA, Meltzer RS. Normal values of prosthetic valve Doppler echocardiographic parameters: a review. *J Am Soc Echocardiogr* 1988;1:201–210; Panidis IP, Ross J, Mintz GS. Normal and abnormal prosthetic valve function as assessed by Doppler echocardiography. *J Am Coll Cardiol* 1986;8:317–326; Chambers J, Fraser A, Lawford P, et al. Echocardiographic assessment of artificial heart valves: British Society of Echocardiography position paper. *Br Heart J* 1994;71[4 Suppl]:6–14.)

valves (Fig. 13.5). Color Doppler imaging may demonstrate transvalvular regurgitation or an eccentric inflow pattern across the affected leaflet.

Hemolysis

Hemolysis is unusual with modern valve prostheses but may develop when blood is subjected to high peak levels of shear stress. These hydrodynamic conditions can occur when blood accelerates or decelerates rapidly during contact with prosthetic material (10). Regurgitant jets associated with hemolysis often exhibit patterns of flow fragmentation, collision, or rapid acceleration on color Doppler flow imaging. Free regurgitant jets or jets that decelerate gradually are less likely to cause hemolysis.

Endocarditis

Prosthetic endocarditis develops in approximately 3% to 6% of patients after valve replacement and is associated with a mortality rate between 20% and 80% (2). TEE is currently the best technique for detecting vegetations, dehiscence, or annular abscess in the diagnosis of prosthetic endocarditis (11) (Fig. 13.15). Imaging the distal side of the prosthetic valve is

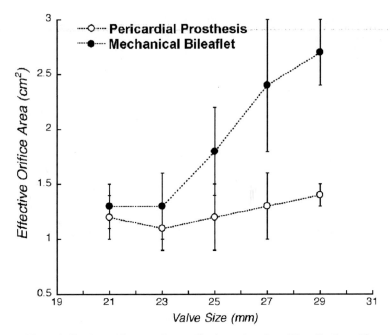

FIG. 13.13. Normal effective orifice area for prosthetic aortic valves. The effective orifice area is determined with the continuity equation (see text). Values are the mean. *Error bars* indicate the standard deviation. (Data from Reisner SA, Meltzer RS. Normal values of prosthetic valve Doppler echocardiographic parameters: a review. *J Am Soc Echocardiogr* 1988;1:201–210; Panidis IP, Ross J, Mintz GS. Normal and abnormal prosthetic valve function as assessed by Doppler echocardiography. *J Am Coll Cardiol* 1986;8:317–326; Chambers J, Fraser A, Lawford P, et al. Echocardiographic assessment of artificial heart valves: British Society of Echocardiography position paper. *Br Heart J* 1994;71[4 Suppl]:6–14.)

made difficult by shadowing of the ultrasound beam, so that it is important to use both ME and TG imaging planes to examine both sides of the prosthesis for vegetations.

Left Ventricular Outflow Tract Obstruction

LVOT obstruction causing subvalvular aortic stenosis is an uncommon but recognized complication of mitral valve replacement (12). After mitral valve replacement by the valve-sparing or chordal-sparing technique, residual mitral valve leaflet or chordal apparatus can cause LVOT obstruction. LVOT obstruction can also be caused by a porcine bioprosthesis in the mitral position with a strut impinging on LV outflow. The TG long-axis view provides a means to image the LVOT after mitral valve replacement and estimate the LVOT pressure gradient with continuous wave Doppler.

SUMMARY

The evaluation of prosthetic heart valves, the diagnosis of prosthetic valve dysfunction, and the detection of complications associated with valve replacement are important clinical applications of TEE.

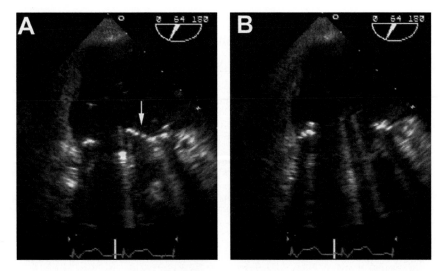

FIG. 13.14. Trapped leaflet, mechanical bileaflet valve in the mitral position. Transesophageal echocardiographic midesophageal mitral valve commissural view in mid diastole provides a cross section to demonstrate the motion of both leaflets in a patient with a mechanical bileaflet valve in the mitral position. **A:** The anterior leaflet of the prosthesis is trapped in the closed position (*arrow*). **B:** Both leaflets are opening completely after surgery to free the trapped leaflet. Color Doppler flow imaging (not shown) demonstrated mitral inflow in diastole through the region of the valve with the open leaflet, but not across the region of the valve with the leaflet trapped in the closed position.

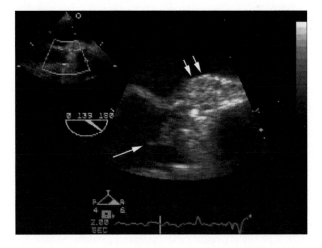

FIG. 13.15. Endocarditis and aortic root abscess, mechanical bileaflet valve, aortic position. Transesophageal echocardiographic midesophageal aortic valve long-axis image demonstrating prosthetic endocarditis in a patient with a mechanical bileaflet valve in the aortic position. A vegetation attached to the prosthetic valve was imaged in the left ventricular outflow tract during diastole (*single arrow*). Thickening of the posterior wall of the aortic root (*double arrows*) suggested aortic root abscess.

REFERENCES

1. Seward JB, Labovitz AJ, Lewis JF, et al. ACC position statement. Transesophageal echocardiography. *J Am Coll Cardiol* 1992;20:506.
2. Vongpatanasin W, Hillis DL, Lange RA. Medical progress: prosthetic heart valves. *N Engl J Med* 1996;335:407–416.
3. Daniel WG, Mugge A, Grote J, et al. Comparison of transthoracic and transesophageal echocardiography for detection of abnormalities of prosthetic and bioprosthetic valves in the mitral and aortic positions. *Am J Cardiol* 1993;71:210–215.
4. Khandheria BK, Seward JB, Oh JK, et al. Value and limitations of transesophageal echocardiography in assessment of mitral valve prostheses. *Circulation* 1991;83:1956–1968.
5. Karalis DG, Chandrasekaran K, Ross JJ, et al. Single-plane transesophageal echocardiography for assessing function of mechanical or bioprosthetic valves in the aortic position. *Am J Cardiol* 1992;69:1310–1315.
6. Chambers J, Fraser A, Lawford P, et al. Echocardiographic assessment of artificial heart valves: British Society of Echocardiography position paper. *Br Heart J* 1994;71[4 Suppl]:6–14.
7. Panidis IP, Ross J, Mintz GS. Normal and abnormal prosthetic valve function as assessed by Doppler echocardiography. *J Am Coll Cardiol* 1986;8:317–326.
8. Reisner SA, Meltzer RS. Normal values of prosthetic valve Doppler echocardiographic parameters: a review. *J Am Soc Echocardiogr* 1988;1:201–210.
9. Guarracino F, Zussa C, Polesel E, et al. Influence of transesophageal echocardiography on intraoperative decision making for Toronto stentless prosthetic valve implantation. *J Heart Valve Dis* 2001;10:31–34.
10. Garcia MJ, Vandervoort P, Stewart WJ, et al. Mechanisms of hemolysis with mitral prosthetic regurgitation. Study using transesophageal echocardiography and fluid dynamic simulation. *J Am Coll Cardiol* 1996;27:399–406.
11. Piper C, Korfer R, Horstkotte D. Prosthetic valve endocarditis. *Heart* 2001;85:590–593.
12. Gallet B, Berrebi A, Grinda JM, et al. Severe intermittent intraprosthetic regurgitation after mitral valve replacement with subvalvular preservation. *J Am Soc Echocardiogr* 2001;14:314–316.

QUESTIONS

1. An important limitation of ultrasound imaging in the evaluation of prosthetic heart valves is
   a. Limited cross-sectional imaging planes
   b. Inability to quantify the severity of valve stenosis
   c. Acoustic shadowing
   d. Poor imaging resolution of structural details
2. The first clinically successful prosthetic valve type was a
   a. Porcine bioprosthesis
   b. Caged-ball mechanical prosthesis
   c. Tilting-disc mechanical prosthesis
   d. Pericardial bioprosthesis
3. Doppler echocardiography with use of the continuity method can estimate the effective orifice area of
   a. A bileaflet mechanical valve in the aortic position
   b. A caged-disc mechanical prosthesis in the mitral position
   c. A caged-ball mechanical prosthesis in the aortic position
   d. A caged-ball mechanical prosthesis in the mitral position
4. A Doppler echocardiographic characteristic of a pathologic regurgitant jet is
   a. Regurgitant jet originating from the hinge points of a mechanical valve
   b. Small regurgitant jet at the central coaptation point of a biologic valve
   c. Regurgitant jets of short duration early in the cardiac cycle during valve closure
   d. Eccentric regurgitant jets that track along the wall of the receiving chamber

5. A relative contraindication to the implantation of a stentless aortic valve is
   a. A native aortic valve annular diameter less than 20 mm
   b. A native aortic valve annular diameter larger than 27 mm
   c. Aortic root abscess
   d. Ascending aortic aneurysm
6. LVOT obstruction can occur after implantation of a
   a. Stented porcine valve in the mitral position
   b. Aortic root allograft
   c. Stentless aortic valve
   d. Mechanical bileaflet valve in the aortic position
7. Prosthetic valve dehiscence produces which of the following echocardiographic findings?
   a. Increased effective orifice area
   b. Vegetations
   c. "Rocking" of the valve prosthesis
   d. Transvalvular regurgitation
8. The best TEE view for assessing valve leaflet motion in a patient with a mechanical bileaflet prosthesis in the aortic position is the
   a. TG long-axis view
   b. ME aortic valve long-axis view
   c. ME long-axis view
   d. ME aortic valve short-axis view
9. A characteristic feature of regurgitant jets causing hemolysis in patients with prosthetic heart valves is
   a. A low-velocity, wide-based regurgitant jet
   b. A high-velocity jet that collides with the valve prosthesis
   c. A free regurgitant jet
   d. Regurgitant jets originating from the hinge points of the occluder mechanism
10. An echocardiographic criterion for the diagnosis of prosthetic endocarditis is
    a. Vegetations on the prosthetic valve
    b. Leaflet calcification
    c. Valve stenosis
    d. Thrombosis of the valve

Right Ventricle, Right Atrium, Tricuspid Valve, and Pulmonic Valve

Gautam M. Sreeram and Jonathan B. Mark

Right ventricular (RV) dysfunction is a common concern in the perioperative period. Inadequate myocardial protection, increases in pulmonary vascular resistance, air embolism to the RV coronary supply, and acute valvular dysfunction can compromise RV performance. This chapter surveys the echocardiographic approaches for evaluating the right side of the heart and its associated valves.

RIGHT VENTRICLE

Anatomy

Echocardiographic evaluation of the RV is complicated by the nongeometric, asymmetric, crescent shape of this chamber. The RV consists of a free wall and a septum that it shares with the left ventricle (LV). The RV free wall can be divided into basal, mid, and apical segments corresponding to the adjacent LV segments seen in the midesophageal (ME) four-chamber view. The RV can also be described in terms of its inflow and outflow tracts, which reflect the separate embryologic origins of these portions of the RV. An encircling muscular band separates the inflow and outflow portions of the RV. Its most apical portion, the moderator band, is often seen with transesophageal echocardiography (TEE). Present in most normal individuals, the moderator band is a muscular trabeculation extending from the lower interventricular septum to the anterior RV wall (Fig. 14.1).

Transesophageal Echocardiographic Views

1. *Midesophageal four-chamber view.* This long-axis view of the RV allows assessment of the apical, mid, and basal segments of the RV. In the four-chamber view, the RV appears triangular in comparison with the elliptic LV, and its length is only two-thirds the length of the LV (see Chapter 2 and Appendices).
2. *Midesophageal right ventricular inflow-outflow view.* This view is often termed the *wraparound view*, owing to the fact that the right atrium (RA), RV, and pulmonary artery (PA) appear to "wrap around" the aortic valve and left atrium, describing a 270-degree arc (see Chapter 2 and Appendices).
3. *Transgastric midpapillary short-axis view.* In addition to allowing monitoring of LV function, this view serves to assess the RV free wall and interventricular septum. (Fig. 14.2).
4. *Transgastric right ventricular inflow view.* This is a long-axis view of the RV similar to the transgastric (TG) two-chamber view of the LV. To acquire this view, one begins with the TG short-axis view of the RV (described earlier) and advances the multiplane angle to approximately 90 degrees, or until the RA and RV are seen in long axis, with the RV inflow and tricuspid valve centered in the image. Alternatively, one develops the TG two-chamber view of the left atrium and ventricle and then rotates the probe clockwise (rightward) until the two right-sided chambers are displayed. Both techniques should result in the same image of the RV inflow tract and the long axis of the RA and RV (Fig. 14.3).

Assessment of Global Right Ventricular Function

Hypertrophy. The normal thickness of the RV free wall is less than half that of the LV and measures less than 5 mm at end-diastole (1). RV hypertrophy is present when the RV free

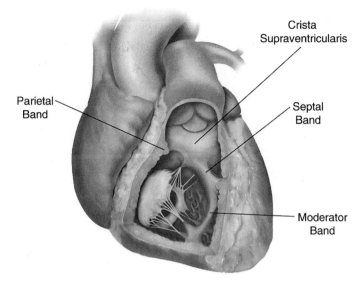

FIG. 14.1. Schematic drawing of anatomic structures in the right ventricle.

wall thickness exceeds 5 mm and may indicate elevated PA pressure or pulmonic stenosis (PS) (2). For example, in patients with chronic cor pulmonale, the RV wall thickness may exceed 10 mm when severe pulmonary hypertension raises PA pressures to systemic levels. Additionally, the intracavitary trabecular pattern is more prominent, particularly at the apex in patients with RV hypertrophy.

Dilation. RV dilation may be seen with RV volume overload or chronic RV pressure overload. Normally, the RV end-diastolic cross-sectional area is approximately 60% of the area of the LV. As the RV dilates, its shape changes from triangular to round. An additional clue to the presence of RV dilation may be found through examination of the cardiac apex, which

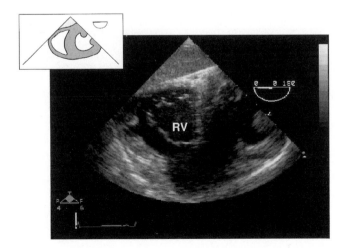

FIG. 14.2. Transgastric midpapillary short-axis view. RV, right ventricle.

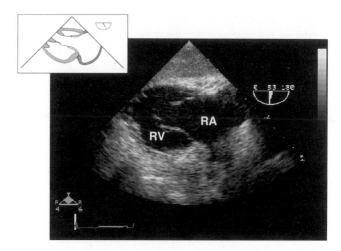

FIG. 14.3. Transgastric right ventricular (*RV*) inflow view.

is formed by the apex of the LV in the ME four-chamber view. *When the RV forms part of the cardiac apex, then RV dilation is present.* With mild RV dilation, the RV area is 60% to 100% of the LV area. With moderate RV dilation, the RV area may equal the LV area, and with severe RV enlargement, the RV area often exceeds the LV area (2) (Fig. 14.4).

Systolic function. The quantitative assessment of RV systolic function is limited by the unique geometry of the RV. Furthermore, variations in chamber shape may occur readily with changes in volume. RV ejection is produced primarily by inward motion of the RV free wall, with lesser contributions from the RV outflow tract (RVOT) and descent of the cardiac base (1). Signs of RV dysfunction include severe hypokinesis or akinesis of the RV free wall, RV enlargement, change in shape of the RV from crescent to round, and flattening or bulging of the interventricular septum from right to left.

Tricuspid annular plane systolic excursion. Long-axis systolic excursion of the lateral aspect of the tricuspid annulus may be used as an indicator of RV systolic function. The

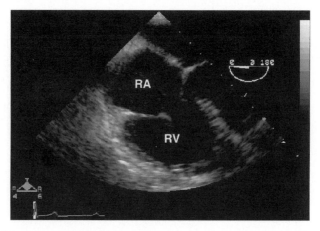

FIG. 14.4. Right ventricular (*RV*) dilation. Note the change in shape of the dilated right ventricle from triangular to round.

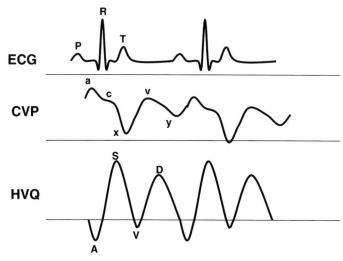

FIG. 14.5. Schematic diagram of the correlation of hepatic vein flow (*HVQ*) with central venous pressure (*CVP*) and electrocardiogram (*ECG*).

normal tricuspid annular plane systolic excursion is 20 to 25 mm toward the cardiac apex, slightly greater than the normal mitral annular plane excursion (3). The tricuspid annulus tilts toward the apex, whereas the mitral annulus moves more symmetrically toward the apex, somewhat like a piston (3).

 Hepatic venous flow patterns. Blood from the hepatic veins flows through the inferior vena cava toward the RA. Examination of the patterns of flow velocity during the different phases of the cardiac cycle with pulsed wave Doppler can reveal important clues about RV function. Normal hepatic venous flow patterns have four phasic components (Figs. 14.5 and 14.6). The initial forward flow toward the RA occurs during systole and is caused by the fall in atrial pressure resulting from atrial relaxation and apical movement of the tricuspid

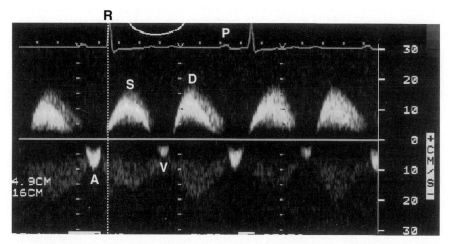

FIG. 14.6. Pulsed wave Doppler image of normal hepatic venous flow with forward flow in systole and diastole and two small retrograde waves (A and V).

valve during RV systole. This corresponds to the x-descent in atrial pressure. Forward flow in diastole is caused by a fall in atrial pressure during early ventricular filling and corresponds to the y-descent in atrial pressure. Two small retrograde waves may be observed, one corresponding to atrial contraction at end-diastole and one appearing at end-systole, before the y-descent in atrial pressure. When RV systolic function is impaired, the systolic inflow wave of hepatic venous flow is attenuated.

Assessment of Regional Right Ventricular Function

RV perfusion is supplied primarily by the right coronary artery, although a small portion of the anterior free wall may be supplied by the conus branch of the left anterior descending artery (4). Regional RV ischemia is difficult to detect with TEE, in part because RV wall motion is more dependent on afterload than that of the LV. Because the thin-walled RV is a volume-pumping chamber, its ejection fraction is extremely sensitive to acute increases in PA pressure. In contrast, the thick-walled LV is a pressure-pumping chamber, and its ejection fraction, although influenced by the systemic arterial pressure, is generally preserved despite marked increases in systemic arterial pressure. Furthermore, the irregularity and asymmetry of the RV make the detection of mild changes in contractility difficult. Akinesis or dyskinesis of the RV is more readily identified and is a very sensitive indicator of RV infarction (5). Less common findings in RV infarction include RV dilation, papillary muscle dysfunction, tricuspid regurgitation, and paradoxic interventricular septal motion (6,7).

Interventricular Septum

Examination of interventricular septal motion can help distinguish RV volume overload from RV pressure overload.

Right ventricular volume overload. RV volume overload may be seen with atrial or ventricular septal defects, tricuspid regurgitation (TR), and pulmonic regurgitation (PR). Although features of RV volume and RV pressure overload may overlap, *RV volume overload more consistently produces dilation of the RV.* Examination of the interventricular septum may yield additional clues to the etiology of RV overload. Normally, the interventricular septum functions as part of the LV and maintains a convex curvature toward the RV throughout the cardiac cycle because its motion is controlled by the center of cardiac muscle mass located in the LV cavity. As the RV dilates or becomes hypertrophic and the RV mass increases to equal that of the LV, the septum flattens, and when RV mass exceeds LV mass, paradoxic septal motion appears. With RV volume overload, septal distortion is maximal at end-diastole, corresponding to the time of peak diastolic overfilling of the RV (8). During systole, the end-diastolic septal flattening reverses, with paradoxic septal motion toward the RV cavity.

Right ventricular pressure overload. RV pressure overload may be seen with pulmonary hypertension or PS. RV pressure overload is characterized primarily by hypertrophy of the RV free wall and, if chronic, hypertrophy of the interventricular septum. *In contrast to RV volume overload, RV pressure overload produces maximal septal distortion at end-systole and early diastole, corresponding to the time of peak systolic afterloading of the RV (9).*

RIGHT ATRIUM

Anatomy

The RA is a thin-walled structure with an irregular shape. The superior vena cava enters the right anterior portion of the superior wall, and the inferior vena cava enters the right posterior portion of the inferior wall. The tricuspid annulus forms the inferior portion of the RA, and the coronary sinus opens into the RA just above this structure. The eustachian valve and Chiari network are two structures associated with the orifice of the inferior vena cava. Failure of regression of the right or inferior valve of the sinus venosus during gestation may result in a persistent eustachian valve. The Chiari network is a fenestrated, strandlike structure within the RA cavity. Although it most often arises from the orifice of the inferior vena cava, the Chiari network may have a primary origin of attachment to the RA free wall, coronary sinus, or interatrial septum.

Transesophageal Echocardiographic Views

TEE evaluation of the RA may be performed from the standard ME four-chamber view and the ME RV inflow-outflow view. The ME bicaval view is also very useful (see Chapter 2 and Appendices), particularly for evaluation of the RA free wall and interatrial septum. The superior-inferior dimension of the RA at end-systole is 4.2 ± 0.4 cm, and the medial-lateral dimension is 3.7 ± 0.4 cm (10).

TRICUSPID VALVE

Anatomy

The tricuspid valve (TV) consists of the valve leaflets, chordae tendineae, papillary muscles, annular ring, and RV myocardium. The TV is trileaflet, with anterior, septal, and posterior leaflets of unequal size (Fig. 14.7). Likewise, there are three papillary muscles; the anterior papillary muscle is the largest and originates from the moderator band as it courses toward the RV free wall. The chordae tendineae connect the papillary muscles to the tricuspid leaflets. The TV annulus is larger and located in a slightly more apical position than the mitral valve annulus. This normal apical displacement of the TV is not present in patients with endocardial cushion defects or primum atrial septal defects and is exaggerated in patients with Ebstein anomaly of the TV.

Transesophageal Echocardiographic Views

TEE evaluation of the TV focuses on the same standard views as those used to evaluate the RV.

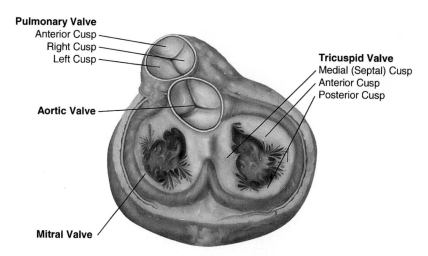

Pulmonary Valve
Anterior Cusp
Right Cusp
Left Cusp

Tricuspid Valve
Medial (Septal) Cusp
Anterior Cusp
Posterior Cusp

Aortic Valve

Mitral Valve

FIG. 14.7. Schematic drawing of tricuspid valve anatomy.

1. ***Midesophageal four-chamber view.*** From the standard ME four-chamber view, slight rightward (clockwise) rotation of the probe moves the TV to the center of the scan plane; advancing and withdrawing the transducer then allows imaging of the entire TV. This view demonstrates the anterior and septal leaflets.
2. ***Midesophageal right ventricular inflow-outflow view.*** This view provides an additional, nearly orthogonal view of the TV. In this scan plane, the plane of the TV orifice is more nearly parallel to the ultrasound beam, so that quantitative measurement of TV flow velocities with continuous wave Doppler is optimized.
3. ***Transgastric views.*** The TG views used to evaluate the RV also provide useful windows for imaging the TV. Rightward (clockwise) rotation of the TEE transducer from the TG mid short-axis view of the LV provides a good view of the TV in short axis, allowing identification of its septal, anterior, and posterior leaflets. The TG RV inflow view provides the best image of the chordae tendineae and RV papillary muscles supporting the TV.

Tricuspid Regurgitation

TR is the most common right-sided valvular lesion in adults. *It is most commonly caused by tricuspid annular dilation secondary to RV enlargement or pulmonary hypertension.*

Two-dimensional echocardiography. Features of TR may include dilation of the RA, RV, and tricuspid annulus, causing incomplete TV closure. TV prolapse may be seen when the valve leaflets are displaced beyond the tricuspid annulus into the RA.

Doppler echocardiography.

Color flow Doppler: The degree of regurgitation is usually assessed with color flow Doppler; severe regurgitation is represented by a large color flow disturbance that fills more than half of the RA. When the regurgitant jet is directed toward the atrial septum, it must be distinguished from normal caval inflow or an atrial septal defect (Fig. 14.8; see Color Plate 26 following page 212).

Pulsed wave Doppler: Assessment of caval or hepatic vein flow by pulsed wave Doppler may reveal abnormal reversed (retrograde) flow in systole, which represents severe TR (Fig. 14.9).

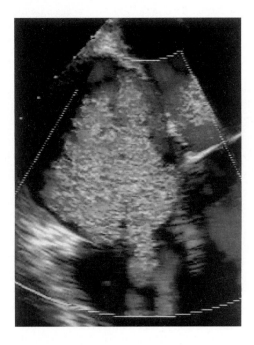

FIG. 14.8. Color flow Doppler image demonstrating severe tricuspid regurgitation. (See Color Plate 26 following page 212.)

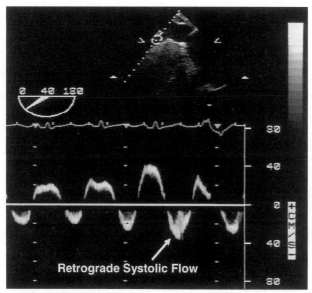

FIG. 14.9. Pulsed wave Doppler image of hepatic venous flow with retrograde systolic flow, indicating severe tricuspid regurgitation.

Use of continuous wave Doppler to determine the pulmonary artery systolic pressure: The jet of TR can also be interrogated with continuous wave Doppler to measure the peak velocity of the regurgitant jet. With the simplified Bernoulli equation, the systolic transvalvular pressure gradient (ΔP) is calculated as $\Delta P = 4\ v^2$, where v is the peak velocity of the TR jet. RV systolic pressure is calculated by adding the tricuspid transvalvular gradient to an estimate of the RA pressure. In the absence of obstruction to RV outflow, this calculated RV systolic pressure provides a good estimate of the PA systolic pressure. Because the vast majority of patients with elevated PA pressure have some degree of TR, even in the absence of clinical signs, this measurement is widely applicable. However, when the calculation is performed, considerable care must be taken to align the ultrasound beam with the regurgitant jet to avoid an underestimation of the pressures (Fig. 14.10; see Color Plate 27 following page 212).

Tricuspid Stenosis

Tricuspid stenosis (TS) is diagnosed by the structural abnormalities of the leaflets and quantified by continuous wave Doppler examination of the trans-tricuspid flow.

Two-dimensional echocardiography. Characteristic features of TS include increased echo density of the thickened leaflets, diastolic leaflet doming, and decreased size of the TV orifice.

Doppler echocardiography. *Because the tricuspid is the largest of the four cardiac valves, flow velocities are the lowest across this valve, typically less than 0.7 m/s* (11). Although normal prosthetic valves in the tricuspid position may demonstrate peak velocities nearly twice normal, velocities greater than 1.5 m/s suggest significant TS, which may be confirmed by noting a deterioration in the effective valve orifice area (12).

Etiology of Tricuspid Valve Disease

Annular dilation. Annular dilation results in decreased leaflet coaptation, which leads to TR. The severity of the regurgitation is directly related to the degree of annular dilation, and the patient may require annuloplasty.

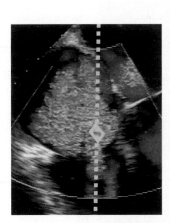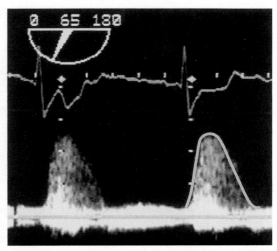

FIG. 14.10. Continuous wave Doppler image of tricuspid regurgitation. A sample calculation of the pulmonary artery systolic pressure follows: $\Delta P = 4(2.6)^2$; Systolic Pulmonary Artery Pressure = 27 + Right Atrial Pressure (15); Systolic Pulmonary Artery Pressure = 42 mm Hg. (See Color Plate 27 following page 212.)

Rheumatic disease. Rheumatic disease is the most common cause of acquired TS and results in fibrosis and scarring of the valve leaflets, leaflet doming, and commissural fusion. Reduced leaflet mobility and a smaller tricuspid orifice impair RV filling. In addition to TS, rheumatic tricuspid disease is characterized by TR, and the mitral valve is almost always involved.

Endocarditis. TV vegetations appear as oscillating, echo-dense masses attached to the leaflets or annulus. Typically, TV vegetations involve the atrial surface of affected leaflets and are larger than left-sided vegetations. Endocarditis may cause leaflet destruction that results in a flail leaflet and TR.

Carcinoid syndrome. Carcinoid tumors typically originate in the ileum and release serotonin, bradykinins, histamine, and prostaglandins. These vasoactive substances can damage the TV and pulmonic valve (PV), but they typically do not affect the left-sided heart valves as a consequence of inactivation of the tumor secretions in the lungs by monoamine oxidase. *Typical features include thickening and fibrosis of the TV and PV with moderate to severe TR, mild TS, and PS* (13). TR is caused primarily by restricted leaflet mobility. In contrast to rheumatic heart disease, carcinoid syndrome does not result in tricuspid leaflet doming or commissural fusion.

Ebstein anomaly. Ebstein anomaly is a congenital condition in which a malformed TV is displaced into the RV cavity. Typically, the anterior leaflet is the least affected, with the septal and posterior leaflets either rudimentary or absent. Ebstein anomaly should be suspected when the long-axis separation between the mitral and tricuspid annular planes exceeds 8 mm/m^2. This marked apical displacement of the TV causes a portion of the morphologic RV to become atrialized (14). Associated features may include impaired RV function, conduction abnormalities, and TR.

PULMONIC VALVE

Anatomy

The PV is a trileaflet valve with anterior, right, and left posterior semilunar cusps. The PV leaflets are thinner than the aortic valve leaflets and are directly connected to the musculature of the RV.

Transesophageal Echocardiographic Views

Because of its anterior position, detailed images of the PV are difficult to obtain with TEE. In fact, complete ultrasound assessment of the PV often requires a transthoracic echocardiographic (TTE) examination. The anteriorly located structures of the right side of the heart are more accessible to TTE imaging, and TTE also provides a greater number of acoustic windows and a greater ability to angulate the ultrasound probe, thereby improving the alignment of the Doppler beam.

1. *Midesophageal right ventricular inflow-outflow view.* The most reliable TEE scan plan for imaging the PV is the ME RV inflow-outflow view. In this imaging plane, the aortic valve provides a useful anatomic guide. The PV can be identified in its normal location adjacent to the commissure separating the right and left coronary cusps of the aortic valve. Because the PV is oriented roughly at a right angle to the aortic valve, it is typically seen in its long axis when the aortic valve is seen in short axis.
2. *Midesophageal aortic valve short-axis view.* In the ME aortic valve short-axis view, the PV may be seen again in long axis adjacent to the aortic valve. Further gradual withdrawal of the probe will display the main PA above the PV and its bifurcation into left and right branches. With the probe at this position high in the esophagus, advancement of the transducer angle to 90 degrees reveals the upper esophageal aortic arch short-axis view. In many patients, the main PA, the PV, and the distal RVOT can be seen beneath the aortic arch. This may be a particularly useful view for detecting PR or quantifying PS with continuous wave Doppler because of the advantageous parallel alignment with blood flow (Fig. 14.11).
3. *Transgastric pulmonic valve view.* From the TG LV midpapillary short-axis view, the probe is rotated to examine the structures of the right side of the heart. The transducer is then rotated to 110 to 140 degrees to obtain a view of the RVOT and PV (Fig. 14.12). This view is useful for obtaining Doppler measurements of cardiac output from the RVOT (15).

Pulmonic Regurgitation

Congenital PR may result from abnormal cusp number or development. Acquired PR often results from pulmonary hypertension and subsequent annular dilation and structural

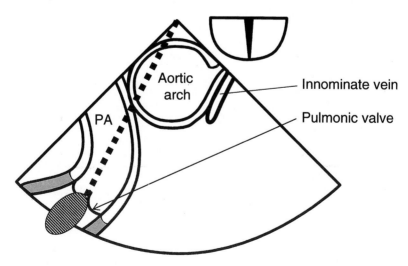

FIG. 14.11. Schematic diagram of image used to evaluate the severity of pulmonic regurgitation or stenosis.

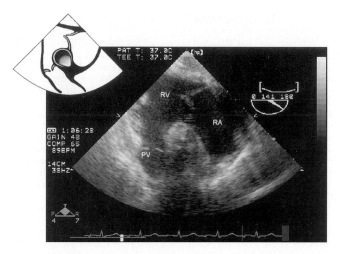

FIG. 14.12. Transesophageal echocardiographic image of the transgastric pulmonic valve view.

distortion. Evaluation of the severity of PR is primarily through the qualitative examination of color flow Doppler mapping. *PA catheters have a minimal effect on the severity of PR or TR* (16).

Pulmonic Stenosis

PS is most commonly congenital but may occasionally result from rheumatic heart disease, carcinoid, or infective endocarditis. The severity of stenosis can be evaluated through qualitative assessments of leaflet motion or Doppler examination.

Two-dimensional echocardiography. Features of PS include abnormal initial systolic leaflet motion and subsequent doming of stenotic leaflets into the PA.

Doppler echocardiography. Doppler features of PS include increased flow velocities through the stenotic valve and turbulence beyond the orifice.

Ross Procedure

In 1967, Donald Ross first described the replacement of a diseased aortic valve with the patient's own PV (i.e., a pulmonary autograft). The TEE examination plays an important role in determining the suitability of candidates for this procedure. The examination should include an assessment for PR and measurement of the annular dimensions of both the pulmonic and aortic valves. *Significant PR or a mismatch in semilunar valve annular dimensions of more than 2 mm is considered a contraindication to this procedure* (17). *Following the Ross procedure, the patient should be evaluated for aortic insufficiency because this is a primary indication of autograft failure.* Additionally, an assessment of LV wall motion may reveal a new septal LV regional wall motion abnormality, which can result from the unintentional ligation of a septal coronary artery branch during dissection and excision of the PV.

SUMMARY

This chapter has explained how TEE provides an extensive evaluation of the right side of the heart and its associated valves. By using the standard TEE views, the echocardiographer can learn to evaluate the right side of the heart as efficiently as the left.

REFERENCES

1. Weyman AE. *Principles and practices of echocardiography.* Philadelphia: Lea & Febiger, 1994:914–915.
2. Otto CM. *Textbook of clinical echocardiography.* Philadelphia: WB Saunders, 2000: 120–122.
3. Hammerstrom E, Wranne B, Pinto FJ, et al. Tricuspid annular motion. *J Am Soc Echocardiogr* 1991;14:131–139.
4. Wilson, BC, Cohn JN. Right ventricular infarction complicating left ventricular infarction secondary to coronary heart disease. *Am J Cardiol* 1978;42:885–894.
5. D'Arcy B, Nanda NC. Two-dimensional echocardiographic features of right ventricular infarction. *Circulation* 1982;65:1967–1973.
6. Sharkey SW, Shelley W, Carlyle PF, et al. M-mode and two-dimensional echocardiographic analysis of the septum in experimental RV infarction: correlation with hemodynamic alterations. *Am Heart J* 1985;110:1210–1218.
7. Judgutt BI, Sussex BA, Sivaram CA, et al. Right ventricular infarction: two-dimensional echocardiographic evaluation. *Am Heart J* 1984;107:505–515.
8. Louie EK, Rich S, Levitsky S, et al. Doppler echocardiographic demonstration of the differential effects of right ventricular pressure and volume overload on left ventricular geometry and filling. *J Am Coll Cardiol* 1992;19:84–90.
9. Jardin F, Dubourg O, Bourdarias J-P. Echocardiographic pattern of acute cor pulmonale. *Chest* 1997;111:209–217.
10. Triulizi MO, et al. Normal adult cross-section echo values: linear dimensions and chamber areas. *Echocardiography* 1984;1:403–426.
11. Perez, JE, Ludbrook PA, Ahumada GG. Usefulness of Doppler echocardiography in detecting tricuspid valve stenosis. *Am J Cardiol* 1985;55:601–603.
12. Feigenbaum H. *Echocardiography,* 5th ed. Philadelphia: Lea & Febiger, 1994:302–307.
13. Pellikka PA, Tajik AJ, Khandheria BK, et al. Carcinoid heart disease: clinical and echocardiographic spectrum in 74 patients. *Circulation* 1993;87:1188–1196.
14. Shiina A, Seward JB, Edwards WD, et al. Two-dimensional echocardiographic spectrum of Ebstein's anomaly: detailed anatomic assessment. *J Am Coll Cardiol* 1984;3: 356–370.
15. Maslow A, Communale ME, Haering JM, et al. Pulsed wave Doppler measurements of cardiac output from the right ventricular outflow tract. *Anesth Analg* 1996;83: 466–471.
16. Goldman ME, Guarino T, Fuster V, et al. The necessity for tricuspid valve repair can be determined intraoperatively by two-dimensional echocardiography. *J Thorac Cardiovasc Surg* 1987;94:542–550.
17. Albertucci M, Karp RB. Aortic valvular allografts and pulmonary autografts. In: Edmunds LH, ed. *Cardiac surgery in the adult.* New York: McGraw-Hill, 1997:911–937.

QUESTIONS

1. Which of the following standard TEE scan planes allows an assessment of ventricular septal motion?
   a. ME bicaval
   b. ME RV inflow-outflow
   c. ME two-chamber
   d. TG midpapillary short-axis
   e. TG RV inflow
2. In patients with RV volume overload, ventricular septal displacement toward the LV is maximal at which point in the cardiac cycle?
   a. End-diastole
   b. End-systole
   c. Mid diastole
   d. Mid systole

3. Which of the following structures is located in the RV?
   a. Chiari network
   b. Crista terminalis
   c. Eustachian valve
   d. Moderator band
4. In patients with RV dysfunction resulting from severe TR, the cardiac apex
   a. Is akinetic
   b. Is formed by the RV
   c. Is displaced toward the base of the heart
   d. Moves paradoxically outward during systole
5. Which of the following standard TEE scan planes allows assessment of TS with continuous wave Doppler?
   a. ME bicaval
   b. ME RV inflow-outflow
   c. TG midpapillary short-axis
   d. TG RV inflow
6. Which of the following features distinguishes Ebstein anomaly from endocardial cushion defects?
   a. Conduction abnormalities
   b. Long-axis position of the TV
   c. PS
   d. TR
7. In the schematic diagram of normal hepatic venous flow shown, which of the following waves is indicated by the asterisk?
   a. A wave
   b. D wave
   c. S wave
   d. V wave

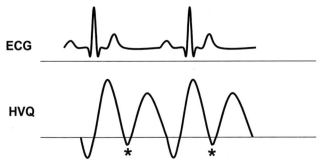

8. Which of the following diagnoses is suggested by the observation of a 5-mm tricuspid annular plane systolic excursion?
   a. RV hypertrophy
   b. RV hypokinesia
   c. TR
   d. TS
9. Compared with the aortic valve, the PV
   a. Has a more rigid annular ring
   b. Has thinner leaflets
   c. Is adjacent to the noncoronary cusp
   d. Is oriented in a parallel scan plane
10. Following a pulmonary autograft (Ross) procedure, which of the following must be sought/evaluated echocardiographically to detect the complications associated with this operation?
    a. Aortic valve stenosis
    b. Mitral valve regurgitation
    c. TS
    d. Ventricular septal function

PART IV

CLINICAL CHALLENGES

Transesophageal Echocardiography for Coronary Revascularization

Stuart J. Weiss and John G. Augoustides

Transesophageal echocardiography (TEE) has evolved to become a critical element in the advanced care of the cardiac surgical patient. Its importance for valvular surgery is widely accepted, but its role for coronary artery bypass grafting is still evolving. TEE is a powerful and versatile tool that can be used to diagnosis the cause of ischemia, acute hemodynamic decompensation, or occult pathology and to facilitate the conduct and management of bypass. Echocardiography can also be used as a hemodynamic monitor to determine cardiac output (CO), stroke volume, pulmonary artery (PA) and right ventricular (RV) systolic pressures. At the current time, it is doubtful that TEE will supplant the PA catheter for hemodynamic monitoring. TEE and the PA catheter have complementary roles in the perioperative setting; the choice depends on factors such as clinician preference, cost, and resource availability. The PA catheter permits continuous measurement of intracardiac pressures and CO, particularly in the postoperative setting, when TEE is often not readily available. Although the PA catheter detects cardiac dysfunction, it often does not diagnose the cause. The forte of TEE is the rapid diagnosis of cardiac dysfunction and analysis that immediately affects both surgical and hemodynamic management, even in the setting of PA catheterization.

INDICATIONS AND APPLICATIONS OF TRANSESOPHAGEAL ECHOCARDIOGRAPHY

TEE is particularly useful during coronary artery bypass grafting (CABG) to assess the clinical significance of dynamic valvular dysfunction, diagnose the cause of ischemia and acute hemodynamic instability, and assist in the conduct of circulatory management and surgery. TEE is the approach most commonly used because the examination does not interfere with the progress of surgery. The value of perioperative echocardiography was evaluated in 1996 by the American Society of Anesthesiologists and the Society of Cardiovascular Anesthesiologists (1). However, these guidelines were based on limited clinical data and need to be reevaluated in light of advances in technology, improvements in surgical and anesthetic techniques, and an expanding base of literature.

A number of studies support an important role of TEE in improving outcome, especially in high-risk patients undergoing coronary revascularization (2). In comparison with historical matched controls, patients evaluated with TEE show decreased rates of mortality and infarction. In our current health care environment, a significant number of patients arrive in the operating room for surgery with an incomplete preoperative evaluation. TEE can serve an important function in the evaluation of patients who are undergoing emergent surgery with an inadequate cardiac evaluation and the potential for undiagnosed cardiac pathology that would affect perioperative management. TEE can assist the surgeon, cardiologist, and anesthesiologist at each stage of CABG surgery (Table 15.1).

CONTRAINDICATIONS AND COMPLICATIONS
OF TRANSESOPHAGEAL ECHOCARDIOGRAPHY

The risk for complications associated with insertion of the TEE probe and performance of the examination is low. In a case series of 7,200 cardiac surgical patients studied at a single institution, the reported incidence of morbidity was 0.2% (severe odynophagia, 0.1%; displacement of the endotracheal tube, 0.3%; upper gastrointestinal hemorrhage, 0.03%; dental injury, 0.03%; esophageal perforation, 0.01%) (3). Although esophageal trauma leading to mediastinitis is rare, it has a significant mortality of approximately 10% (4). Therefore, esophageal pathology (e.g., web, stricture, diverticulum, cancer) and prior esophageal

TABLE 15.1. USES OF TRANSESOPHAGEAL ECHOCARDIOGRAPHY IN PATIENTS UNDERGOING CORONARY ARTERY BYPASS GRAFTING

To supplement an incomplete cardiac workup
Confirm diagnosis and evaluate cardiac function for patients undergoing emergent surgery
Provide an updated examination of cardiac and valvular function
Evaluate potential target sites of coronary revascularization by administration of contrast
 agents (evaluate coronary perfusion) or dobutamine (stress test to evaluate viability)
To assist the surgeon in the conduct of circulatory management
Positioning/placement of:
 Aortic cross-clamp
 Coronary sinus catheter
 Intraaortic balloon pump
 Femoral venous cannula
 Ventricular assist device cannula
 MIDCAB (endoaortic catheter, venous cannula, pulmonary artery drainage catheter,
  coronary sinus catheter)
To diagnose cause of acute cardiovascular compromise
To diagnose impact of previously unrecognized pathology on surgical procedure
Valvular pathology:
 Aortic insufficiency distension of the ventricle during cardiopulmonary bypass
 Mitral regurgitation: dynamic MR ischemic
Patent foramen ovale/atrial septal defect
Emboli, thrombus, or mass
Persistent left superior vena cava
Onset of regional wall motion abnormalities
Aortic dissection
Atherosclerotic disease
To facilitate the conduct of circulatory management or surgical procedure
Redo sternotomy
Conduct of bypass: assess left ventricle chamber size for distention
Plan management strategies for separation from cardiopulmonary bypass for patients with
 poor cardiac function
Separation from cardiopulmonary bypass (titration of volume and pharmacologic support)

---

surgery are contraindications to insertion of the TEE probe. In such cases, surface scanning with a hand-held probe should be considered.

SURFACE SCANNING: EPICARDIAL AND EPIAORTIC SCANNING

The alternative to TEE is surface scanning with a hand-held probe. Surface scanning of the heart (epicardial imaging) and aorta (epiaortic imaging) is the procedure of choice when TEE is contraindicated or the acoustic window for TEE is inadequate. *Because the air-filled trachea is interposed, TEE provides only limited imaging of the ascending aorta. Epiaortic scanning is being increasingly used to detect severe atheromatous disease, a significant risk factor for poor neurologic outcome.*

Surface scanning with a hand-held probe requires considerable patience and experience if optimal results are to be obtained (Fig. 15.1). The ultrasound probe is inserted in a sterile sheath filled with saline solution and positioned such that a column of fluid acts as a "standoff" between the structure of interest and the ultrasound crystal. This standoff enhances the imaging of structures in the near field (i.e., the anterior surface of the ascending aorta). Alternatively, a standoff device can be purchased or made to improve visualization of the near field. The probes typically feature 5- to 10-MHz transducers with two-dimensional and Doppler capability. Although surface scanning is suitable for most applications that

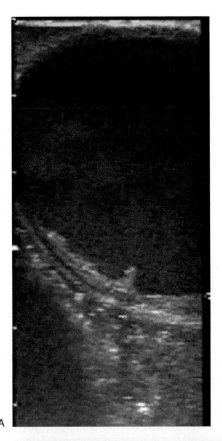

A

FIG. 15.1. Ultrasound imaging of the aorta is useful for detecting and assessing the severity of atherosclerotic disease. **A:** A high-frequency ultrasound probe that is placed in a sterile sheath is used to examine the ascending aorta before aortic cannulation and cross-clamping. A mobile plaque can be visualized in the posterior aspect of the aorta. **B:** A transesophageal echocardiographic probe can be used to evaluate the severity of disease in the descending thoracic aorta. A large plaque (P) is visualized just distal to the left subclavian artery.

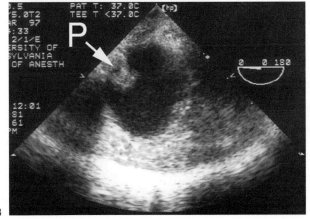

B

require TEE, *the major applications of surface scanning include assessing the severity of aortic atherosclerotic disease, confirming the patency of coronary grafts, elucidating the anatomy of intramyocardial coronary vessels, and diagnosing acute aortic dissections.*

BASIC APPROACH TO THE TRANSESOPHAGEAL ECHOCARDIOGRAPHIC EXAMINATION

The indication for the study should determine the direction and focus of the perioperative TEE examination. Regardless of the indication, each study should proceed in a routine and organized manner in which each structure of the heart and great vessels is examined in several imaging planes (5). The initial examination before cardiopulmonary bypass (CPB) is usually a more thorough standardized approach, whereas the post-CPB, "post-intervention" examination is commonly focused on a full assessment of the intervention and possible complications thereof. Digital cine loops of pre-CPB cardiac function should be recorded for readily available review and comparison with the post-CPB examination findings. Excessive focus of the pre-CPB examination on one aspect may jeopardize patient care as a consequence of missed or incorrect diagnoses. Unexpected findings are not uncommon and may have a significant impact on perioperative management. For example, the diagnosis of persistent left superior vena cava is a contraindication to retrograde cardioplegia, and the finding of previously unrecognized dynamic mitral valvular insufficiency might alter surgical management. The strategy of progressing through a standardized protocol will decrease the chances of missing important findings (Table 15.1). A complete TEE examination should include a written report for the medical record and a review of the findings with the cardiac surgeon. The process of writing a report provides a mechanism for critically reviewing the recorded study and making sure that all relevant images and measurements have been acquired.

TRANSESOPHAGEAL ECHOCARDIOGRAPHIC ASSESSMENT OF VENTRICULAR FUNCTION

Two-Dimensional Measurements of Ventricular Size

TEE is a versatile monitor of cardiac function in that it can provide either a rapid qualitative assessment of chamber size and function or quantitative measures of chamber size, intracardiac pressures, and hemodynamic indices, such as stroke volume and CO (Table 15.2). Left ventricular (LV) function is first evaluated from the midesophageal (ME) four-chamber long-axis and two-chamber views; the TEE probe should then be advanced into the stomach to obtain a series of transgastric (TG) short-axis views. The ME views permit rapid qualitative evaluation of all four cardiac chambers but are used less commonly for quantitative planimetry because of apical foreshortening. The TG short-axis ventricular views are most commonly used to monitor global and regional function because the image planes are relatively easy to maintain (Fig. 15.2). Experienced echocardiographers use these views to quantify global ventricular function, the ejection fraction, and the adequacy of the LV preload. In a study of Cheung et al. (6), TEE was highly sensitive for detecting changes in LV function and preload following controlled decreases in the circulating blood volume. The changes in the LV end-diastolic area accurately reflected the decrement in LV preload and PA pressures. This application is very helpful in titrating volume administration during separation from CPB or periods of bleeding.

Planimetry can quantify changes in LV area (LV end-diastolic area [EDA] and end-systolic area [ESA]). The fractional area change (FAC) is then calculated as follows: FAC = 100 × (EDA − ESA)/EDA. The TEE-derived changes in LV area are accurate and reproducible but may not directly correlate with changes in LV volume. Assumptions based on LV areas measured in one plane may not reliably reflect LV volume, particularly in patients with regional wall motion abnormalities (RWMAs) and LV aneurysms. Geometric algorithms can be used to calculate LV volume; they typically require multiple measurements in several imaging planes. The correlation of end-diastolic and end-systolic volumes with the ejection fraction is clinically acceptable but consistently underestimates the true changes in ventricular

TABLE 15.2. ASSESSMENT OF CARDIAC FUNCTION BY TRANSESOPHAGEAL ECHOCARDIOGRAPHY

Preload
    LV end-diastolic area
    LV end-diastolic pressure (estimated from AI jet)
    LA pressure (estimated from pulmonary vein flow)
Contractility
    Fractional area change (calculated)
    Ejection fraction (visual estimate)
    Segmental wall motion
    Fractional shortening
    Tissue Doppler
Quantitative hemodynamics
    Stroke volume/cardiac output
    Systemic vascular resistance
    RV systolic pressure
Diastolic function
    Mitral inflow velocities
    Pulmonary vein blood flow velocities

LV, left ventricle; LA, left atrium; AI, aortic insufficiency; RV, right ventricle.

volume because of foreshortening of LV length in the four-chamber view. *Because performing planimetry and the aforementioned calculations is time-consuming, their application is usually limited to off-line analysis.*

Until recently, TEE was limited in regard to the continuous processing and reporting of reliable quantitative numeric parameters. However, the development of continuous automated border detection is a technologic advance that can be applied in research and clinically. Proprietary algorithms are used to discriminate the endocardial interface and thus continually measure changes in the chamber area. The difference between the LV end-diastolic area and the LV end-systolic area is continuously calculated to yield an on-line FAC (see Fig. 3.5). Perrino et al. (7) demonstrated good correlation between automated measurement of

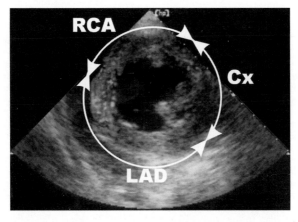

FIG. 15.2. The transgastric short-axis view is routinely used intraoperatively to assess left ventricular function and diagnose myocardial ischemia. Myocardial function at the midpapillary level reflects the vascular distribution of the three major coronary arteries: the left anterior descending (*LAD*), circumflex (*Cx*), and right coronary (*RCA*) arteries.

ventricular dimensions and off-line manual measurements of these parameters by experienced echocardiographers. However, the proprietary technology of automated border detection has not gained wide clinical popularity as a continuous monitor because of technical limitations related to ventricular wall resolution and artifacts related to movement of the heart.

Quantitative Assessment of Left Ventricular Function: Cardiac Output

Two-dimensional and Doppler echocardiography are used to evaluate stroke volume and CO. This is accomplished by measuring the transit of blood through an area of known size (e.g., the mitral valve, LV outflow tract, or PA). Although the transmitral inflow velocity is easy to obtain, its agreement with measurements obtained by thermodilution is unacceptable because of inaccuracy in measuring the area of the mitral valve orifice (8). Savino et al. (9) describe a better correlation with the use of the transpulmonic flow. This approach may be limited by the difficulty of consistently interrogating the transpulmonic blood flow and measuring the dimensions of the proximal PA. The alternative method is to measure the transit of blood through the LV outflow tract or aortic valve in the TG long-axis and deep TG long-axis views (10) (see Fig. 6.3). Combining the TEE-derived CO with the mean arterial pressure and the mean central venous pressure can yield the systemic vascular resistance. These measures of stroke volume, CO, and systemic vascular resistance are particularly useful when PA catheter measurements are not available.

Assessment of Intracardiac Pressures

TEE measures important intracardiac pressures by quantifying the pressure gradient across a regurgitant valve (Table 15.2). The flow velocity of the regurgitant jet (v) is measured with Doppler echocardiography. The pressure gradient (ΔP) across the regurgitant valve is then calculated with the simplified Bernoulli equation: $\Delta P = 4v^2$. The accuracy of the measurements depends on the presence of valvular insufficiency and correct alignment of the regurgitant jet. Like the TEE measurements of CO, these measurements are laborious and not automated. Consequently, the PA catheter currently is still preferred over TEE for the on-line measurement of intracardiac pressures.

MONITORING OF ISCHEMIA

Predictive Value of Regional Wall Motion Abnormalities for Myocardial Infarction

The clinical application of TEE to detect and monitor myocardial ischemia gained considerable attention in the early 1980s (11). TEE can diagnose and characterize myocardial ischemia by a more sensitive method than either the electrocardiogram or pulmonary artery catheter. Canine studies documented that the reduction in coronary blood flow occurs in rapid association with the decrease in regional myocardial function and precedes any ischemic changes on the electrocardiogram (12,13). The TG short-axis view is the one most commonly used to monitor and diagnose ischemia because it reflects the distribution of all three major coronary vessels (Fig. 15.2).

In two classic studies by Roizen et al. (14) and Smith et al. (15), the occurrence of postoperative myocardial infarction was increased in patients who exhibited new RWMAs during CABG or aortic vascular surgery. The incidence of postoperative infarction was more strongly associated with the new RWMAs than with new electrocardiographic changes. *Although TEE may be sensitive in diagnosing ischemia, a new RWMA does not always predict myocardial infarction.* In the study of Leung et al. (16), a myocardial infarction was subsequently diagnosed in only one of eight patients in whom a new, persistent RWMA had developed. This apparent discrepancy is consistent with the concept of "myocardial stunning," in which an acute episode of myocardial ischemia can result in wall motion abnormalities that later resolve without any permanent injury. Alternatively, new RWMAs may be related to loading conditions of the ventricle, electrolyte abnormalities, blood viscosity, level of

TABLE 15.3. STRATEGY FOR MANAGEMENT OF A NEW REGIONAL WALL MOTION ABNORMALITY AFTER SEPARATION FROM CARDIOPULMONARY BYPASS

Increase the coronary perfusion pressure
Restore normal conduction pathways (sinus rhythm, A-pace)
Normalize electrolytes and arterial blood gases
Inspect coronary grafts
    Visual inspection and stripping
    Doppler flow examination
    Echo contrast examination
Return to cardiopulmonary bypass

---

inotropic support, hypothermia, cardiac pacing, and bundle branch conduction abnormalities. *Any apparent dyskinesis that is attributable to conduction abnormalities can be differentiated from ischemia by closely evaluating the area in question for the presence of myocardial thickening.*

Strategy for the Management of a New Regional Wall Motion Abnormality after Cardiopulmonary Bypass

The appearance of new RWMAs after bypass is common, but the interpretation is complicated by factors such as infusion of inotropic drugs, inadequate recovery from cardioplegia, conduction abnormalities, and transient ischemia resulting from the distal coronary embolization of air or debris. Although some investigators have suggested that the detection of new RWMAs warrants further surgical intervention, no prospective study is available to support such an aggressive approach. The additional morbidity/mortality associated with the resumption of bypass to place another graft would likely outweigh the potential benefit in most cases. A more rational, conservative approach may include the following: increasing the coronary perfusion pressure to flush any emboli or residual cardioplegic agents, restoring normal conduction pathways, normalizing the arterial blood gases and electrolytes, and inspecting the coronary grafts to confirm patency (Table 15.3). New RWMAs, such as ventricular septal wall motion abnormalities, are often related to conduction disturbances caused by ventricular pacing or bundle branch block. Atrial pacing commonly restores the normal ventricular conduction pathway and contractile synchrony of the ventricular septum. If atrial pacing is not possible, the most common bundle branch conduction abnormalities usually resolve within the first postoperative day. In addition, the surgeon can assess graft patency and flow by visual inspection to confirm the absence of graft kinking or torsion, by stripping the vein graft to confirm refill, by palpation, and by use of a Doppler flow probe. Decreased flow in an arterial conduit can result from poor distal runoff, a compromised anastomosis, or vasospasm that can be effectively treated by infusing a calcium channel antagonist such as nicardipine. Differentiation between poor perfusion and stunned myocardium is more difficult. A possible strategy is the administration of a contrast agent to determine coronary flow patterns. If the area demonstrates flow of the contrast agent, the RWMA may resolve with time. The absence of contrast agent suggests a technical problem at the anastomosis or distal obstruction in the native coronary. Such information can help guide any possible surgical intervention. The technique of contrast perfusion can also be performed before bypass. If a specific area is likely to be infarcted, as demonstrated by the absence of contrast flow and significant wall thinning, surgical interventions are not likely to be of value. This technique is uncommonly applied in routine operative practice, and its impact remains to be determined.

ACUTE CARDIAC DYSFUNCTION: ASSESSMENT AND MANAGEMENT

Cardiac dysfunction may develop at any time during the perioperative period. *The prompt, accurate diagnosis of the cause of hemodynamic instability is one of the major applications, if not the forte, of TEE.* Ultrasound examination of the heart and great vessels can provide a

TABLE 15.4. ECHOCARDIOGRAPHIC FINDINGS IN HYPOTENSION
AND CARDIAC DYSFUNCTION

	LVEDA	LVESA	FAC	CO
Decreased LV preload	↓	↓	0	↓
Decreased LV afterload	0	↓↓	↑↑	↑
Increased LV afterload	↑	↑	↓	↓
LV dysfunction	↑	↑↑	↓↓	↓
RV dysfunction	↓	↓	↓/0	↓
Acute mitral regurgitation				
LV distention	↑↑	0/↑	↓	↓

LVEDA, left ventricular end-diastolic diameter; LVESA, end-systolic diameter; FAC, fractional area change; CO, cardiac output; RV, right ventricle.

quick assessment of the primary factors related to hypotension: preload, afterload, myocardial contractility, valvular function, and integrity of the aorta. TEE can significantly affect the surgical and anesthetic management, especially in high-risk patients or in patients with acute hemodynamic collapse. The reader is reminded that post-CPB cardiac function must be interpreted in the context of the pre-bypass examination findings and the occurrence of any significant bypass events.

The echocardiographic examination quickly provides data that guides pharmacologic therapy and volume resuscitation. In several studies, echocardiography significantly modified both surgical and hemodynamic decision making during the perioperative period (17). The echocardiographic findings associated with common causes of hypotension and cardiac dysfunction are presented in Table 15.4.

Hypovolemia

Hypovolemia, a common cause of perioperative hypotension, is often related to the obstruction of venous inflow as a consequence of pre-bypass cannula placement, volume reequilibration after separation from bypass, and bleeding. Hypovolemia can be differentiated from low systemic vascular resistance by assessing the LV chamber size and contractility. The assessment of LV chamber size by TEE has been shown to be a sensitive measure of LV preload. In the study of Cheung et al. (6), the quantitative analysis of changes in the TG short-axis area could reliably detect even a 2.5% decrease in intravascular volume.

Dynamic Mitral Regurgitation

The development of mitral regurgitation may be associated with hypotension, increased pulmonary pressures, RV failure, and decreased CO. Excessive volume resuscitation or increased afterload can result in LV distention with incomplete coaptation of the mitral leaflets and a central jet of regurgitation. Alternatively, ischemia or LV dysfunction can lead to papillary muscle dysfunction or LV distention. Significant mitral regurgitation may require mitral valve surgery or hemodynamic management, such as adjusting the systemic vascular resistance, administering inotropic agents, or decreasing the LV preload.

Right Ventricular Dysfunction

RV dysfunction is another common cause of perioperative hypotension. The ME four-chamber view allows a rapid assessment of ventricular chamber size and function. RV dysfunction is associated with RV dilation, tricuspid regurgitation, abnormal septal wall motion, and decreased LV chamber size. The management of RV dysfunction includes checking for ischemia

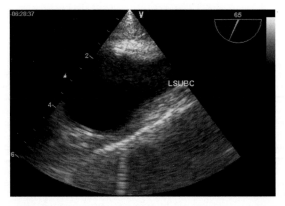

FIG. 15.3. The descending aorta short-axis view demonstrating the takeoff of the left subclavian artery (*LSUB*). An intraaortic balloon pump should not be visualized in this view but 2 cm distally for optimal placement.

in the distribution of the right coronary artery, hyperventilation to decrease pulmonary vascular resistance, administration of inotropic agents that also decrease pulmonary vascular resistance (e.g., milrinone, dobutamine), and titration of pulmonary vasodilators (nitric oxide, prostaglandin E_1, or nitroglycerin).

Intraaortic Balloon Counterpulsation

Severe global LV dysfunction may require more aggressive management, including the institution of intraaortic balloon counterpulsation (IABP). TEE is often used to confirm proper location of the guidewire and positioning of the IABP. The cross section of the descending thoracic aorta can be visualized by positioning the TEE probe at the ME level and rotating it counterclockwise. The image depth is then decreased to approximately 6 cm, and the probe is slowly withdrawn until the origin of the left subclavian artery and distal aortic arch are visualized (Fig. 15.3). The pulsatile hyperrefractile IABP is advanced to a location 1 to 2 cm distal to the origin of the left subclavian artery. If the cardiac dysfunction is refractory to such interventions, TEE can also be used to assist the surgeon in placing a mechanical ventricular assist device.

TRANSESOPHAGEAL ECHOCARDIOGRAPHY FOR PREVENTING LEFT VENTRICULAR DISTENTION

Distention of the LV during bypass results in increased chamber pressure that decreases coronary perfusion and stretches myocardial fibers. If unrecognized or untreated, LV distention can result in severe cardiac dysfunction that complicates attempts at separation from CPB. LV distention may be caused by excessive return from the bronchial and thebesian veins or by unsuspected aortic regurgitation during the administration of antegrade cardioplegia.

Distention of the RV is usually obvious to the observer because of its anterior location. In contrast, LV distention may not be visually appreciated in the surgical field because it is located posteriorly. TEE can be used to evaluate the chamber size serially by imaging the LV in the TG short-axis and ME four chamber views. If LV distention or a gradual increase in the pulmonary pressures is noted, the conduct of bypass is altered by placing a drainage cannula in the PA or superior pulmonary vein to aspirate blood and decompress the ventricle.

ROLE OF TRANSESOPHAGEAL ECHOCARDIOGRAPHY IN VASCULAR CANNULATION

Imaging the Ascending Aorta

Atherosclerotic disease of the ascending aorta is a significant risk factor for stroke and a poor neurologic outcome after CABG (18–20). Assessment of the aorta is feasible with both TEE and epiaortic imaging. Palpation by the surgeon is not sensitive in detecting atherosclerotic disease except for hard calcific plaques (21). TEE is an excellent modality with which to examine the descending thoracic aorta and aortic arch, but the acoustic window of the mid and distal ascending aorta is inadequate. *TEE fails to image 42% of the ascending aorta because visualization is obstructed by the air-filled trachea and left main bronchus* (21). In comparison, epiaortic scanning provides excellent imaging of these areas and is significantly more sensitive than TEE in detecting clinically significant atherosclerotic disease in the ascending aorta. In a study of 81 cardiac surgical patients, epicardial imaging detected 14 of 15 patients with significant atherosclerotic disease, whereas TEE identified only 5 of 15 patients (22).

The ascending aorta is best imaged by epicardial scanning with the transducer placed in a sterile sheath filled with saline solution (Fig. 15.1). The surgeon usually performs the manipulation with the assistance of the echocardiographer. The examination should proceed in the following fashion:

1. The scanning depth is set to about 5 cm, and the probe is positioned at the level of the aortic valve to produce a cross-sectional image.
2. The probe is then slowly advanced distally to the arch, with care taken to identify atheroma on the anterior surface at the sites of cannulation and cross-clamping.
3. The longitudinal image can be obtained by manually rotating the transducer about 90 degrees until the long axis of the aorta is visualized, after which the probe is again slowly advanced along the aorta.

The epiaortic examination should determine the plaque thickness in millimeters and its mobility and location. The presence of mobile plaque or a plaque thickness greater than 5 mm indicates severe atheromatous disease and is a risk factor for poor outcome.

Management Strategy for Aortic Atheromatous Disease

The detection of significant pathology warrants consideration of modifying the aortic cannulation to reduce the risk for cerebral atheroembolism. The possible modifications of surgical technique include the following: avoiding bypass with off-pump CABG, alternating the aortic cannulation and cross-clamp sites, using endoaortic balloon occlusion, avoiding a side-biting aortic clamp by performing both distal and proximal coronary anastomoses within a single ischemic period, and performing coronary revascularization under hypothermic circulatory arrest (23–27). In the presence of severe aortic pathology, the surgeon may consider elective aortic atherectomy or replacement of the ascending aorta and arch. *We recommend that epiaortic scanning of the aorta be performed in patients who are considered at increased risk for neurologic complications.* The patients most likely to benefit are those with a history of stroke or prior CABG surgery, an age past 70 years, diabetes mellitus, hypertension, peripheral vascular disease, or a diagnosis of significant atheromatous disease by TEE examination or surgical palpation (18–20). The main objection to the use of this technology is the additional training, equipment, and time required to perform an examination adequately. Such concerns should diminish as individual surgeons gain more experience and the technology enters the mainstream of clinical practice.

Administration of Antegrade Cardioplegia

Antegrade cardioplegia is the most common method of cardiac preservation during bypass. It is usually administered by cannulating the ascending aorta. The delivery of cardioplegia depends on a competent aortic valve to pressurize the aortic root and drive the agent into the coronary vessels. *The presence of aortic valvular regurgitation not only compromises myocardial preservation but can result in LV distention, an important cause of post-CPB LV dysfunction.* It may be difficult for the surgeon to diagnose significant aortic regurgitation clinically because the LV is located posteriorly and therefore not easily visible. The prompt diagnosis of significant aortic regurgitation by TEE can alter the conduct of surgery as follows: administration of antegrade cardioplegia via a hand-held cannula after aortotomy, use of retrograde cardioplegia, decompression of the LV, or replacement of the aortic valve. Aortic regurgitation is best detected and characterized by using the ME long-axis view of the aortic valve. The severity of regurgitation is determined by comparing the diameter of the regurgitant jet with the diameter of the outflow tract (see Chapter 11). The diagnosis of anything more than mild aortic regurgitation should prompt the aforementioned considerations.

Administration of Retrograde Cardioplegia

Retrograde cardioplegia is routinely performed during CABG surgery as an adjunct to antegrade cardioplegia. This technique is often used in the presence of severe LV hypertrophy, severe proximal coronary artery disease, aortic regurgitation, or pathology within the aortic root that may compromise the delivery of antegrade cardioplegia. An incision is made in the right atrium, and the coronary sinus cannula is directed into the ostium of the coronary sinus, which lies inferiorly and medially in the right atrium adjacent to the tricuspid valve. Placement is commonly confirmed by palpating the catheter in the coronary sinus as it courses along the atrioventricular groove. Catheter malposition, which can be difficult to detect, puts the patient at risk for myocardial ischemia during bypass. Positioning the catheter may be difficult because of variations in the anatomy, such as eustachian valves, a thickened Chiari network, or thebesian valves. Another anatomic variant that complicates the administration of retrograde cardioplegia is the presence of a persistent left superior vena cava that empties the left central venous circulation into the coronary sinus instead of the superior vena cava via the innominate vein. Although the incidence of this congenital variant is low, timely detection is important to prevent the misdirection of cardioplegia into the left arm away from the heart. In addition, misdirection of the cannula through the tricuspid valve into the RV or insufficient advancement of the cannula negates the benefit of cardioplegia.

Echocardiography is useful to assist the surgeon in positioning the catheter. The stippled appearance of the balloon at the tip of the retrograde catheter can be easily identified as it is engaged in the ostium of the coronary sinus. The ostium of the coronary sinus is best viewed by slight retroflexion of the probe in the ME four-chamber view. The final position of the catheter can be confirmed by the presence of the thin hollow cannula within the lumen of the coronary sinus (Fig. 15.4).

Femoral Venous Cannulation

The surgical placement of a femoral venous cannula can be facilitated with the use of TEE, first to confirm the location of the guidewire in the right atrium and later to verify adequate positioning of the cannula tip at the junction of the atrium and superior vena cava. The best view to visualize the cannula is the ME bicaval imaging plane. Slight rotation of the probe or readjustment of the angle should enable visualization of the echogenic cannula wall. Obstruction of the venous drainage can often be corrected by slightly advancing or withdrawing the catheter, which often abuts the venous wall or interatrial septum.

Femoral Arterial Cannulation

Femoral arterial cannulation is often used in cases of previous sternotomy, aortic dissection, or MIDCAB (endoaortic catheter, venous cannula, PA drainage catheter, coronary sinus catheter) surgery. After the surgeon has accessed the femoral artery, a guidewire is threaded

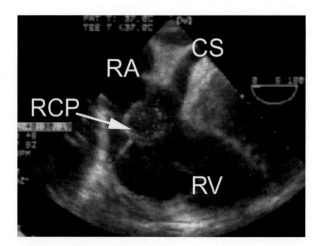

FIG. 15.4. A modified midesophageal four-chamber view can be used to visualize the coronary sinus. Transesophageal echocardiography can be used to assist the surgeon in positioning the retrograde cardioplegia cannula in the coronary sinus (*CS*). The *arrow* points to the balloon of the retrograde cannula (*RCP*), right atrium (*RA*), and right ventricle (*RV*). The ostium of the coronary sinus is best viewed by slightly retroflexing the probe in the midesophageal four-chamber view.

proximally into the descending aorta. Because it is very echogenic, the wire can easily be seen in the thoracic aorta. It is important to confirm the absence of an aortic dissection and correct placement of the cannula by visualizing the bypass blood flow with color flow Doppler.

TRANSESOPHAGEAL ECHOCARDIOGRAPHY IN PORT ACCESS SURGERY

In an effort to avoid median sternotomy and minimize invasiveness, a limited thoracotomy exposure is now being used for coronary revascularization. In this approach, the percutaneous cannulation for CPB and coronary artery anastomoses are performed through a series of small ports in the chest wall. The catheter-based Port Access system (Heartport, Redwood City, California) is based on a modified extracorporeal circulation and a combination of five intravascular cannulas (coronary sinus catheter, PA drainage catheter, intraaortic occlusive balloon, venous drainage catheter, and arterial drainage catheter).

Coronary Sinus and Pulmonary Catheters

The coronary sinus and pulmonary catheters are inserted percutaneously by the anesthesiologist via the right jugular venous approach. TEE or fluoroscopy can be used as a complementary technique to assist in positioning these cannulas. The PA drainage catheter decompresses the heart by aspirating blood from the PA. This catheter is inserted through a 9F introducer and advanced to a position distal to the pulmonic valve. Correct placement is confirmed by visualizing the catheter in the PA with TEE and by detecting a change in the pressure wave form as it is advanced distally. The PA is best visualized by slightly anteflexing and withdrawing the probe in the ME view. Confirmation of adequate drainage with this catheter is confirmed by using TEE to evaluate distention of the cardiac chambers. This is best achieved by monitoring the TG LV short-axis and ME four-chamber views.

Endoaortic Clamp

The endoaortic clamp is a triple-lumen balloon-tipped catheter that is introduced through the femoral arterial cannula and advanced into the ascending aorta. TEE is used to guide placement of the balloon catheter centrally in a position just distal to the sinuses of Valsalva. The ME long-axis view of the aortic valve is the best view for endoclamp positioning and monitoring during balloon inflation. The anesthesiologist must not only confirm correct initial positioning but also monitor to detect balloon migration. Migration of the balloon proximally can damage the aortic valve and distally can occlude blood flow to the arch vessels, resulting in cerebral ischemia. TEE is also used to monitor the delivery of antegrade cardioplegia through the lumen within the cannula and to detect LV distention.

TRANSESOPHAGEAL ECHOCARDIOGRAPHY FOR THE DIAGNOSIS OF OCCULT DISEASE

The detection of anatomic variants or incidental findings is fairly common (Table 15.5). No prospective outcome studies have addressed the issue of altering surgery based on unanticipated echocardiographic findings. Some findings, such as a pleural effusion, do not affect the progress of the intended surgery, whereas others markedly alter surgical management. The implications of significant atheromatous disease in the ascending aorta and persistent left vena cava have already been discussed.

Thrombus

The detection of intracardiac thrombus by TEE is infrequent but may alter the surgical management. Thrombus in the left atrial appendage can be managed by minimizing manipulation of the heart or plication of the appendage. Mobile fresh thrombus, especially in the left side of the heart, merits surgical extraction. Thrombus can increase the risk for postoperative complications, and its detection is likely to alter postoperative management with the initiation of long-term anticoagulation.

Patent Foramen Ovale

The management of an unsuspected patent foramen ovale, which has an incidence of 20% to 25% in adult cardiac surgical patients, can affect the anticipated surgical plan and long-term neurologic prognosis (28). Closure of an incidental patent foramen ovale should be considered in a patient with a history of stroke or when an open chamber procedure is performed in conjunction with CABG surgery. A patent foramen ovale is most reliably detected when the interatrial septum is interrogated with both color flow Doppler and imaging after contrast

TABLE 15.5. TRANSESOPHAGEAL ECHOCARDIOGRAPHY FOR THE DIAGNOSIS OF INCIDENTAL DISEASE

Incidental findings	Clinical considerations
Patent foramen ovale	Shunting, risk for paradoxical embolism
Persistent left superior vena cava	Contraindication for retrograde cardioplegia
Atherosclerotic disease	Modify cannulation/cross-clamping of aorta
Aortic regurgitation	Inadequate antegrade cardioplegia, distention of left ventricle
Valvular disease	Valve repair or replacement
Intracardiac thrombus	Risk for embolism, alter surgical management
Pleural effusion	Drainage of effusion

injection in the ME four-chamber and bicaval views (29). The contrast agent is made by agitating 10 mL of saline that is forcefully injected back and forth through a three-way stopcock into another syringe. The excess air is then removed and the solution injected as the interatrial septum is interrogated by TEE. The passage of contrast bubbles in the left atrium within five cardiac cycles confirms the diagnosis patent foramen ovale.

Pleural Effusions

Pleural effusions are often present in patients undergoing CABG surgery as a result of decompensated coronary artery disease, coexisting valvular disease, or other pathology. Large effusions that cause significant atelectasis result in decreased ventilatory capacity and increased alveolar-to-arterial oxygen gradients. The left pleural space is best imaged by counterclockwise rotation of the TEE probe to image the short axis of the descending thoracic aorta. An effusion surrounds the aorta, displacing normal parenchyma of the lung.

Mitral Regurgitation

The presence of significant mitral regurgitation may merit surgical intervention. It is important to assess the severity and dynamic nature of mitral valvular disease under conditions that best mimic the preoperative state and to consider the patient's preoperative symptoms and cardiac function. Coronary revascularization alone may significantly decrease mitral regurgitation as a consequence of improved coronary perfusion and ventricular function. The surgical plan should be modified by the surgeon and cardiologist with input from the echocardiographer.

TRANSESOPHAGEAL ECHOCARDIOGRAPHY IN OFF-PUMP CORONARY ARTERY BYPASS GRAFTING

Off-pump CABG (OPCAB) surgery is increasing in popularity because it avoids the morbidity of CPB. During the critical time when the heart is surgically positioned for distal coronary anastomosis, hemodynamic instability and coronary ischemia can develop. One of the factors critical to the success of this procedure is that the anesthesiologist remains vigilant and communicates with the cardiac surgeon. Effective communication and gradual positioning of the heart greatly facilitate the maintenance of stable hemodynamics. Because this surgical procedure is relatively new, the national consensus in regard to monitoring with TEE is still emerging. The application of TEE in OPCAB surgery may vary within an institution and is generally physician-specific.

Hemodynamic Compromise during Off-Pump Coronary Artery Bypass

Hemodynamic compromise during OPCAB can be caused by hypovolemia (bleeding, manual compression of the heart, chamber distortion during positioning), ischemia (coronary air or debris), valvular dysfunction, or arrhythmias (secondary to ischemia or mechanical perturbation).

Regional Wall Motion Abnormalities in Off-Pump Coronary Artery Bypass

New RWMAs are common but may not indicate ongoing ischemia. As discussed previously, these can be attributed to altered volume status, positioning, and stabilization devices that distort the anatomy to reduce the excursion of affected myocardium. Positioning the heart to enable the anastomosis of distal left coronary grafts may cause torsion and compression of the right atria and ventricle, impeding venous return. This problem can be alleviated in part by administering fluid, placing the patient in a slight Trendelenburg position, opening the pericardium to the right side of the chest, and using a positioning device that is affixed to the apex of the heart and shifts the heart into a less compromising position.

Mitral Regurgitation in Off-Pump Coronary Artery Bypass

Distortion of the heart during anastomosis of the right or posterior coronary arteries can also exacerbate mitral regurgitation. The mechanism is most likely distortion of the mitral valve annulus and supportive structures that interferes with leaflet coaptation. In some cases, the mitral regurgitation may cause sufficient hemodynamic compromise that conversion to circulatory bypass is required.

Patent Foramen Ovale in Off-Pump Coronary Artery Bypass

Positioning the heart during OPCAB can also be associated with profound hypoxemia that results from right-to-left intracardiac shunting through a patent foramen ovale (30). The patent foramen ovale may be unmasked by an acute increase in pressure in the right side of the heart that occurs during positioning. Repositioning the heart should permit closure of the shunt and resolution of the hypoxia. However, in the case of refractory hypoxia, it may be necessary to perform the surgery with CPB and also close the patent foramen ovale (30).

SUMMARY

The major role of echocardiography in patients undergoing coronary revascularization is as a versatile diagnostic device that can dramatically alter the conduct and management of a surgical procedure. It is unlikely that echocardiography will supplant the traditional PA catheter because the PA catheter offers the advantage of providing continuous quantitative assessment of overall cardiac function and loading conditions throughout the perioperative period. However, advances in echocardiography have markedly expanded its applications and importance in cardiac surgery. As explained in this chapter, the potential indications for this technology include both monitoring and diagnosis. The multiple modalities (two-dimensional imaging, color flow mapping, spectral Doppler imaging, and use of contrast agents) provide for both the qualitative and quantitative assessment of cardiac function and pathophysiology. In the future, the increased availability of equipment, trained personnel, and technologic advances will foster an expanded role of echocardiography in selected groups of cardiac surgical patients.

REFERENCES

1. Practice guidelines for perioperative transesophageal echocardiography. A report by the American Society of Anesthesiologists and the Society of Cardiovascular Anesthesiologists Task Force on Transesophageal Echocardiography. *Anesthesiology* 1996;84:986.
2. Savage RM, Lytle BW, Aronson S, et al. Intraoperative echocardiography is indicated in high-risk coronary artery bypass grafting. *AnnThorac Surg* 1997;64:368.
3. Kallmeyer IJ, Collard CD, Fox JA, et al. The safety of intraoperative transesophageal echocardiography: a case series of 7200 cardiac surgical patients. *Anesth Analg* 2001;92:1126.
4. Cheung EH, Craver JM, Jones EL, et al. Mediastinitis after cardiac valve operations: impact on survival. *J Thorac Cardiovasc Surg* 1985;90:517.
5. Shanewise JS, Cheung AT, Aronson S, et al. ASE/SCA guidelines for performing a comprehensive intraoperative multiplane transesophageal echocardiography examination:

recommendations of the American Society of Echocardiography Council for Intraoperative Echocardiography and the Society of Cardiovascular Anesthesiologists Task Force for Certification in Perioperative Transesophageal Echocardiography. *Anesth Analg* 1999;89:870.

6. Cheung AT, Savino JS, Weiss SJ, et al. Echocardiographic and hemodynamic indexes of left ventricular preload in patients with normal and abnormal ventricular function. *Anesthesiology* 1994;81:376–387.

7. Perrino AC, Luther MA, O'Connor TZ, et al. Automated echocardiographic analysis. Examination of serial intraoperative measurements. *Anesthesiology* 1995;83:285.

8. Muhiudeen IA, Kuecherer HF, Lee E, et al. Intraoperative estimation of cardiac output by transesophageal pulsed Doppler echocardiography. *Anesthesiology* 1991;74:9.

9. Savino JS, Troianos CA, Aukburg S, et al. Measurement of pulmonary blood flow with transesophageal two-dimensional and Doppler echocardiography. *Anesthesiology* 1991;75:445.

10. Darmon PL, Hillel Z, Mogtader A, et al. Cardiac output by transesophageal echocardiography using continuous-wave Doppler across the aortic valve. *Anesthesiology* 1994;80:796.

11. Smith JS, Cahalan MK, Benefiel DJ, et al. Intraoperative detection of myocardial ischemia in high-risk patients: electrocardiography versus two-dimensional echocardiography. *Circulation* 1985;72:1015.

12. Battler A, Froelicher VF, Gallagher KP, et al. Dissociation between regional myocardial dysfunction and ECG changes during ischemia in the conscious dog. *Circulation* 1980;62:735.

13. Gallagher KP, Kumada T, Koziol JA, et al. Significance of regional wall thickening abnormalities relative to transmural myocardial perfusion in anesthetized dogs. *Circulation* 1980;62:1266.

14. Roizen MF, Beaupre PN, Alpert RA, et al. Monitoring with two-dimensional transesophageal echocardiography. Comparison of myocardial function in patients undergoing supraceliac, suprarenal-infraceliac, or infrarenal aortic occlusion. *J Vasc Surg* 1984; 1:300.

15. Smith JS, Cahalan MK, Benefiel DJ, et al. Intraoperative detection of myocardial ischemia in high-risk patients: electrocardiography versus two-dimensional transesophageal echocardiography. *Circulation* 1985;72:1015.

16. Leung JM, O'Kelly B, Browner WS, et al. Prognostic importance of post-bypass regional wall-motion abnormalities in patients undergoing coronary artery bypass graft surgery. SPI Research Group. *Anesthesiology* 1989;71:16.

17. Deutsch HJ, Curtius JM, Leischik R, et al. Diagnostic value of transesophageal echocardiography in cardiac surgery. *Thorac Cardiovasc Surg* 1991;39:199.

18. Gardner TJ, Horneffer PJ, Manolio TA, et al. Stroke following coronary artery bypass grafting: a ten-year study. *Ann Thorac Surg* 1985;40:574.

19. Roach GW, Kanchuger M, Mora Mangano C, et al. Adverse cerebral outcomes after coronary bypass surgery. *N Engl J Med* 1996;335:1857.

20. Newman MF, Kirchner JL, Phillips-Bute B, et al. Longitudinal assessment of neurocognitive function after coronary artery bypass surgery. *N Engl J Med* 2001;344:395.

21. Konstadt SN, Reich DL, Quintana C, et al. The ascending aorta: how much does transesophageal echocardiography see? *Anesth Analg* 1994;78:240.

22. Konstadt SN, Reich DL, Kahn R, et al. Transesophageal echocardiography can be used to screen for ascending aortic atherosclerosis. *Anesth Analg* 1995;81:225.

23. Paul D, Hartman G. Foley balloon occlusion of the atheromatous ascending aorta: the role of transesophageal echocardiography. *J Cardiothorac Vasc Anesth* 1998;12:61.

24. Cohn LH, Rizzo RJ, Adams DH, et al. Reduced mortality and morbidity for ascending aortic aneurysm resection regardless of cause. *Ann Thorac Surg* 1996;62:463.

25. Byrne JG, Aranki SF, Cohn LH. Aortic valve operations under deep hypothermic circulatory arrest for the porcelain aorta: 'no touch' technique. *Ann Thorac Surg* 1998;65:1313.

26. Kouchoukos NT, Wareing TH, Daily BB, et al. Management of the severely atherosclerotic aorta during cardiac operations. *J Card Surg* 1994;9:490.

27. Grossi EA, Kanchuger MS, Schwartz DS, et al. Effect of cannula length on aortic arch flow: protection of the atheromatous aortic arch. *Ann Thorac Surg* 1995;59:710.

28. Louie EK, Konstadt SN, Rao TL, et al. Transesophageal echocardiographic diagnosis of

right to left shunting across the foramen ovale in adults without prior stroke. *J Am Coll Cardiol* 1993;21:1231.

29. Konstadt SN, Louie EK, Black S, et al. Intraoperative detection of patent foramen ovale by transesophageal echocardiography. *Anesthesiology* 1991;74:212.

30. Akhter M, Lajos TZ. Pitfalls of undetected patent foramen ovale in off-pump cases. *Ann Thorac Surg* 1999;67:546.

QUESTIONS

1. All of the following statements regarding TEE for CABG surgery are true **except**
   a. TEE is more sensitive than ECG for the detection of ischemia.
   b. TEE can play an important role during cardiac surgery by influencing circulatory and surgical management.
   c. The morbidity associated with TEE is low.
   d. TEE completely images the ascending and descending thoracic aorta.
2. Epiaortic imaging in CABG surgery
   a. Does not offer any significant benefit beyond that of TEE
   b. Images the ascending aorta better than TEE
   c. Is contraindicated in the case of a friable or atherosclerotic aorta
   d. Always requires the use of a "standoff" to improve resolution in the far field
3. The TEE examination for CABG surgery
   a. Should focus only on the specific surgical indication of ischemia detection
   b. Is classified as a "group 1 indication" according to the American Society of Anesthesiologists/Society of Cardiovascular Anesthesiologists guidelines
   c. Should be reviewed with the attending cardiac surgeon
   d. Has been shown to significantly improve the clinical outcome of off-pump surgery
4. TEE assessment of ventricular function
   a. Requires only the "classic" TG short-axis view
   b. Is independent of afterload
   c. Uses the volumetric determination of FAC
   d. Is dependent on ventricular preload
5. The TEE measurement of CO
   a. Cannot be performed in cases of high blood flow velocity
   b. Is most commonly achieved by interrogating blood flow through the mitral valve
   c. Shows good agreement with measurements determined by thermodilution
   d. Is dependent on the absence of valvular stenosis
6. Which of the following statements is the most accurate?
   a. TEE provides for the continuous on-line measurement of intracardiac pressures.
   b. The TEE-derived measurement of CO is often inaccurate because of LV foreshortening.
   c. A change in PA pressure is a more sensitive diagnostic indicator of cardiac ischemia than a new RWMA.
   d. TEE and PA catheterization function as complementary technologies during CABG surgery.
7. New RWMAs that develop after separation from bypass during CABG surgery
   a. May respond to the administration of calcium channel antagonist
   b. Are diagnostic of myocardial ischemia
   c. Support the further intervention of returning to bypass and performing another coronary anastomosis
   d. Result in myocardial infarction
8. Which of the following is the most appropriate statement?
   a. TEE often inaccurately assesses LV preload because of LV foreshortening.
   b. An increase in FAC should not be equated with an increase in contractility.
   c. With TEE, it is difficult to distinguish a low systemic vascular resistance syndrome from a pulmonary embolism.
   d. The septal wall motion abnormality that is observed after bypass is most commonly related to transient ischemia.

9. TEE is used for all the following **except**
   a. Confirming the absence of significant aortic valvular insufficiency
   b. Diagnosing LV distention
   c. Guiding arterial cannulation of the ascending aorta
   d. Assisting in placement of a coronary sinus catheter
10. Which of the following is the most appropriate statement?
    a. The diagnosis of a patent foramen ovale has more important implications for CABG surgery that uses CPB than for off-pump surgery.
    b. TEE assists with positioning the endoaortic clamp during port access procedures.
    c. Incidental findings of the intraoperative TEE examination have no effect on cardioplegia techniques.
    d. The presence of bubbles emerging from the coronary sinus following an injection of contrast in a peripheral vein is of minimal importance in conducting bypass surgery.

Transesophageal Echocardiography of the Thoracic Aorta

Kim J. Payne, William M. Yarbrough, John S. Ikonomidis, and Scott T. Reeves

In few diseases is an accurate and timely diagnosis more important than in those of the thoracic aorta. This chapter guides the reader through the classification systems used for thoracic aortic aneurysms and dissections, their echocardiographic manifestations, and the surgical decision-making process. Emphasis is placed on obtaining a quick and accurate examination, with particular attention given to the echocardiographic findings diagnostic of aortic disease. The chapter concludes with a discussion of associated thoracic disease states, including intramural hematoma and atheroma.

CLASSIFICATION SYSTEMS

Diseases of the thoracic aorta include aortic aneurysms, aortic dissections, intramural hematomas, giant penetrating ulcers, and significant atherosclerosis that can present problems at the time of cardiac surgery.

Aortic Aneurysms

Aortic aneurysms can be classified according to their location in the ascending aorta, aortic arch, descending thoracic aorta, or any combination thereof. Any patient with a thoracic aortic aneurysm larger than 5 cm in diameter should be considered for operative repair because of the considerable risks for rupture. A further corollary is that any patient with an aneurysmal segment of the aorta that attains a luminal diameter more than two times that of a normal aortic segment, which can usually be estimated in an unaffected area at the level of the aortic arch or the abdominal aorta vessels, should be considered for surgery. Patients with connective tissue disease, such as Marfan syndrome or Ehlers-Danlos syndrome, may be considered for surgery at an earlier time.

The Crawford classification delineates four types of thoracoabdominal aneurysms (1) (Fig. 16.1). Type I originates in the proximal descending thoracic aorta and ends above the renal arteries. Type II begins in the proximal descending thoracic aorta and terminates below the renal arteries. Type III originates in the distal descending aorta, conveniently identified as being below the level of the thoracic incision in the sixth intercostal space. Type IV involves most of the abdominal aorta. Figure 16.2 illustrates the distribution, frequency, and morphology of thoracic aortic aneurysms.

Aortic Dissections

Thoracic aortic dissections are classified by either of two schemes. The Stanford classification (2) separates aortic dissections into type A, in which the dissection involves the ascending aorta, and type B, in which the dissection is confined to the descending thoracic aorta. The DeBakey system (3) classifies dissections as type I, in which the dissection starts in the ascending aorta and involves variable portions of the descending aorta; type II, in which the dissection is confined to the ascending aorta; and type III, in which the dissection originates distal to the left subclavian artery and either involves only the descending thoracic aorta (III-A) or extends into the abdominal segment of the descending aorta (III-B) (Fig. 16.3).

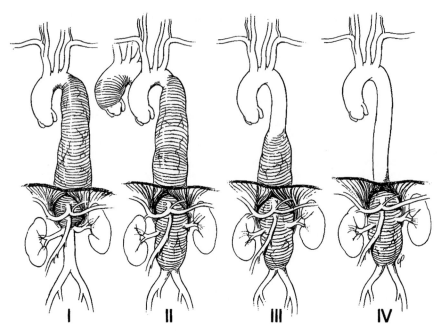

FIG. 16.1. Crawford classification of thoracoabdominal aortic aneurysms according to extent of involvement of the thoracoabdominal aorta. Crawford type I, most or all of the descending thoracic aorta and the suprarenal abdominal aorta; type II, most or all of the descending thoracic aorta and most or all of the abdominal aorta; type III, distal descending thoracic aorta and varying segments of the abdominal aorta, including the renal and visceral arteries; type IV, most or all of the abdominal aorta. (From Crawford ES, Svensson LG, Hess HE, et al. A prospective randomized study of cerebrospinal fluid drainage to prevent paraplegia after high-risk surgery on the thoracoabdominal aorta. *J Vasc Surg* 1991;13:37, with permission.)

Intramural Hematomas

Intramural hematomas of the thoracic aorta are classified the same way as thoracic aortic dissections.

Giant Penetrating Ulcers

Giant penetrating ulcer disease of the thoracic aorta is still a relatively poorly defined condition that is generally classified in relation to the anatomic location of the lesion (i.e., ascending aorta, arch, or descending thoracic aorta).

DIAGNOSTIC MODALITIES FOR AORTIC DISSECTION

The mortality rate for acute aortic dissection can be as high a 1% per hour among untreated patients during the first 48 hours (4). A quick and accurate diagnosis is imperative if one is to improve survival and initiate the appropriate surgical or medical therapy. Until recently, aortography was the gold standard for evaluating patients with suspected aortic dissection (5). Currently, multiple imaging modalities, including computed tomography (CT) (6–8), transesophageal echocardiography (TEE) (5–12), and magnetic resonance imaging (MRI) (6–9),

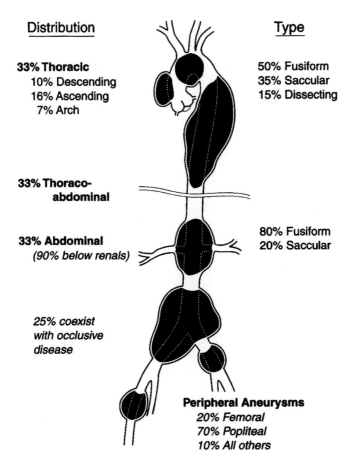

Distribution

33% Thoracic
10% Descending
16% Ascending
7% Arch

**33% Thoraco-
abdominal**

33% Abdominal
(90% below renals)

*25% coexist
with occlusive
disease*

Type

50% Fusiform
35% Saccular
15% Dissecting

80% Fusiform
20% Saccular

Peripheral Aneurysms
20% Femoral
70% Popliteal
10% All others

FIG. 16.2. Distribution frequency and morphology of type A aortic aneurysms. (From Estafanous FG, Barash PG, Reves JG, eds. *Cardiac anesthesia principles and clinical practice,* 2nd ed. Philadelphia: Lippincott Williams & Wilkins, 2001:785, with permission.)

have been shown to be useful. The relative advantages of each modality are presented in Table 16.1. One must consider availability, time required to perform the study, safety, and cost when considering the four different modalities.

Aortography

Aortography requires the visualization of a double lumen or intimal flap to be completely diagnostic. Indirect signs that suggest acute dissection include thickening of the aortic wall, aortic insufficiency, ulcerlike projections along the aortic wall, abnormalities of branch vessels, an abnormal position of a catheter in the aorta, and compression of a true aortic lumen by a false lumen (5). As Table 16.1 shows, aortography may be the least sensitive of the modalities currently available (7). Furthermore, it is difficult to perform on an emergent basis because adequate personnel must be available in the hospital, the patient must be transferred to the interventional suite, and intravenous contrast, which can be detrimental in patients with renal insufficiency, must be used.

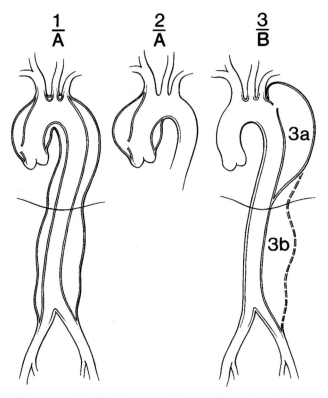

FIG. 16.3. The Stanford (A and B) and DeBakey (I, II, III) classification systems for thoracic aorta dissections. (From Crawford ES, Crawford JL. *Diseases of the aorta.* Baltimore: Williams & Wilkins, 1984:174, with permission.)

TABLE 16.1. DIAGNOSTIC PERFORMANCE OF IMAGING MODALITIES IN THE EVALUATION OF SUSPECTED DISSECTION

Diagnostic performance	Angiography	CT	MRI	TEE
Sensitivity	++	++	+++	+++
Specificity	+++	+++	+++	++/+++
Site of intimal tear	++	+	+++	++
Presence of thrombus	+++	++	+++	+
Presence of aortic insufficiency	+++	−	+	+++
Pericardial effusion	−	++	+++	+++
Branch vessel involvement	+++	+	++	+
Coronary artery involvement	++	−	−	++

CT, computed tomography; MRI, magnetic resonance imaging; TEE, transesophageal echocardiography; +++, excellent; ++, good; +, fair; −, not detected. Modified from Cigarro JE, Isselbacher EM, DeSanctis RW, et al. Diagnostic imaging in the evaluation of suspected aortic dissection: old standards and new directions. *N Engl J Med* 1993;328:35, with permission.

Computed Tomography

CT requires the identification of two distinct lumina with a visible intimal flap. CT is more sensitive than aortography but is still less sensitive than MRI and TEE. CT rarely identifies the intimal flap entry site. CT also cannot reliably identify aortic insufficiency or coronary artery involvement (6–8).

Magnetic Resonance Imaging

MRI is the most sensitive and specific methodology currently available for evaluating aortic dissection. Unfortunately, an MRI examination is contraindicated for the many patients with pacemakers, certain types of aneurysm clips, or orthopedic hardware. Patients with acute aortic dissection are often hemodynamically unstable, require intravenous antihypertensive agents, and are intubated, so that proper management in the MRI scanner is further complicated (6–9).

Transesophageal Echocardiography

TEE is becoming the standard modality for the acute evaluation of a suspected acute aortic dissection. It is widely available, noninvasive, and cost-effective, and it can be performed quickly at the bedside. *One must demonstrate an undulating intimal flap in the aorta in two different views to make the diagnosis.* The skill of the reader is paramount in making an accurate diagnosis with TEE. The study usually requires only 5 to 20 minutes to complete. The distal ascending aorta and proximal aortic arch may be poorly visualized with TEE because of the juxtaposition of the air-filled trachea and left main bronchus, which can lead to false-negative results. Visualization of this area has improved with the use of newer technologies, such as multiplane probes. TEE is also extremely helpful in detecting aortic insufficiency, pericardial effusion, and coronary artery involvement. In addition, other information, such as the left ventricular (LV) ejection fraction and parameters of valvular function, can easily be obtained (5–12).

Because it is safe, quick, accurate, and convenient and can be performed at the bedside, even in an unstable patient, we feel that TEE should be considered first when a patient is being evaluated for possible acute aortic dissection. For patients with chronic dissection and those requiring postoperative evaluation, MRI appears to be the test of choice (6–9).

EXAMINATION TECHNIQUES

Because of the close proximity of the thoracic aorta to the esophagus, TEE is the preferred echocardiographic approach. Figure 16.4 illustrates the changing relationship of the thoracic aorta to the esophagus along its course from the upper thorax to the diaphragm. At the level of the distal arch, the aorta is anterior to the esophagus, whereas at the level of the diaphragm, the aorta is posterior to the esophagus. This changing anatomic relationship makes it difficult for the echocardiographer to designate the anterior and posterior and the left and right orientation of the descending thoracic aorta. *To communicate the location of a lesion to the surgeon, we find it useful to relate its location to known anatomic landmarks. We measure the distance of lesions in the ascending aorta from the aortic valve, and the distance of those in the descending aorta from the left subclavian artery.* It is also useful to record the distance of a lesion from the incisors to guide follow-up examinations in the echocardiography suite; however, the usefulness of this measurement in directing the surgeon to lesions within the aorta is limited.

As is discussed later, two areas are of primary concern in acute aortic dissection. These are the area just distal to the aortic valve in the region of the sinotubular junction, where acute ascending aortic dissections tend to occur, and the area just distal to the left subclavian artery, where descending dissections originate. A complete thoracic aortic examination is necessary to delineate both the aneurysm and the acute dissection pathology. These two

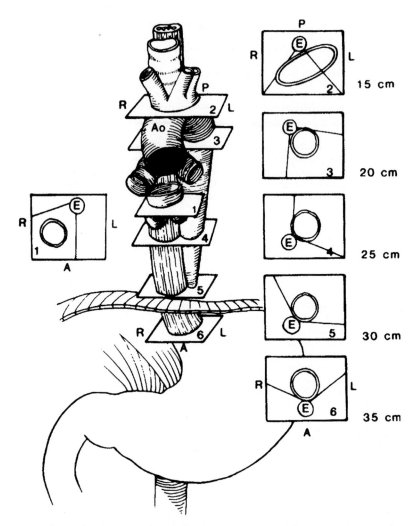

FIG. 16.4. Relationship between the esophagus and aorta at different levels of the thoracic esophagus. (From Estafanous FG, Barash PG, Reves JG, eds. *Cardiac anesthesia principles and clinical practice,* 2nd ed. Philadelphia: Lippincott Williams & Wilkins, 2001:785, with permission).

high-risk areas must be carefully examined. One must remember also that the air-filled trachea is interposed between the esophagus and the distal ascending aorta and proximal aortic arch. *The distal ascending aorta may not be visualized clearly, even with multiplane TEE technology* (13).

Examination of the Ascending Thoracic Aorta

The examination technique that follows focuses on rapidly determining whether an aortic dissection is present. The examination of the thoracic aorta is begun at a probe depth of 30 to 35 cm from the incisors. At 0 degree, the midesophageal (ME) five-chamber view is

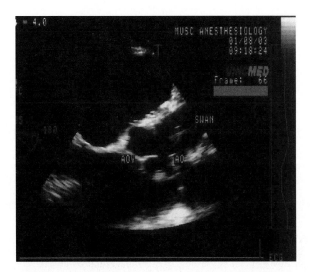

FIG. 16.5. Transesophageal echocardiographic image demonstrating a linear streak in the middle of the proximal ascending aorta, representing an image artifact caused by a Swan-Ganz catheter.

identified. The angle is rotated first to 40 to 60 degrees for the ME aortic valve short-axis view and then to 90 to 120 degrees to identify the ME aortic valve long-axis view. The long-axis view allows interrogation of the proximal ascending aorta and measurement of the diameter of the sinus of Valsalva and sinotubular junction. To optimize this view, one generally rotates the handle toward the patient's right side. By gradually advancing the probe from the ME aortic valve long-axis view, one can frequently visualize an additional 2 to 3 cm of the ascending aorta. It is paramount that this view be carefully examined to detect proximal ascending aortic dissections. *Extreme care must be taken if a Swan-Ganz catheter is in place because it frequently appears as an artifact within the ascending aorta at this level* (Fig. 16.5). If a question arises regarding the diagnosis of an intimal flap verses an artifact, our motto is *"when in doubt, pull the Swan out!"* The angle is now gradually decreased to 60 degrees and then 0 degree as the probe is gradually withdrawn from the patient's mouth. This demonstrates the ME ascending aorta short-axis view, in which the ascending aorta lies adjacent to the pulmonary artery and its right main branch.

Examination of the Descending Thoracic Aorta

Attention is now turned to the descending thoracic aorta. Again, one starts with the ME four- or five-chamber view, and the probe is manually rotated to the left until the circular short-axis image of the descending thoracic aorta is located in the center of the near field. This view is called the *descending aorta short-axis view*. It can be more easily seen by adjusting the depth settings on the machine to 6 to 8 cm to increase the size of the aorta on the display screen. By advancing and withdrawing the probe within the esophagus, one can evaluate the entire descending thoracic aorta and a portion of the upper abdominal aorta from this position. The probe is advanced within the esophagus starting at the level of the distal arch and is gradually rotated farther to the left to keep the descending aorta in view. Once the stomach is entered, the ability to evaluate the descending abdominal aorta is lost. At this level, one gradually withdraws the probe while watching the descending aorta until the left subclavian artery is reached. Further withdrawal demonstrates the upper esophageal aortic arch long-axis view. One then rotates the probe 90 degrees to obtain the upper esophageal aortic arch short-axis view.

The probe is again advanced into the stomach until the descending aorta short-axis view is visualized. The probe is then rotated 90 degrees, and the descending aortic long-axis view is now demonstrated. The probe is withdrawn until the left subclavian artery is identified.

With careful inspection of the aorta in at least two planes and the use of colored Doppler, most pathology of the ascending and descending aorta can be identified by this technique. Once the examination of the thoracic aorta is complete, attention can be turned to other matters of concern, such as pericardial effusion, aortic insufficiency, and LV function.

TRANSESOPHAGEAL ECHOCARDIOGRAPHIC EVALUATION OF AORTIC DISSECTION

Surgeons' Questions (What They Need to Know)

The goals of intraoperative TEE for the evaluation of aortic dissection include the following:

1. Confirmation of the preoperative diagnosis.
2. Determination of the dissection entry site, including differentiation of true and false lumina.
3. Intraoperative monitoring of the patient's volume status by assessing the LV chamber area and ventricular wall motion during the operative procedure and by determining whether aortic insufficiency is present. In cases of circulatory arrest, it is critical to know whether aortic insufficiency is present to detect ventricular distention if an aorta cross-clamp is not planned. Also, short-axis monitoring for LV distention when fibrillation occurs allows early chamber decompression through vent insertion, either via the LV apex or a pulmonary vein.
4. Examination to detect complications.
5. Confirmation of the integrity of the surgical repair.

Characteristics of Aortic Dissection

In aortic dissection, an accumulation of blood dissects the intima from the media. On TEE examination, most cases are associated with an intimal flap, seen as a mobile linear echo within the vascular lumen (4,14–17) (Fig. 16.6). The intimal flap is the most important

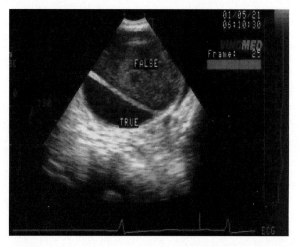

FIG. 16.6. True and false lumina of acute aortic dissection. Note spontaneous echo contrast within the false lumen.

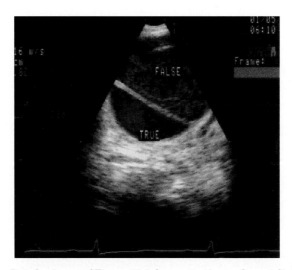

FIG. 16.7. A color Doppler image of Figure 16.6 demonstrating early systolic flow within the true lumen. (See Color Plate 28 following page 212.)

evidence of an aortic dissection (15,18). An intimal flap and flow within the true and false lumina on either side of the flap are highly sensitive features of aortic dissection (14,17,18) (Fig. 16.7; see Color Plate 28 following page 212). Additional TEE findings consistent with aortic dissection include the following: (a) complete thrombosis of the false lumen, (b) central displacement of intimal calcification with bright echogenic densities within the aorta, and (c) separation of the intimal layers from the thrombus (14,17,19).

Location and Entry Sites

TEE is a valuable tool for evaluating the location of an intimal tear entry site. The entry site of an intimal tear is defined as a disruption in the continuity of the flap, often identified by color flow Doppler (20) (Fig. 16.8). With color Doppler, small intimal tears can be identified that may not be visualized by two-dimensional echocardiography. A turbulent jet of bright mosaic color can be seen flowing from the true to the false lumen (7,21,22) (Fig. 16.9; see Color Plate 29 following page 212).

The intimal tear occurs in the ascending aorta 1 to 3 cm above the right or left sinus of Valsalva in approximately 70% of cases. In the remaining 20% to 30% of cases, the intimal flap is located at the site of the ligamentum arteriosum in the descending thoracic aorta (4,7,21). The exact location of a tear can be estimated by the depth of probe insertion in relation to a major anatomic landmark, such as the sinus of Valsalva or the left subclavian artery. In some cases, the primary tear cannot be accurately identified because multiple tears are present or TEE visualization of the distal ascending aorta "blind spot" is poor. In a study by Adachi et al. (23), the entry site was identified in 88% patients with acute dissection. Type B dissection entry sites were identified in 90% of cases, and type A dissections in 83% of cases.

The dissection of the medial layer may be localized or split longitudinally. In the ascending aorta and arch, the plane of dissection usually courses along the greater curvature, whereas in the descending thoracic aorta, the dissection plane is usually localized lateral to the true lumen, although it may spiral along the longitudinal axis (21).

As previously noted, the location and extent of the dissection flap are used to determine the type of aortic dissection. Identification and localization of the primary tear are important to the success of the surgical repair (24). Surgical resection of the primary entry site may decrease the incidence of late reoperation and complications (25).

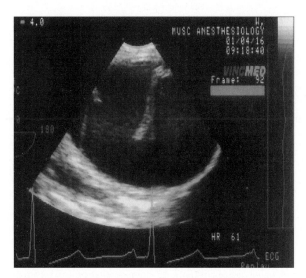

FIG. 16.8. Entry site of an intimal tear within the descending thoracic aorta.

False versus True Lumen

Identification of the true and false lumina by TEE is critical to the assessment of aortic dissection (17,20). It may be difficult to differentiate the true from the false lumen, especially when the dissection involves the entire aorta and the intimal flap separates the lumen into halves (17).

Multiple indirect findings differentiate true from false lumina on TEE (17,19,20,26,27). The true lumen usually expands during systole and is compressed during diastole (15). The true lumen has a thin, less echogenic inner layer, whereas the false lumen has a bright echogenic layer adjacent to the aortic lumen (Fig. 16.6). Spontaneous echo contrast and

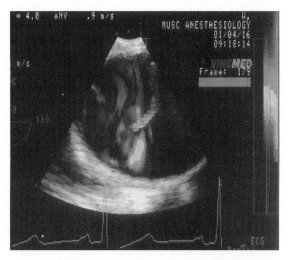

FIG. 16.9. A color flow image of Figure 16.8 demonstrating flow from the true lumen to the false lumen through the entry site. (See Color Plate 29 following page 212.)

variable amounts of thrombus are frequently present in the false lumen as a consequence of the stagnant flow (Fig. 16.6). The false lumen is usually larger that the true lumen, especially in chronic dissections (17,19,20,26,27).

Color flow Doppler imaging provides additional information regarding aortic flow patterns in dissection. The true lumen is identified by forward systolic flow, whereas flow in the false lumen is complicated and variable. With large, proximal entry tears, flow in the nearby segments of the false lumen may be the same in direction and timing as flow in the true lumen (27). With small distal tears, flow in the false lumen less closely resembles flow in the true lumen; it may be in the opposite direction and peak later in the cardiac cycle because of the delay of flow into the false lumen (15).

Multiple communications between the true and false lumina can frequently be identified by pulsed wave and color flow Doppler. Some communications represent entry sites with flow from the true toward the false lumen during systole, whereas others represent exit sites with bidirectional flow (20,22,27–29).

Thrombosis of the False Lumen

Thrombosis of the false lumen is an indirect finding of aortic dissection and requires further evaluation by TEE (15,20,22,26) (Fig. 16.10). A thrombus can be identified as a mass within the vascular true or false lumen that is separate from the intimal flap and aortic wall (29). A thickening of the aortic wall in excess of 15 mm has been considered a sign of dissection, suggesting thrombosis of a false channel, and can make the intimal flap difficult to identify (15). Many areas of the false lumen may show spontaneous echo contrast with stagnant flow and often exhibit partial thrombosis. These thrombosed segments tend to develop in areas remote from high-velocity large entry or exit sites.

The differentiation of a descending thoracic aortic aneurysm with laminated clot from a completely thrombosed false lumen is an important function of TEE. In a patient with a thrombosed false lumen, persistent small and limited areas with a sluggish, swirling flow pattern are typically seen, consistent with a false lumen rather than intraluminal clot. The presence of thrombus in the ascending aorta suggests thrombosis of the false lumen of an aortic dissection.

Aortic Insufficiency

A TEE evaluation of aortic value structure and function is integral in the assessment of aortic dissection; aortic insufficiency is associated with 50% to 70% of proximal dissections and

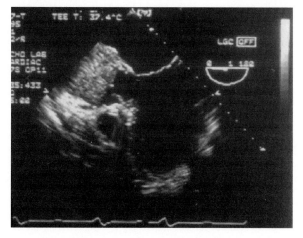

FIG. 16.10. A proximal aortic hematoma that could cause significant aortic insufficiency.

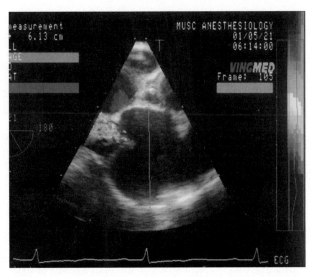

FIG. 16.11. Ascending aortic aneurysm with dilation in the proximal ascending aorta resulting in poor coaptation of the aorta valve leaflets and a central jet of aortic regurgitation. (See Color Plate 30 following page 212.)

10% of descending thoracic aortic dissections, and its presence carries important surgical implications (30). TEE is more sensitive than aortography in detecting mild aortic insufficiency (31). Aortic insufficiency is diagnosed with color flow Doppler (see Chapter 11). We have found that the ratio of the regurgitant jet height to the LV outflow tract width is the most useful method for grading aortic insufficiency as mild (1%–24%), moderate (25%–46%), moderate-severe (47%–64%), or severe (>65%) (28).

TEE can also demonstrate the causes of aortic insufficiency, thereby facilitating surgical decision making. The mechanisms of aortic insufficiency in the face of aortic dissection include the following: (a) dilation of the aortic root with widening of the aortic annulus and disturbance of aortic valve cusp coaptation (Fig. 16.11; see Color Plate 30 following page 212); (b) disturbance of cusp closure by hematoma at the annulus (Fig. 16.10); (c) destruction of annular support of the cusps with subsequent cusp prolapse; and (d) prolapse of the dissection flap into the aortic valve orifice and LV outflow tract with interference of aortic cusp motion (20,32) (Fig. 16.12).

Aortic insufficiency has a negative effect on outcome in aortic dissection and may dictate the surgical approach. Preservation of the native aortic valve with repair and resuspension is possible in 86% of type A dissections, especially if the aortic valve leaflets appear normal (33). Specific involvement of the aortic annulus by Marfan syndrome or annuloaortic ectasia may dictate aortic valve replacement because of the limited long-term durability of aortic valve reconstruction. As previously noted, the presence of aortic insufficiency necessitates the use of either ostial or retrograde cardioplegia during cardiopulmonary bypass.

Involvement of the Coronary Arteries

The coronary arteries are involved in 10% to 20% of cases of acute aortic dissection (4,32). Although angiography is the gold standard for assessing the coronary anatomy, TEE has been shown to be a reliable tool for evaluating the proximal coronary anatomy, especially in the critical setting of aortic dissection (32). The coronary arteries can be visualized as two parallel lines originating from the aortic lumen in short axis in the ME aortic valve short-axis view (7). The relationship of the dissection flap to the proximal left and right coronary

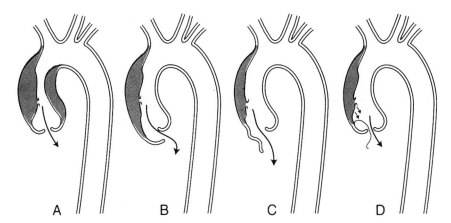

FIG. 16.12. Mechanism of aortic regurgitation in proximal aortic dissection. **A:** An extensive or circumferential tear dilates the aortic root and annulus, causing failure of coaptation of the aortic valve leaflets. **B:** With asymmetric dissection, pressure from the false lumen depresses one aortic leaflet below the coaptation line of the other leaflets. **C:** The annular support is disrupted, resulting in a flail aortic leaflet. **D:** Prolapse of a mobile intimal flap through the aortic valve during diastole, which permits leaflet coaptation. (From Braunwald E, ed. *Heart disease: a textbook of cardiovascular medicine,* 5th ed, vol 2. Philadelphia: WB Saunders, 1997:1557, with permission.)

arteries, the extent of dissection into the coronary arteries, and the degree of coronary blood flow obstruction caused by the flap should be evaluated by TEE.

Ballard et al. (32) detected coronary artery involvement with TEE in six of seven surgically documented cases of coronary artery dissection. Adequate views of the ostia and proximal vessels were obtained in 88% of the left main coronary arteries and 50% of the right coronary arteries. Although no studies have shown that coronary artery bypass grafting affects the ultimate outcome in patients with aortic dissection, coronary involvement in patients with proximal aortic dissection is an indication for urgent surgery (34). *TEE, which enables a rapid diagnosis and a relative sensitive assessment of the proximal coronary anatomy, is the test of choice for defining the coronary anatomy in the setting of aortic dissection* (24,32,34).

Left Ventricular Function

The TEE evaluation of aortic dissection also includes an assessment of LV function. The heart represents an end organ that may experience significant ischemia during aortic dissection and subsequent coronary dissection. Global dysfunction may be secondary to diffuse ischemia with dissection of both coronary arteries or to aortic insufficiency–related LV decompensation. Segmental wall motion abnormalities are an additional sign of coronary artery involvement in the dissection.

Pericardial and Pleural Effusion

In an aortic dissection, the aortic wall may rupture through the adventitia at the site of the dissection. Proximal extension of the dissection with rupture at the aortic root may result in cardiac tamponade as blood enters the pericardium. From the descending thoracic aorta, blood will enter the left pleural space, leading to hemothorax. Uncontained rupture into the mediastinum or pleural space causes sudden death, whereas ruptures contained by the aortic adventitia result in pseudoaneurysm formation or hematoma. Echo-free spaces around the aorta are a sign of penetration and periaortic hematoma. Mediastinal hematomas are identified when the distance from the esophagus to the left atrium or aorta increases and a pleural effusion develops (29).

Intraoperative Assessment of Aortic Graft Repair

After surgical repair, TEE assessment of the integrity of the aortic graft and detection of a residual flow signal in the false lumen provide vital information to the surgical team. The absence of a false luminal blood flow signal after repair indicates successful closure of the communication between the true and false lumina. This may reduce the risk for subsequent dissection and rupture, thereby improving the long-term prognosis (19,32).

Limitations of Transesophageal Echocardiography

Although the TEE evaluation of aortic dissection is sensitive and specific, it has notable limitations. Whereas the proximal ascending aorta and descending thoracic aorta are easily visualized by TEE, the distal ascending aorta may be inadequately visualized because of the interposed air-filled trachea. Longitudinal plane imaging has significantly improved imaging of the distal ascending aorta; however, in a study by Konstadt (35), a variable portion of the distal ascending aorta (4.5–10.7 cm) could not be visualized.

Side branch involvement of the brachiocephalic arch vessels and thoracoabdominal aortic branches is not visualized by TEE (24). To obtain supplementary information regarding these arteries, angiography may be required.

Transesophageal Echocardiographic Artifacts

All ultrasound imaging techniques can produce artifacts when ultrasound is reflected back and forth between strongly reflective surfaces. These multiple-path artifacts introduce apparent boundaries and structures into an image when no structures actually exist. A multitude of tissue-fluid and tissue-air interfaces produce an ideal setting for imaging artifacts during a TEE examination of the heart and aorta (24).

Artifacts involving the ascending aorta are an important clinical problem in the evaluation of aortic dissection because whether or not the ascending aorta is involved determines the need for surgery. In a study by Appelbe et al. (36), linear artifacts were detected in the ascending aorta in 44% of the cases, leading to false-positive results and a decreased specificity of TEE. Linear artifacts in the ascending aorta are caused by reverberation of the aortic wall in the presence of arteriosclerosis, a sclerotic aortic root, or calcific aortic disease, and they produce echo images that resemble an intimal flap (7,20). Linear artifacts are also commonly encountered at the level of the left atrium in the presence of a dilated aorta. Side lobe artifacts from the aortic valve can also simulate an intimal flap. A linear artifact of the ascending aorta can be distinguished from an intimal flap by (a) indistinct borders of the artifact, (b) lack of the rapid oscillatory movement associated with an intimal flap, (c) extension of the artifact through the aortic wall as a straight line, and (d) the ability to extrapolate the linear artifact to the starting point of the transducer (36,37). In the presence of an artifact, color Doppler imaging will demonstrate homogeneous color on both sides of the linear echo, without any transverse or communicating jets.

Artifacts also occur in the transverse and descending aorta. In the study of Appelbe et al. (36), "mirror image" artifacts of the transverse and descending aorta were present in more than 80% of patients. These artifacts appear as a reduplication of the aortic lumen. The mirror image is caused by a highly reflective aorta-lung interface and is easy to distinguish from a true anatomic structure. The mirror image occurs at a predictable distance related to the width of the aorta, and the double-lumen appearance of the aorta disappears where the lung is not adjacent to the aorta.

SPECIAL CONSIDERATIONS IN THE EVALUATION OF TYPE III (STANFORD B) DISSECTIONS

The approach to a descending thoracic aortic dissection depends on the location of the primary intimal tear and the status of the patient. Surgery is considered for those patients who present with complications of the dissection, such as impending rupture, intractable pain, expanding size of the aorta, and signs of poor visceral or limb perfusion; it is also considered for young persons with connective tissue diseases who present with dissections at an early age. In these situations, TEE can be very helpful in identifying the exact location of the primary intimal tear at the time of operation. Identification of a normal proximal segment of aorta indicates that the patient can be safely cross-clamped. Currently, however, patients who have type B aortic dissections with primary intimal tears close to the left subclavian artery or extension of the dissection to the left subclavian artery or distal aortic arch should be treated with circulatory arrest. Under these circumstances, TEE is useful for identifying pathology and also for careful monitoring of the LV diameter in the short-axis view. During cooling for circulatory arrest, when the ventricle fibrillates, it is important to monitor for dilation of the LV secondary to aortic insufficiency. If this is identified, it is necessary to place an LV vent through the apex of the LV or across the mitral valve through a pulmonary vein. Currently, it is felt that avoidance of cross-clamping of the dissected aorta facilitates visualization for a proximal anastomosis and may reduce the incidence of residual aortic dissection and pseudoaneurysm formation at the anastomotic site following surgery.

INTRAMURAL HEMATOMA

Intramural hematoma is felt to be a noncommunicating aortic dissection that does not fall within the traditional DeBakey classification system. Intramural hematomas most often involve the ascending or descending aorta and are characterized by a thickened aortic wall without an intimal flap or dissection entry site. The false lumen is felt to be secondary to rupture of the vasa vasorum that results in massive hemorrhage into the vessel wall. The natural history of this disease is such that 60% of patients progress to either rupture or dissection within 1 year (38–40). Aortic rupture usually occurs within several days in patients who have ascending aortic involvement; therefore, rapid diagnosis and surgical treatment are imperative. In patients with a descending thoracic aorta intramural hematoma, the decision between surgical therapy and medical management with a strict antihypertensive regimen and frequent imaging follow-up remains controversial.

The initial TEE classification of intramural hematoma was described by Mohr-Kahaly (41). Intramural hematoma is characterized by circular or crescentic thickening of the aorta wall of more than 7 mm, central displacement of intimal calcification, a longitudinal extent of 1 to 20 cm, a layered appearance, and the absence of an intimal tear or dissection membrane. The thickness is measured from the internal border of the intima to the outer edge of the adventitia. Harris (39) further clarified the TEE findings by noting that an intramural hematoma involving the ascending aorta typically measures 7 ± 2 mm, whereas a hematoma in the descending aorta is much thicker, measuring 15 ± 6 mm. Most of the patients had a crescent-shaped intramural hematoma involving one wall predominantly that compressed the aortic lumen. Compression of the normal circular lumen of the aorta resulted in a major-minor axis ratio of the aortic lumen of $1.3\% \pm 0.2\%$ (39).

THORACIC AORTIC PLAQUE

Stroke continues to be a serious complication of cardiac surgery, occurring in approximately 1% to 5% of patients. The ability to detect atheroma within the thoracic aorta and alter the surgical approach is an important part of most strategies for stroke prevention (42). Royse (43) proposed dividing the thoracic aorta into six zones corresponding to sites of surgical manipulation. Zones 1 through 3 are the proximal, mid, and distal ascending aorta. Zones 1 and 2 are the sites of incision for aortic valve replacement. Figure 16.13 shows a zone 1

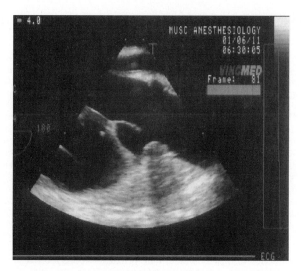

FIG. 16.13. A grade 3 anterior atheroma in zone 1.

atheroma. Zone 2 is also the site for proximal coronary artery bypass graft anastomosis and can be used for antegrade cardioplegia cannulation. Zone 3 is where the aortic cross-clamp is usually placed. Zone 4 includes the proximal arch and is typically the site where the aortic cannula is manipulated. Zone 5, which includes the distal arch, and zone 6, which includes the proximal descending aorta, are not typically manipulated during cardiac surgery (43). However, in these areas, atheroma can be dislodged by the aortic cannula or an endoluminal device, such as an intraaortic balloon pump. In the study of Royse (43), adequate imaging by TEE was obtained in zone 3 in only 58% of patients, and in zone 4 in 42% of patients. These findings are consistent with the work of Konstadt (35,44), who showed that as much as 42% of the length of the ascending aorta is not adequately visualized with TEE. Manual surgical palpation detects only 50% of important atheromas identified by epiaortic ultrasonography (43).

TEE has been proposed as an intraoperative screening tool to identify patients who should undergo epiaortic scanning before cannulation for cardiopulmonary bypass. When moderate to severe atheroma is identified in zones 5 and 6 by TEE, the incidence of moderate to severe atheroma in zones 1 through 4 is high. Therefore, epiaortic scanning should be performed. If all visualized zones (1, 2, 5, and 6) are negative for atheroma, epiaortic scanning of zones 4 and 5, the TEE potential blind spots, is not necessary.

In 1992, Katz (45) published a five-point grading system for aortic atheroma (Table 16.2). Figure 16.14 shows a grade 4 atheroma. Patients with a mobile (grade 5) atheroma had a

**TABLE 16.2. GRADING OF THORACIC
AORTA ATHEROMA**

Grade	Description
1	Normal aorta
2	Extensive intimal thickening
3	Protrudes <5 mm into aortic lumen
4	Protrudes >5 mm into aortic lumen
5	Mobile atheroma

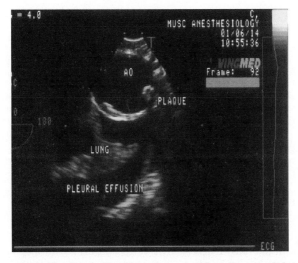

FIG. 16.14. Atheroma in the descending thoracic aorta. Note the consolidated lung with a significant pleural effusion.

25% incidence of stroke, whereas stroke occurred in only 2% of patients without a mobile atheroma. It is therefore important to consider alternative surgical approaches for patients who have a significant protruding atheroma and especially patients with mobile components (45).

Severe ascending aortic calcification or atherosclerosis makes aortic cannulation and cardiopulmonary bypass dangerous and makes it difficult to construct aortic graft anastomoses. This problem has two potential solutions. One involves circulatory arrest with deep hypothermia, which usually requires replacement of a portion of the aorta. A second solution is a less complex operation that avoids cardiopulmonary bypass. Patients who are considered for coronary artery bypass grafting exclusively who present with a calcified ascending aorta can be managed with an off-pump approach. Through a median sternotomy, both the left internal and right internal mammary arteries can be used as conduits. Saphenous vein grafts or radial artery grafts can be taken off either of these conduits or separately anastomosed proximally to side branches of the aortic arch, such as the innominate artery.

SUMMARY

TEE plays an important role in the management of aortic pathology. Its ability to diagnose aortic aneurysm, dissection, and aortic atheroma rapidly and reliably has improved patient outcomes.

REFERENCES

1. Svensson LG, Crawford ES. Aortic dissection and aortic aneurysm surgery: clinical observations, experimental investigations, and statistical analyses. Part II. *Curr Probl Surg* 1992;29:915–1057.
2. DeBakey ME, Henly WS, Cooley DA, et al. Surgical management of dissecting aneurysms of the aorta. *J Thorac Cardiovasc Surg* 1965;49:130–149.

3. Daily PO, Trueblood HW, Stinson EB, et al. Management of acute aortic dissections. *Ann Thorac Surg* 1970;10:237–247.
4. Hirst AE Jr, Johns VJ Jr, Kime SW Jr. Dissecting aneurysm of the aorta: a review of 585 cases. *Medicine (Baltimore)* 1985;37:217–279.
5. Chirillo F, Cavillini C, Longhini C, et al. Comparative diagnostic valve of transesophageal echocardiography and retrograde aortography in the evaluation of thoracic aortic dissection. *Am J Cardiol* 1994;74:590–595.
6. Sommer T, Fehske W, Holzknecht N, et al. Aortic dissection: a comparative study of diagnosis with spiral CT, multiplanar transesophageal echocardiography, and MR imaging. *Radiology* 1996;199:347–352.
7. Cigarroa JE, Isselbacher EM, DeSanctis RW, et al. Diagnostic imaging in the evaluation of suspected aortic dissection. *N Engl J Med* 1993;328:35–43.
8. Barbant SD, Eisenberg MJ, Schiller NB. The diagnostic value of imaging techniques for aortic dissection. *Am Heart J* 1992;124:541–543.
9. Masani ND, Banning AP, Jones RA, et al. Follow-up of chronic thoracic aortic dissection. Comparison of transesophageal echocardiography and magnetic resonance imaging. *Am Heart J* 1996;131:1156–1163.
10. Willens HJ, Kessler KM. Transesophageal echocardiography in the diagnosis of diseases of the thoracic aorta. *Chest* 1999;116:1172–1179.
11. Adachi H, Omoto R, Kyo S, et al. Emergency surgical intervention of acute aortic dissection with the rapid diagnosis by transesophageal echocardiography. *Circulation* 1991;84[Suppl III]:III-14–III-19.
12. Keren A, Kim CB, Hu BS, et al. Accuracy of biplane and multiplane transesophageal echocardiography in diagnosis of typical acute aortic dissection and intramural hematoma. *J Am Coll Cardiol* 1996;28:627–636.
13. Shanewise JS, Cheung AT, Aronson S, et al. ASE/SCA guidelines for performing a comprehensive intraoperative multiplane transesophageal echocardiography examination: recommendations of the American Society of Echocardiography Council for Intraoperative Echocardiography and the Society of Cardiovascular Anesthesiologists Task Force for Certification in Perioperative Transesophageal Echocardiography. *Anesth Analg* 1999;89:870–884.
14. Erbel R, Engberding R, Daniel W, et al. Echocardiography in diagnosis of aortic dissection. *Lancet* 1989;1(8636):457–461.
15. Iliceto S, Nanda NC, Rizzon P, et al. Color Doppler evaluation of aortic dissection. *Circulation* 1987;75:748–755.
16. Matthew T, Nanda NC. Two-dimensional and Doppler echocardiographic evaluation of aortic aneurysm and dissection. *Am J Cardiol* 1984;54:379–385.
17. Erbel R, Mohr-Kahaly S, Oelert H, et al. Diagnostic strategies in suspected aortic dissection: comparison of computed tomography, aortography, and transesophageal echocardiography. *Am J Card Imaging* 1990;4:157–172.
18. Erbel R, Borner N, Steller D, et al. Detection of aortic dissection by transesophageal echocardiography. *Br Heart J* 1987;58:45–51.
19. Mohr-Kahaly S, Erbel R, Rennollet H, et al. Ambulatory follow-up of aortic dissection by transesophageal two-dimensional and color-coded Doppler echocardiography. *Circulation* 1989;80:24–33.
20. Hashimoto S, Kumada T, Osakada G, et al. Assessment of transesophageal Doppler echocardiography in dissecting aortic aneurysm. *J Am Coll Cardiol* 1989;14:1253–1261.
21. Erbel K, Mohr-Kahaly S, Rennullet H, et al. Diagnosis of aortic dissection: the value of transesophageal echocardiography. *Thorac Cardiovasc Surg* 1987;35[Special Issue 1]:126–133.
22. Dagli SV, Nanda NC, Roitman D, et al. Evaluation of aortic dissection by Doppler color flow mapping. *Am J Cardiol* 1985;56:497–498.
23. Adachi H, Kyo S, Takamoto S, et al. Early diagnosis and surgical intervention of acute aortic dissection by transesophageal color flow mapping. *Circulation* 1990;82[Suppl IV]:IV-19–IV-23.
24. Taams MH, Gussenhoven WJ, Schippers LA, et al. The value of transesophageal

echocardiography for diagnosis of thoracic aortic pathology. *Eur Heart J* 1988;9:1308–1316.

25. Heinemann M, Laas J, Karck M, et al. Thoracic aortic aneurysms after acute type A aortic dissection: necessity for follow-up. *Ann Thorac Surg* 1990;49:580–584.

26. Bansal RC, Shah PM. Transesophageal echocardiography. *Curr Probl Cardiol* 1990;15:643–720.

27. Erbel R, Mohr-Kahaly S, Rennollet H, et al. Diagnosis of aortic dissection: the value of transesophageal echocardiography. *Thorac Cardiovasc Surg* 1987;35:126–133.

28. Perry GJ, Helmcke F, Nanda NC, et al. Evaluation of aortic insufficiency by Doppler color flow mapping. *J Am Coll Cardiol* 1987;9:952–959.

29. Erbel R, Oelert H, Meyer J, et al. Effect of medical and surgical therapy on aortic dissection evaluated by transesophageal echocardiography. *Circulation* 1993;87:1604–1615.

30. Slater EE, DeSanctis RW. The clinical recognition of dissecting aortic aneurysm. *Am J Med* 1976;60:625–633.

31. Hunt D, Baxley WA, Kennedy JW, et al. Quantitative evaluation of cine aortography in the assessment of aortic regurgitation. *Am J Cardiol* 1973;31:696–700.

32. Ballard RS, Nanda NC, Gatewood R, et al. Usefulness of transesophageal echocardiography in assessment of aortic dissection. *Circulation* 1991;84:1903–1914.

33. Mazzucotelli JP, Deleuze PH, Baufreton C, et al. Preservation of the aortic valve in acute aortic dissection: long-term echocardiographic assessment and clinical outcome. *Ann Thorac Surg* 1993;55:1513–1517.

34. DeBakey ME, McCollum CH, Crawford ES, et al. Dissection and dissecting aneurysm of the aorta: twenty-year follow-up of five hundred twenty-seven patients treated surgically. *Surgery* 1982;92:1118–1134.

35. Konstadt SN, Reich DL, Kahn R, et al. Transesophageal echocardiography can be used to screen for ascending aortic atherosclerosis. *Anesth Analg* 1995;81:225–228.

36. Appelbe AF, Walker PG, Yeoh JK, et al. Clinical significance and origin of artifacts in transesophageal endocardiography of the thoracic aorta. *J Am Coll Cardiol* 1993;21:754–760.

37. Nienaber CA, Spielman RP, Von Kodolitsch Y, et al. Diagnosis of thoracic aortic dissection: magnetic resonance imagery versus transesophageal echocardiography. *Circulation* 1992;85:434–447.

38. Robbins RC, McManus RP, Mitchell RS, et al. Management of patients with intramural hematoma of the thoracic aorta. *Circulation* 1993;88:1–10.

39. Harris KM, Braverman AC, Gutierrez FR, et al. Transesophageal echocardiography and clinical features of aortic intramural hematoma. *J Thorac Cardiovasc Surg* 1997;114:619–626.

40. Kang DH, Song JK, Song MG, et al. Clinical and echocardiographic outcomes of aortic intramural hemorrhage compared with acute aortic dissection. *Am J Cardiol* 1998;81:202–206.

41. Mohr-Kahaly S, Erbel R, Kearney P, et al. Aortic intramural hemorrhage visualized by transesophageal echocardiography: findings and prognostic implications. *J Am Coll Cardiol* 1994;23:658–664.

42. Ribakove GH, Katz ES, Galloway AC, et al. Surgical implications of transesophageal echocardiography to grade the atheromatous aortic arch. *Ann Thorac Surg* 1992;53:758–763.

43. Royse C, Royse A, Blake D, et al. Screening the thoracic aorta for atheroma: a comparison of manual palpation, transesophageal and epiaortic ultrasonography. *Ann Thorac Cardiovasc Surg* 1998;4:347–350.

44. Konstadt SN, Reich DL, Quintana C, et al. The ascending aorta: how much does transesophageal echocardiography see? *Anesth Analg* 1994;78:240–244.

45. Katz ES, Tunick PA, Rusinek H, et al. Protruding aortic atheromas predict stroke in elderly patients undergoing cardiopulmonary bypass: experience with intraoperative transesophageal echocardiography. *J Am Coll Cardiol* 1992;20:70–77.

QUESTIONS

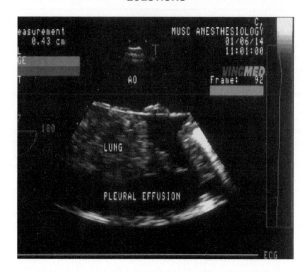

1. Figure 16.15 (above) shows a descending aorta long-axis view of an atheroma. This plaque is consistent with grade
   a. 1
   b. 2
   c. 3
   d. 4
   e. 5
2. The appropriate response for the patient in Question 1 is
   a. Doing nothing
   b. Surgical manual palpation of the ascending aorta in the area of the aortic cross-clamp
   c. Completely evaluating zones 1, 2, 5, and 6, and if no lesions above grade 3 are identified, proceeding with aortic cannulation in the normal fashion
   d. Completely examining zones 1, 2, 5, and 6, and if an atheroma of grade 4 or 5 is found, then performing epiaortic ultrasonography of zones 3 and 4
3. The following characteristics indicate an intramural hematoma **except**
   a. A circular or crescentic thickening in the aortic wall larger than 7 mm
   b. Central displacement of intimal calcification
   c. A layered appearance
   d. Longitudinal extent of 1 to 20 cm
   e. A very fine intimal tear
4. Which statement most closely explains the relationship between TEE and the ascending distal aorta and proximal arch?
   a. Multiplane TEE can clearly visualize the entire ascending aorta and proximal arch.
   b. A blind spot is caused by the trachea overlying the ascending aorta.
   c. A blind spot is caused by the trachea and left main bronchus overlying the ascending aorta and proximal arch.
   d. A blind spot is caused by the trachea, left main bronchus, and right main bronchus overlying the ascending aorta and proximal arch.

5. Causes of aortic insufficiency secondary to aortic dissection include all of the following **except**
   a. An extensive or circumferential tear dilates the aortic root and annulus, causing failure of coaptation of the aortic valve leaflets.
   b. With asymmetric dissection, pressure from the false lumen depresses one aortic leaflet below the coaptation line of the other leaflets.
   c. The annular support is disrupted, resulting in a flail aortic leaflet.
   d. Prolapse of a mobile intimal flap through the aortic valve during systole prevents leaflet coaptation.
   e. All of the above.
6. All of the following statements about the diagnostic performance of imaging modalities in the evaluation of suspected aortic dissections are true **except**
   a. TEE is as sensitive as angiography, CT, and MRI.
   b. TEE is the most sensitive modality for detecting a thrombus within an aortic dissection.
   c. TEE is extremely sensitive in detecting aortic insufficiency.
   d. Angiography is not useful in determining whether a patient has a pericardial effusion.
7. Which of the following statements about the DeBakey and Stanford classification criteria for aortic dissections is false?
   a. The DeBakey classification comprises three types.
   b. Stanford type A includes both DeBakey type I and DeBakey type III.
   c. The Stanford criteria were developed to determine whether a patient requires medical or surgical management.
   d. A DeBakey type III-B dissection is a type III dissection that extends below the diaphragm.
8. The surgical goals of intraoperative TEE in the evaluation of aortic dissection include which of the following?
   a. Confirmation of the preoperative diagnosis
   b. Determination of the dissection entry site, including the differentiation of true from false lumina
   c. Evaluation of ventricular distention and aortic insufficiency if circulatory arrest is planned.
   d. Assessment of the surgical repair
   e. All of the above
9. Which of the following is/are TEE manifestations of acute aortic dissection?
   a. Intimal flap
   b. Complete thrombus of the false lumen
   c. Central displacement of intimal calcification, evidenced as a bright echogenic area within the aorta
   d. Separation of intimal layers secondary to thrombus
   e. All of the above
10. Which of the following statements is false?
    a. Aortic insufficiency is present in up to 70% of patients with a proximal dissection.
    b. Aortic insufficiency is present in 10% of patients with a dissection of the descending thoracic aorta.
    c. Preservation of the native aortic valve with repair and resuspension is possible in more 80% of patients with a type A dissection.
    d. Coronary artery involvement by acute aortic dissection is rare, occurring in fewer than 5% of patients.

17

Transesophageal Echocardiography in the Intensive Care Unit

Emilio B. Lobato and Felipe Urdaneta

Paralleling the increased application of transesophageal echocardiography (TEE) in intra-operative cardiac evaluation has been its widespread utilization in the intensive care unit (ICU) to evaluate hemodynamically unstable patients. This chapter examines the unique advantages of TEE and discusses its use in many of the common diagnostic dilemmas confronting the intensivist.

COMPARISON OF TRANSESOPHAGEAL ECHOCARDIOGRAPHY WITH OTHER DIAGNOSTIC AND MONITORING MODALITIES

Transesophageal Echocardiography versus Transthoracic Echocardiography

Echocardiography in intensive care settings is well described (1). Transthoracic echocardiography (TTE) is the easiest and least invasive way to image cardiac structures. However, in many critically ill patients, low-quality images are obtained because the acoustic windows are suboptimal. The examination is estimated to be inadequate in approximately 50% of patients on mechanical ventilation and 60% of all ICU patients (2). Acoustic windows are frequently suboptimal in patients who are morbidly obese, have multiple chest tubes or extensive dressings, or are receiving mechanical ventilation (Table 17.1). TEE, although more invasive, often provides images of better quality and resolution than TTE because the acoustic windows from the esophagus to the heart and great vessels are unobstructed. In addition, the TEE probe can be left in place for many hours for the continuous monitoring of cardiac function, and its position can be readily reproduced to provide repeated comparisons. At present, only oral probes are available, which are poorly tolerated for continuous monitoring. However, newer, smaller probes placed transnasally for long-term use are currently being evaluated.

In many conditions, even with the best-quality TTE imaging, the diagnostic yield of TEE is greater. Conditions in which TEE is superior to TTE are listed in Table 17.2. TEE is by far more sensitive for the detection of left atrial thrombi, small vegetations, periprosthetic valvular insufficiency, aortic dissection, and central pulmonary emboli. In patients receiving mechanical ventilation and positive end-expiratory pressure, LV function is more easily and more accurately assessed with TEE. This diagnostic superiority is particularly important when mechanical ventilation is applied in patients with hemodynamic instability. *TEE provides unexpected diagnoses that are missed by TTE in up to 40% of cases* (3,4). The clinical impact of TEE on therapeutic decision making is substantial, frequently leading to changes in medical or surgical management.

Transesophageal Echocardiography versus Pulmonary Artery Catheterization

Pulmonary artery (PA) catheterization is often utilized in critically ill patients. The evaluation of left ventricular (LV) preload and function and the measurement of cardiac output (CO) are considered essential for appropriate hemodynamic management. The PA occlusion pressure remains the most commonly used variable to assess LV preload; however, the values can be misleading. In the ICU setting, factors such as positive end-expiratory pressure and changes in ventricular compliance can be associated with elevation of the PA occlusion pressure independently of LV volume. Similarly, LV function is evaluated indirectly based on the relationship of the PA occlusion pressure to the CO. As was noted previously, TEE rapidly visualizes the LV, providing direct estimates of ventricular dimensions and function. *Data obtained with TEE frequently differ from PA catheterization assessments of the LV preload*

TABLE 17.1. CHALLENGES TO TRANSESOPHAGEAL ECHOCARDIOGRAPHIC IMAGES IN CRITICAL CARE

Obesity
Mediastinal drainage tubes
Chest dressings
Inability to position patient on left side
Chronic obstructive pulmonary disease
Positive end-expiratory pressure
Ribs, calcified rib cartilages

and systolic function and can lead to a change in therapy 40% to 60% of patients when utilized (5,6). In patients with preexisting myocardial dysfunction and cardiomegaly, changes in the LV end-diastolic area and concomitant measurements of the PA occlusion pressure may serve to determine the optimal LV preload and provide a better titration of inotropic agents.

In addition, TEE measurement of the CO in critically ill patients, with Doppler analysis of the LV outflow, has been found to correlate well with bolus thermodilution (7). The ability to provide continuous CO measurements is compromised because minimal movement of the probe will significantly alter results.

PROBE INSERTION

Although relatively safe in experienced hands, TEE is a semiinvasive procedure that is not without risk. Critically ill patients represent a heterogeneous population, and an individualized approach to the TEE examination is required. The use of mechanical ventilation and the patient's hemodynamic and respiratory status and level of consciousness are important factors that must be considered. Placement of a TEE probe in an uncooperative patient can be associated with esophageal trauma, increased cardiovascular stress, hypoxia, and dysrhythmias. Emesis and aspiration are real concerns, particularly in nonfasting patients without an endotracheal tube.

Preparation

1. ***Fasting.*** If possible, the patient should be fasting for at least 4 hours before the procedure.
2. ***History.*** A history of esophageal/gastric pathology or dysphagia should be evaluated.
3. ***Monitoring.*** The electrocardiography apparatus, pulse oximeter, and blood pressure monitors should be placed.
4. ***Sedation.*** Passage of the TEE transducer tip through the oropharynx is not infrequently cumbersome; an adequate level of sedation ensures better patient cooperation. The choice of sedatives must be tailored to the patient's respiratory and hemodynamic status to

TABLE 17.2. SITUATIONS IN WHICH TRANSESOPHAGEAL IS SUPERIOR TO TRANSTHORACIC ECHOCARDIOGRAPHY

Mechanical ventilation
Cardiac tamponade
Diagnosis of vegetations and complications of endocarditis
Central pulmonary emboli
Exclusion of a cardiac source of embolism
Evaluation of a mediastinal hematoma
Diagnosis of ascending or descending thoracic aortic dissection
Structural and functional evaluation of native valves, including
    postoperative assessment of mitral repair
Acute hemodynamic instability

decrease the likelihood of hypoxemia or hypotension. Small intravenous doses of benzodiazepines or opiates are commonly used, and pharmacologic reversal (naloxone, flumazenil) can be instituted if necessary. *Excessive sedation resulting in a lack of patient cooperation is problematic because swallowing on command is necessary to facilitate probe insertion.*

5. ***Prevention of the gag reflex.*** Topical anesthesia of the oropharynx effectively decreases the gag reflex. Lidocaine or benzocaine spray is applied to the posterior pharynx, or the patient is instructed to gargle with viscous lidocaine. A drying agent such as glycopyrrolate may decrease the possibility of salivary aspiration; however, it can be associated with tachyarrhythmias.

6. ***Tracheal intubation.*** Sedation, paralysis, and tracheal intubation may be necessary in patients with severe respiratory distress or cardiovascular collapse in whom TEE must be performed urgently or emergently.

7. ***Nasogastric suction.*** If a nasogastric tube is present, the stomach contents should be suctioned before the examination. *Nasogastric tubes usually do not interfere with insertion of the transducer or the quality of the images;* however, on occasion, they must be removed.

8. ***Patient positioning.*** Patients are commonly placed in a semirecumbent, left lateral decubitus position with the head slightly flexed to facilitate probe placement and drainage of secretions. Supine positioning is most commonly used for intubated patients.

Technique

1. Place a mouth guard to protect the TEE probe unless the patient is edentulous.
2. Thoroughly lubricate the tip of the transducer with ultrasonic gel.
3. Check for free movement of the tip and *maintain in the unlocked position.*
4. With the patient's mouth open, gently depress the tongue with the index finger, place the transducer over the finger in the midline, and gently advance it posteriorly toward the esophagus.
5. Instruct the patient to swallow.
6. Advance the transducer into the esophagus. As you advance, slight resistance from the cricoid sphincter may have to be overcome before the probe enters the esophagus. However, significant resistance to advancement typically signifies that the probe has deviated from the midline and rests within the pyriform sinus. Withdraw the probe and make adjustments in the patient's position and flexion of the probe to advance it into the esophagus.
7. Intubated patients frequently require sedation and muscle relaxants. *On occasion, direct laryngoscopy, deflation of the endotracheal tube cuff, or both are necessary to facilitate passage of the transducer.*
8. Once the probe is advanced to approximately 30 cm from the incisors, the examination can begin.

CONTRAINDICATIONS AND COMPLICATIONS TO TRANSESOPHAGEAL ECHOCARDIOGRAPHY

Contraindications to TEE include significant esophageal or gastric pathology (e.g., tumors, strictures). Esophageal varices are not an absolute contraindication, especially when TEE is urgently indicated. However, bleeding can occur, particularly in the presence of coagulation abnormalities. In patients with cervical spinal disease or injury, manipulation of the neck must be avoided to prevent disastrous consequences.

Overall, complications associated with TEE are rare, averaging 0.5% in the general population (8,9). Table 17.3 lists the types and incidence of the complications most often encountered during TEE. A multicenter study of more than 10,000 TEE examinations reported a procedural mortality of 0.01%. Cardiac, pulmonary, and bleeding events requiring interruption of the procedure occurred in 0.18% of cases (9).

It is logical to assume that in critically ill patients, TEE-associated complications may be more frequent as a consequence of their severe illness and unstable state. However, the incidence of complications remains low, albeit slightly higher than in patients who are not critically ill. A review of 943 TEE examinations performed in several ICUs reported a

TABLE 17.3. COMPLICATIONS IN 15,381
TRANSESOPHAGEAL EXAMINATIONS

Complication	Percentage (%)
Hypoxia	0.6
Hypotension	0.5
Hypertension	0.2
PSVT	0.2
NSVT	<0.1
Hematemesis	0.1
Laryngospasm	0.1
Esophageal tear	<0.02
Death	<0.02

PSVT, paroximal supraventricular tachycardia; NSVT, nonsustained
ventricular tachycardia.
Modified from Oh JK, Seward JB, Tajik AJ. Transesophageal echocardiography. In: Oh JK, Seward JB, Tajik AJ, eds. *The echo manual* 2nd
ed. Philadelphia: Lippincott Williams & Wilkins, 1999:23–36.

complication rate of 1.7%, with arrhythmias and hypotension occurring most frequently (7).
Serious complications developed in only two patients (0.2%). Difficulties with probe insertion
have been reported in only 1.4% of patients (7). Thus, with appropriate monitoring, TEE is
a safe technique, even in the patients who are most compromised.

DISADVANTAGES AND LIMITATIONS

Transducer Size

The adult TEE probe is a modified gastroesophageal endoscope measuring about 100 cm
in length and 1 cm in width. The transducer, located at the tip, measures between 10 and
16 mm. Because of its size, it can create significant discomfort. Occasionally, attempts at
probe insertion are unsuccessful, and one should desist or risk esophageal perforation. Although the probe can be safely left in place to provide continuous monitoring, many of these
patients require high levels of sedation, so that its usefulness as a monitoring tool is limited.
New, miniaturized TEE probes can be inserted transnasally and left in place for prolonged
periods of time. They currently are being tested for image quality and patient acceptance,
and it is hoped that they will be available in the near future.

Limited Acoustic Windows

The TEE views of some anatomic structures are limited. These include the following:

1. Superior portion of the ascending aorta (because of interference from the left main
   bronchus): frequent
2. Left branch of the pulmonary artery: frequent
3. LV apex: occasional.

In addition, proper alignment of the LV outflow tract and ascending aorta during Doppler
spectral analysis to measure the CO or the aortic valve area can be technically demanding.

Time-Consuming Analysis

1. Off-line quantitative measurements of LV function (preload, afterload, and fraction of
   area of change) require meticulous interpretation and considerable time.

2. Real-time assessment with automatic border detection techniques may be limited by the inability to visualize the entire endocardium.

COMMON INDICATIONS FOR TRANSESOPHAGEAL ECHOCARDIOGRAPHY IN CRITICAL CARE

The indications for TEE examinations are varied and continue to increase (Table 17.4). Not surprisingly, the use of TEE varies according to the type of ICU. In medical ICUs, most patients were examined by TEE to rule out endocarditis; in coronary and surgical ICUs, aortic dissection and valvular assessment were the primary indications; and in neurosurgical ICUs, a cardiac source of embolism was the principal indication (10).

Hemodynamic Instability

The evaluation of hemodynamic instability is one of the most common and important indications for TEE in the ICU. Because the patient is usually hypotensive, an accurate diagnosis expedites therapy and helps to prevent an adverse event or death. Frequently, the physical examination findings are limited; placement of a PA catheter is time-consuming, and the information obtained is often ambiguous and incomplete. TEE is a fast and accurate method to ascertain whether the hemodynamic instability is cardiac or noncardiac in origin. The lack of a blood pressure response to a fluid challenge leaves the clinician in doubt about whether to repeat the fluid challenge or obtain further diagnostic information. TEE can provide the necessary information less invasively and faster than a PA catheter (11–13).

Assessment of ventricular function. Knowledge of the cardiac volume status and pump function are major priorities in ICU care. By providing rapid visualization of the left and right ventricles, TEE can aid both in the diagnosis and in monitoring the response to therapy. A recommended rapid examination to assess ventricular function follows.

Assessment of the left ventricular end-diastolic area: One starts at the transgastric (TG) mid short-axis view to evaluate the LV preload and global systolic function. Determination of the LV preload is of primary importance in critically ill patients. The LV end-diastolic area, obtained from this view, allows the rapid identification of LV volume depletion or overload. It provides a better estimate of LV preload than the PA occlusion pressure (14,15). The range of normal values for the LV end-diastolic area is wide; thus, determination of the optimal preload may require a fluid challenge to assess changes.

Estimation of the left ventricular ejection fraction: A visual estimation of LV global systolic function (LV ejection fraction) is performed in the same view.

Assessment of regional wall motion abnormalities: An analysis of segmental wall motion in multiple views (TG mid short-axis, midesophageal [ME] four-chamber, ME two-chamber, and ME long-axis views) completes the assessment of LV function.

Assessment of right ventricular function: Right ventricular (RV) function is evaluated with the ME views. A visual assessment of ventricular dilation and systolic function provides a

TABLE 17.4. INDICATIONS FOR TRANSESOPHAGEAL ECHOCARDIOGRAPHY IN THE INTENSIVE CARE UNIT

Assessment of left ventricular function	Complications of myocardial infarction
Hemodynamic instability	Pericardial effusion
Assessment of valvular function	Evaluation of heart transplant donors
Suspected endocarditis	Hemodynamic management
Determination of source of systemic embolism	Evaluation of chest trauma
Pulmonary emboli	

qualitative impression of RV function. The PA systolic pressure can be estimated by Doppler analysis of a tricuspid regurgitant jet if present.

Additional evaluation: The above sequence often allows an initial diagnosis and treatment. A more comprehensive TEE examination can be completed as therapy continues.

Evaluation of valvular function. TEE is invaluable in the assessment of valvular function. It can detect significant mitral regurgitation and unsuspected severe aortic valve disease in patients with unexplained heart failure (16). Besides providing a diagnosis and establishing the severity of disease, TEE can provide clues to its cause by detecting abnormal ventricular function, ruptured chordae, valvular perforation, abnormal masses, and vegetations (17).

Following prosthetic valve replacement, TEE can identify perivalvular regurgitation, especially in the mitral position. Perivalvular leaks from the aortic valve are not as easily detected because of acoustic shadowing of the LV outflow tract. Jets of perivalvular regurgitation must be differentiated from the normal cleansing regurgitation present in mechanical prostheses. TEE can also detect mitral and aortic bioprosthetic dysfunction secondary to degeneration and rupture of the cusps as the predominant mechanism of heart failure.

The echocardiographic evaluation of valve function is discussed in detail in Part 3 of this book.

Evaluation of hypotension. Table 17.5 summarizes the causes of hypotension and lists the associated TEE findings.

TABLE 17.5. CONDITIONS ASSOCIATED WITH HYPOTENSION

Condition	Useful views	TEE findings
Pericardial tamponade	Four-chamber view, short- and long-axis transgastric	Effusion Diastolic collapse of the atrium Exaggerated variation on E- or S-wave velocities with inspiration
Aortic dissection	Five-chamber view, aortic valve and ascending and descending aorta	Intimal flap No flow on false lumen (color Doppler) Aortic regurgitation Pericardial effusion
Pulmonary embolus	Four-chamber pulmonary artery and RVOT views	Echogenic density in pulmonary artery Dilated RA and RV Small LA and LV TR and PR jets Flow through PFO
Hypovolemia	LV short-axis transgastric LV long-axis transgastric	↓EDA ↑FAC "Kissing" papillary muscles
Decreased systolic function	LV short-axis transgastric LV long-axis transgastric	↑EDA ↑ESA ↓FAC
Severe valvular regurgitation or stenosis	Appropriate valvular plane	Doppler methods Planimetry
Vasodilation	Short-axis transgastric	Normal EDA ↑FAC Absence of severe valvular regurgitation

RA, right atrium; RV, right ventricle; LA, left atrium; LV, left ventricle; PR, pulmonary regurgitation; TR, tricuspid regurgitation; PFO, patent foramen ovale; EDA, end-diastolic area; ESA, end-systolic area; FAC, fractional area of change; RVOT, right ventricular outflow tract.

Endocarditis

Indications for transesophageal echocardiography. Suspected infective endocarditis is a rather common indication for a TEE examination in the ICU. Critically ill patients are at high risk for bacteremia caused by indwelling catheters or colonized endotracheal tubes. TEE is cost-effective in ICU patients in comparison with other modalities when the probability of endocarditis exceeds 2% (7,19). *Because critically ill patients often present with nonspecific signs and symptoms, the threshold for performing TEE should be low.*

Clinical implications of the transesophageal echocardiographic findings. The hallmark lesions are vegetations, which are generally attached to valves (Fig. 17.1) but can also adhere to a wall in areas of denuded endocardium. The appearance is that of an echo-dense, often pedunculated mass exhibiting a variable range of motion. Multiplane TEE is credited with a 90% to 100% sensitivity in detecting left-sided vegetations, and a special benefit in detecting small vegetations in patients with a prosthetic valve (20). For right-sided vegetations, it may not offer a substantial benefit in comparison with conventional TTE. *However, TEE is the procedure of choice to identify complications such as abscess, perforation, mycotic aneurysms, and fistulae.* In addition, it offers important prognostic information. The size of vegetations, location (mitral vs. aortic), mobility, and number of valves affected all are related to the likelihood of complications (systemic embolization, congestive heart failure, failure to respond to treatment, death) (21). TEE may also assist in the decision to perform surgery, particularly when a prosthetic valve is involved.

When native endocarditis is suspected, a negative TEE examination result makes this diagnosis very unlikely. If the patient has a prosthetic valve, it is wise to repeat the examination when the clinical picture remains consistent with the presumptive diagnosis. Other echocardiographic findings, including myxomatous changes, Lambl excrescences in the aortic valve (small oscillating masses on the aortic side of the valve cusps), thrombus formation, and suture material, can be confused with infective endocarditis. Degenerative changes of the bioprosthesis are usually seen as prolapsing masses and can also be confused with vegetations. Finally, it must be remembered that vegetations may occur in the absence of infection, such as those associated with marantic endocarditis, systemic lupus erythematosus, and tumors.

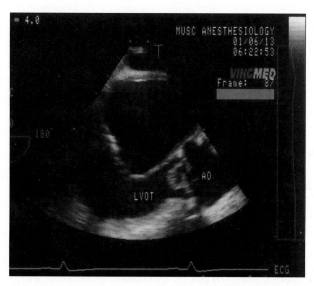

FIG. 17.1. Midesophageal aortic valve long-axis view demonstrating large aortic valve (*AO*) vegetation.

Aortic Dissection

Imaging caveats. TEE is ideal for evaluating the thoracic aorta because of the proximity of the esophagus to the aorta. One must remember, however, that the air-filled trachea is interposed between the esophagus and the distal ascending aorta and proximal aortic arch. This area is not clearly visualized, even with multiplane technology. Fortunately, an isolated dissection in this area is rare. Multiplane TEE is a useful diagnostic modality in patients with suspected aortic dissection, having 99% sensitivity and better than 90% specificity (17). TEE should be the procedure of choice for an ICU patient because it can be performed safely and rapidly at the bedside.

Transesophageal echocardiographic examination. The goals of perioperative TEE in the evaluation of aortic dissection include the following: (a) establishing the diagnosis, (b) localizing primary and secondary entry sites, (c) differentiating the true from the false lumen, (d) evaluating the aortic valve for insufficiency, (e) establishing involvement of the coronary arteries, and (f) ruling out associated conditions such as pericardial infusions and tamponade.

Localization of the intimal flap: *The diagnosis is established by identifying an intimal flap (a mobile linear echo within the vascular lumen) in at least two planes.* Figure 17.2 demonstrates an intimal flap within the descending aorta. Color flow Doppler can identify flow within the true and false lumina on either side of an intimal flap and is also highly sensitive for detecting aortic dissection. We find it most useful to begin in the stomach with the descending aorta short-axis view. Typically, the depth setting is reduced to enlarge the size of the aorta on the display monitor. The transducer is gradually withdrawn while an intimal flap is sought until the ME ascending aorta short-axis view is obtained. *Special care must be taken in evaluating the aorta near the left subclavian artery (ligamentum arteriosum area) because approximately 30% of acute dissections originate at this location.* The transducer is then rotated to approximately 90 degrees to obtain the ME ascending aorta long-axis view, and the probe is gradually advanced to achieve the descending aorta long-axis view, with careful observation throughout its path to detect an intimal flap.

Once the descending aorta has been evaluated, the ME aortic valve long-axis view is obtained to interrogate the proximal ascending aorta. *More than 70% of dissections exhibit*

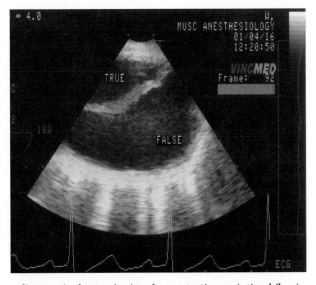

FIG. 17.2. Descending aortic short-axis view demonstrating an intimal flap in a patient with a type B aortic dissection.

an intimal tear originating in the ascending aorta 1 to 3 cm above the right or left sinus of *Valsalva.* The surgeon will need to know the location of the entrance site. We use anatomic landmarks to assist in the surgical identification. In the ascending aorta, we use the distance in centimeters from the aortic valve. Within the descending aorta, we use the distance from the left subclavian artery.

Identification of true and false lumina: The true lumen can be identified by expansion during systole and compression during diastole. M-mode is extremely helpful in identifying and timing these events (22). Thrombus or spontaneous echo contrast may be present in the false lumen as a consequence of stagnant flow. In chronic dissections, the false lumen is typically much larger (23–25). Small secondary tears and any exit sites must be identified to facilitate repair.

Evaluation of coronary artery involvement: Coronary artery involvement is evaluated by observing acute regional wall motion abnormalities.

Evaluation of cardiac tamponade: Cardiac tamponade is suspected and evaluated when a pericardial effusion is present. The echocardiographic manifestations of cardiac tamponade are discussed in Chapter 7 and later in this chapter.

Unexplained Hypoxemia

In some ICU patients, the degree of hypoxemia appears disproportionate to the severity of their illness. In patients with elevated right atrial pressure, TEE may diagnose an intracardiac shunt through a patent foramen ovale (Fig.17.3; see Color Plate 31 following page 212) or an atrial septal defect. Right-to-left intracardiac shunting can be demonstrated by means of color flow Doppler or contrast echocardiography with agitated saline solution as a contrast agent or a commercially available agent. When right-to-left intracardiac shunting occurs through a patent foramen ovale, left atrial contrast is observed within three cardiac cycles, and the density does not match that of the right side (7). In contrast, in intrapulmonary shunting, right-sided opacification frequently diminishes while the intensity of left-sided contrast continues to increase (18). In intrapulmonary shunting, contrast is frequently seen entering the left atrium via the pulmonary veins. A diagnosis of intracardiac shunting leads to changes in management, such as the elimination of positive end-expiratory pressure or the placement of catheter-based septal closure devices.

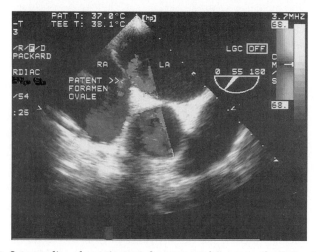

FIG. 17.3. Intracardiac shunt (patent foramen ovale) across the intraatrial septum. (See Color Plate 31 following page 212.)

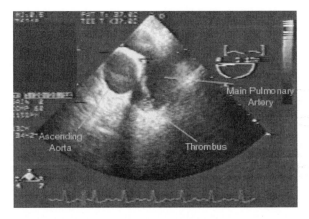

FIG. 17.4. Upper esophageal view showing main pulmonary artery bifurcation with an echo-dense structure (thrombus).

Embolism

Pulmonary embolism. Acute pulmonary embolism carries a high mortality. In the ICU, it remains difficult to diagnose, so that one must have a high index of suspicion. Successful imaging of acute pulmonary emboli within the main or right pulmonary artery has been extensively described (26–28) (Fig. 17.4). The left pulmonary artery, however, is rarely seen beyond a few centimeters because of interposition of the left main bronchus. Pruszczyk et al. (28) have delineated the following echo manifestations of thrombus in an effort to minimize false-positive diagnoses of pulmonary embolism.

1. An unequivocal thrombus should have distinct borders and an echo density different from that of blood in the adjacent vascular walls.
2. The thrombus may protrude into the arterial lumen and thus alter the blood flow by Doppler imaging.
3. The thrombus must be imaged in more than one plane.
4. The thrombus may have a distinct movement separate from that of the vascular wall and blood flow.

Although TTE is routinely used to screen patients with suspected pulmonary embolism, TEE is indicated if TTE is nondiagnostic, hemodynamic instability is present, or RV overload is identified (to confirm central pulmonary or intracardiac thromboemboli). Central thromboemboli are frequently demonstrated in patients with associated hemodynamic compromise. In these cases, TEE has a sensitivity of 80% and a specificity of approximately 100% (28). Although a negative TEE examination cannot rule out pulmonary embolism, positive TEE findings confirm the decision to institute either thrombolytic or surgical therapy.

Systemic embolism. TEE is useful in determining the source of emboli in patients with stroke, transient ischemic attack, or emboli in the extremities or viscera (29). Findings include atrial and ventricular thrombi, vegetations, tumors, and atrial septal aneurysms. Spontaneous echo contrast ("smoke") in the atrium, particularly in patients with atrial fibrillation, indicates a low-flow state that may lead to thrombus formation (see Fig. 10.10). In ICU patients with atrial fibrillation, TEE is often necessary to rule out the presence of thrombi before cardioversion when a long period of anticoagulation is not possible.

Mobile atheromatous plaques in the aorta are a frequent source of emboli that are readily identified by TEE (30). TEE can assess plaque mobility and overall load. Arteriosclerosis of the aorta is a marker of diffuse disease and commonly associated with carotid and peripheral vascular disease. Hence, a thorough workup (e.g., carotid ultrasound) should be performed to evaluate the common sites of embolism and ensure that appropriate treatment is instituted.

Myocardial Infarction

In patients with myocardial infarction, particularly patients in cardiogenic shock, TEE can provide useful information regarding the extent of myocardial involvement and suspected complications (16). Acute valvular insufficiency, secondary to either chordal or papillary muscle rupture and the presence of mural thrombi, is best evaluated with TEE. Other mechanical complications, such as ventricular septal defect and ventricular pseudoaneurysm, are readily diagnosed with TEE. The latter condition is also associated with characteristic color flow Doppler findings of antegrade flow into the pseudoaneurysm during early systole and retrograde flow in early diastole. This flow pattern is helpful in differentiating a pseudoaneurysm from a true aneurysm or a loculated pericardial effusion (16).

One limitation of TEE is that the ventricular apex is sometimes poorly visualized, and thus infarction, aneurysms, or thrombi in that location may not be obvious. In these situations, apical views with TTE may be required.

Blunt Chest Trauma

Injury patterns. In patients with severe chest wall injury, a complete assessment of cardiac structures and function may not be possible with TTE, as previously discussed. The most common abnormality following blunt chest trauma is myocardial contusion. The RV wall, because of its proximity to the sternum, is the most vulnerable structure and is involved in approximately 25% of patients. The LV is also involved in more than 15% of patients. Findings on TEE include ventricular dilation and poor systolic function (31).

Assessment of valvular function is also important because occasionally lacerations of the valvular annuli or ruptured chordae can be seen. Because of higher pressures on the left side of the heart, the aortic and mitral valves are at greater risk for damage.

Cardiac tamponade and pericardial effusion. Pericardial effusion resulting from hemopericardium and cardiac tamponade can easily be diagnosed with TEE. *The most sensitive two-dimensional manifestation of cardiac tamponade is RV collapse during diastole in a patient with a pericardial effusion.* Right atrial collapse frequently occurs in late diastole. Left atrial and ventricular collapse can occur, especially if LV pressures are low. This phenomenon is frequently encountered following cardiac surgery when a loculated pericardial effusion or thrombus impedes left atrial or ventricular filling.

The Doppler manifestations of cardiac tamponade consist of a significant increase in the early diastolic E-wave velocity across the tricuspid valve during inspiration in a spontaneously breathing patient. Because the patient's heart can be considered to be encased in a concrete box, the resulting increase in RV inflow creates a reciprocal decrease in LV inflow and therefore a fall in the early diastolic E-wave velocity across the mitral valve during inspiration. The opposite occurs in the tricuspid and mitral E-wave velocities during expiration. Diastolic pulmonary venous forward flow decreases during inspiration and increases during expiration. Finally, during expiration, hepatic venous flow is reduced in both diastole and systole (32,33).

SUMMARY

TEE is easily performed in the ICU setting with a wide margin of safety. In the ICU, TEE is frequently superior to TTE, particularly in mechanically ventilated patients. It also provides a better assessment of heart function than the PA catheter. TEE is most useful in patients with hemodynamic instability when accurate information must be obtained rapidly. Because of its ability to provide high-resolution images and a superior diagnostic yield, TEE has become indispensable in ICU care.

REFERENCES

1. Parker MM, Cunnion RE, Parillo JE. Echocardiography and nuclear cardiac imaging in the critical care unit. *JAMA* 1985;254:2935–2939.
2. Vignon P, Mentec H, Terre S, et al. Diagnostic accuracy and therapeutic impact of transthoracic and transesophageal echocardiography in mechanically ventilated patients in the ICU. *Chest* 1994;106:1829–1834.
3. Pearson AC, Castello R, Labovitz AJ. Safety and utility of transesophageal echocardiography in the critically ill patient. *Am Heart J* 1990;119:1083–1089.
4. Hwang JJ, Shyu KG, Chen JJ, et al. Usefulness of transesophageal echocardiography in the critical care unit. *Chest* 1993;104:861–866.
5. Benjamin E, Griffin K, Leibowitz AB, et al. Goal-directed transesophageal echocardiography performed by intensivists to assess LV function: comparison with pulmonary artery catheterization. *J Cardiothorac Vasc Anesth* 1998;12:10–15.
6. Poelaert JI, Trouerbach J, De Buyzere M, et al. Evaluation of transesophageal echocardiography as a diagnostic and therapeutic aid in a critical care setting. *Chest* 1995; 107:774–779.
7. Heidenreich PA. Transesophageal echocardiography in the critical care patient. *Cardiol Clin* 2000;18:789–805.
8. Seward JB, Khandheria BK, Oh JK, et al. Transesophageal echocardiography: technique, anatomic correlations, implementation, and clinical applications. *Mayo Clin Proc* 1988;63:649–680.
9. Daniel WG, Erbel R, Kasper W, et al. Safety of transesophageal echocardiography. A multicenter study of 10,419 examinations. *Circulation* 1991;83:817–821.
10. Alam M. Transesophageal echocardiography in critical care units: Henry Ford Hospital experience and review of the literature. *Prog Cardiovasc Dis* 1996;38:315–328.
11. Oh JK, Seward JB, Khandheria BK, et al. Transesophageal echocardiography in critically ill patients. *Am J Cardiol* 1990;66:1492–1495.
12. Slama MA, Novara A, Van de Putte P, et al. Diagnostic and therapeutic implications of transesophageal echocardiography in medical ICU patients with unexplained shock, hypoxemia, or suspected endocarditis. *Intensive Care Med* 1996;22:916–922.
13. Chenzbraun A, Pinto FJ, Schnittger I. Transesophageal echocardiography in the intensive care unit: impact on diagnosis and decision making. *Clin Cardiol* 1994;17:438–444.
14. Greim CA, Roewer N, Apfel G, et al. Relation of echocardiographic preload indices to stroke volume in critically ill patients with normal and low cardiac index. *Intensive Care Med* 1997;23:411–416.
15. Swenson JD, Harkin C, Pace NL, et al. Transesophageal echocardiography: an objective tool defining maximum ventricular response to intravenous fluid therapy. *Anesth Analg* 1996;83:1149–1153.
16. Foster E, Schiller NB. Transesophageal echocardiography in the critical care patient. *Cardiol Clin* 1993;11:489–503.
17. Keren A, Kim CB, Hu BS, et al. Accuracy of biplane and multiplane transesophageal echocardiography in diagnosis of typical acute aortic dissection and intramural hematoma. *J Am Coll Cardiol* 1996;28:627–636.
18. Dansky HM, Schwinger ME, Cohen MV. Using contrast material-enhanced echocardiography to identify abnormal pulmonary arteriovenous connection in patients with hypoxemia. *Chest* 1992;102:1690–1692.
19. Heidenreich PA, Masoudi FA, Maini B, et al. Echocardiography patients with suspected endocarditis: a cost-effectiveness analysis. *Am J Med* 1999;107:198–208.
20. Shanewise JS, Martin RP. Assessment of endocarditis and associated complications with transesophageal echocardiography. *Crit Care Clin* 1996;12:411–427.
21. Sanfilippo AJ, Picard MH, Newell JB, et al. Echocardiographic assessment of patients with infectious endocarditis: prediction of risk for complications. *J Am Coll Cardiol* 1991;18:1191–1199.
22. Iliceto S, Nanda NC, Rizzon P, et al. Color Doppler evaluation of aortic dissection. *Circulation* 1987;75:748–755.
23. Erbel R, Engberding R, Daniel W, et al. Echocardiography in diagnosis of aortic dissection. *Lancet* 1989;1:457–460.

24. Erbel R, Mohr-Kahaly S, Oelert H, et al. Diagnostic strategies in suspected aortic dissection: comparison of computed tomography, aortography, and transesophageal echocardiography. *Am J Card Imaging* 1990;4:157–172.
25. Mohr-Kahaly S, Erbel R, Rennollet H, et al. Ambulatory follow-up of aortic dissection by transesophageal two-dimensional and color-coded Doppler echocardiography. *Circulation* 1989;80:24–33.
26. Lengyel M. Should transesophageal echocardiography become a routine test in patients with suspected pulmonary thromboembolism? *Echocardiography* 1998;15:779–785.
27. Steiner P, Lund GK, Debatin JF, et al. Acute pulmonary embolism: value of transthoracic and transesophageal echocardiography in comparison with helical CT. *AJR Am J Roentgenol* 1996;167:931–936.
28. Pruszczyk P, Torbicki A, Pacho R, et al. Noninvasive diagnosis of suspected severe pulmonary embolism: transesophageal echocardiography versus spiral CT. *Chest* 1997;112:722–728.
29. Mariano MC, Gutierrez CJ, Alexander J, et al. The utility of transesophageal echocardiography in determining the source of arterial embolization. *Am Surg* 2000;66:901–904.
30. Montgomery DH, Ververis JJ, McGorisk G, et al. Natural history of severe atheromatous disease of the thoracic aorta. A transesophageal echocardiographic study. *J Am Coll Cardiol* 1996;27:95–101.
31. Garcia-Fernandez MA, Lopez-Perez JM, Perez-Castellano N, et al. Role of transesophageal echocardiography in the assessment of patients with blunt chest trauma: correlation of echocardiographic findings with the electrocardiogram and creatine kinase monoclonal antibody measurements. *Am Heart J* 1998;135:476–481.
32. Tsang TSM, Oh JK, Seward JM. Diagnosis and management of cardiac tamponade in the era of echocardiography. *Clin Cardiol* 1999;22:446–452.
33. Merce J, Sagrista-Sauleda J, Permanyer-Miralda G, et al. Imaging/diagnostic testing. Correlation between clinical and Doppler echocardiographic findings in patients with moderate and large pericardial effusion: implications for the diagnosis of cardiac tamponade. *Am Heart J* 1999;138:759–764.

QUESTIONS

1. Limitations of TEE in the ICU include all of the following **except**
   a. Poor visualization of the aortic arch
   b. Patient discomfort
   c. Foreshortening of the LV apex
   d. Inability to evaluate the RV
2. Current indications for TEE in a critically ill patient are
   a. Evaluation of the LV preload
   b. Assessment of the severity of aortic stenosis
   c. Unexplained heart failure
   d. All of the above
3. In patients with suspected infective endocarditis, TEE
   a. Is cost-effective in comparison with TTE
   b. Can detect small pedunculated masses of the mitral valve
   c. Allows identification of the organism
   d. Always detects tricuspid valve vegetations
   e. **a** and **b**
4. TEE findings in acute pulmonary embolus include all of the following **except**
   a. Dilated right atrium
   b. Echogenic mass in the right PA
   c. Tricuspid regurgitation
   d. Pulmonary filling defect

5. In patients with an unexplained cerebrovascular accident, TEE can reveal all the following **except**
   a. Patent foramen ovale
   b. Mural thrombus
   c. Carotid atheroma
   d. Spontaneous echo contrast in the left atrium
6. The PA catheter is superior to TEE in the measurement of
   a. LV preload
   b. LV contractility
   c. Mixed venous oxygen level
   d. Intermittent CO
7. In a patient with unexplained hypotension after cardiac surgery, common TEE findings include
   a. Decreased LV end-diastolic area
   b. Compression of the right cardiac chambers
   c. New regional wall motion abnormalities
   d. All of the above
8. Common reasons why TTE is often nondiagnostic in critically ill patients are
   a. Mechanical ventilation with positive end-expiratory pressure
   b. Chest dressings
   c. Inability to lie on the left side
   d. All of the above
9. The following hemodynamic measurements are possible with TEE **except**
   a. PA systolic pressure
   b. CO
   c. Oxygen extraction ratio
   d. Systemic vascular resistance
10. Complications associated with TEE include all the following **except**
    a. PA perforation
    b. Hypertension
    c. Supraventricular tachycardia
    d. Hematemesis

Transesophageal Echocardiography for Congenital Heart Disease in the Adult

Kathryn Rouine-Rapp and Wanda C. Miller-Hance

Lesions in adults with congenital heart disease (CHD) range from simple to complex. The objectives of intraoperative transesophageal echocardiography (TEE) for patients with CHD include characterization of the primary pathology, identification of associated defects, assessment of hemodynamics, evaluation of ventricular function, and detection of residual pathology.

INCIDENCE OF CONGENITAL HEART DISEASE

The incidence of CHD in the United States is estimated to be 6.2 per 1,000 live births. Approximately 85% of such infants are expected to survive to adulthood. At least 10% of cases of CHD in adults are diagnosed during a visit to a clinic that specializes in the care of adults with this type of heart disease.

PREVALENCE OF CONGENITAL HEART DISEASE IN ADULTS

At present, approximately 800,000 adults in the United States have CHD. This number is increasing by an estimated 5% per year, and for the first time, the numbers of adults and children with CHD are equal.

SURVIVAL PATTERNS

The survival of adults with CHD depends on multiple factors. Survival rates according to year of birth and complexity of the lesion are given in Table 18.1. Definitive surgical repair at an earlier age and improvements in the postoperative care of patients with complex defects are expected to lead to continued increases in survival.

CLASSIFICATION OF CONGENITAL HEART DISEASE

Several classification schemes have been proposed for CHD. Lesions have been characterized according to level of complexity, presence or absence of cyanosis, and primary physiologic alteration.

Simple versus Complex Lesions

Isolated lesions, such as intracardiac communications, are considered simple. Complex lesions include severe malformations of the cardiovascular structures and malpositions of the heart and visceral organs (heterotaxy syndromes).

Acyanotic versus Cyanotic Lesions

In this scheme, congenital cardiac malformations are divided into two groups based on whether the primary functional disorder includes cyanosis (i.e., hypoxemia). Cyanotic

TABLE 18.1. SURVIVAL RATE TO YEAR 2000

Year of birth	Complexity of congenital heart disease		
	Simple	Moderate	Complex
1940–1959	90%	55%	10%
1960–1979	95%	65%	50%
1980–1989	95%	90%	80%

Adapted from the Bethesda Conference Report. *J Am Coll Cardiol* 2001;37: 1161–1196, with permission.

conditions are those with restrictive pulmonary blood flow in the presence of intracardiac shunting or complete arterial and venous admixture. Cyanosis is less likely to occur in individuals with pulmonary overcirculation secondary to isolated intracardiac communications.

Shunts and Obstructive, Regurgitant, and Mixed Lesions

The classification algorithm based on the physiologic spectrum of CHD comprises four major categories: shunts, obstructions to flow, regurgitant pathology, and mixed lesions. Shunt lesions may occur within the heart (intracardiac) or outside the heart (extracardiac). The direction and magnitude of the shunt depend on the size of the communication and the relative resistances of the pulmonary and systemic circulations. Obstructive lesions may affect blood inflows or outflows and vary in severity. Regurgitant lesions are rarely found in isolation. They occur secondary to the primary pathology. In mixed lesions, which account for a significant number of cyanotic heart defects, the systemic and pulmonary venous returns are completely mixed.

SIMPLE LESIONS

Atrial Septal Defects

Anatomy. The four types of atrial septal defect (ASD) are ostium secundum, ostium primum, sinus venosus, and coronary sinus defects (Fig 18.1). They account for approximately 30% of all cases of CHD detected in adults. *Ostium secundum defects* are located in the region of the fossa ovalis and account for 70% of all ASDs (Fig 18.2). Associated abnormalities include mitral valve prolapse and mitral regurgitation. *Ostium primum defects* (also known as *partial atrioventricular [AV] septal defects*) are located in the lower portion of the interatrial septum. They account for 15% to 25% of ASDs and frequently are associated with a cleft in the anterior leaflet of the mitral valve and mitral regurgitation. *Sinus venosus defects* occur adjacent to the entrance of the superior vena cava (most common) or inferior vena cava (Fig. 18.1). They account for 5% to 10% of ASDs and often are associated with anomalous drainage of the pulmonary veins. *Coronary sinus defects* are very rare and result from a communication between the left atrium and coronary sinus. They typically are associated with a persistent left superior vena cava.

Physiology. The physiologic consequences are determined by the size of the defect and the degree of left-to-right shunting. The defect size, ventricular compliance, and pulmonary artery (PA) pressures determine the magnitude of the shunt. In a patient with a large defect leading to a substantial shunt, atrial enlargement, dilation of the right ventricle (RV) and PAs, and pulmonary hypertension can develop. With time, RV compliance may decline and failure ensue. Atrial arrhythmias may occur, especially after the third decade of life. Although most adult patients with ASDs have mild-to-moderate pulmonary hypertension, severe elevation of the PA pressure develops in 5% to 10% of older patients. The surgical mortality risk is greater in patients who undergo surgical repair after the age of 24 years

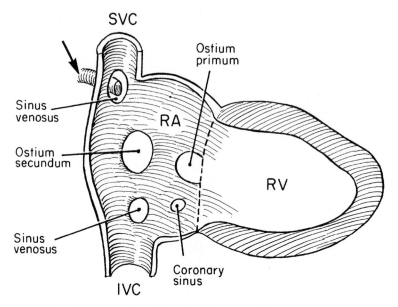

FIG. 18.1. Atrial septal defects. Location of atrial septal defects. Centrally located ostium secundum and inferiorly located ostium primum sinus venosus defects near the superior vena cava (*SVC*) or the inferior vena cava (*IVC*), and associated anomalous pulmonary venous connection (*arrow*) and coronary sinus defect. RA, right atrium; RV, right ventricle. (From Perloff JK. *The clinical recognition of congenital heart disease,* 4th ed. Philadelphia: WB Saunders, 1994:295, with permission.)

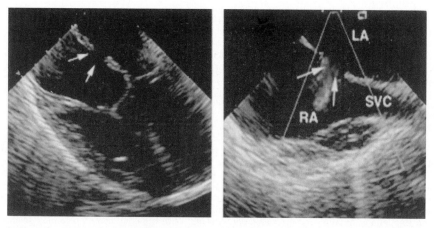

FIG. 18.2. Secundum atrial septal defect. **Left:** Central defect in the atrial septum (*arrows*), typical of a secundum atrial septal defect, seen in the midesophageal four-chamber view. **Right:** Defect in the long-axis plane (midesophageal bicaval view). LA, left atrium; RA, right atrium; SVC, superior vena cava.

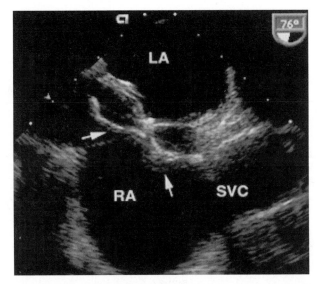

FIG. 18.3. Atrial septal defect closure device. Transesophageal imaging (midesophageal bicaval view) during placement of an atrial septal defect closure device (*arrows*). LA, left atrium; RA, right atrium; SVC, superior vena cava.

and in whom the PA systolic pressure exceeds 40 mm Hg. Some secundum defects are suitable for closure in the cardiac catheterization laboratory with a transcatheter closure device (Fig. 18.3).

Intraoperative transesophageal echocardiographic evaluation

Two-dimensional examination: Goals of the two-dimensional TEE examination include the following:

1. Defining the defect location and size
2. Determining right-sided chamber and vessel dimensions
3. Examining the mitral valve for prolapse or cleft
4. Evaluating the pulmonary venous connections
5. Assessing the ventricular function.

Color flow Doppler examination: Color flow Doppler is used to assess flow across the defect and detect tricuspid or mitral valve regurgitation. The detection of a small interatrial shunt may be enhanced by the intravenous injection of agitated saline solution (contrast). The hemodynamic assessment includes the use of spectral Doppler for measuring the tricuspid regurgitant jet velocity to estimate the PA systolic pressure. In the absence of significant valvular disease, velocities across the AV valves or outflow tracts can be used to estimate shunt magnitude.

Examination after repair: The intraoperative TEE examination following surgical repair includes the detection of residual interatrial shunts, evaluation of valve competence, and assessment of ventricular function.

Ventricular Septal Defect

Anatomy. The ventricular septum is comprised of a small membranous and a large muscular component that is divided into inlet, trabecular, and outlet regions. The components of the ventricular septum are represented in Figure 18.4.

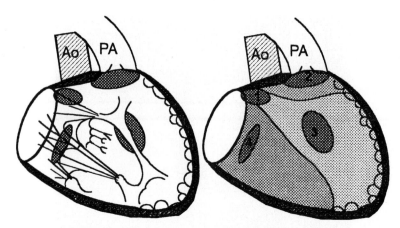

FIG. 18.4. Components of the ventricular septum. Components of the ventricular septum and major ventricular septal defect locations. **Left:** The defects relative to the right ventricular surface of the interventricular septum and attachments of the tricuspid valve. **Right:** The defects and their locations are perimembranous (*1*), doubly committed subarterial in the outlet portion of the ventricular septum (*2*), and muscular defects in the trabecular (*3*) and (*4*) inlet portions of the ventricular septum. (From Moller JH, Hoffman JIE. *Pediatric cardiovascular medicine.* Philadelphia: Churchill Livingstone, 2000:290, with permission.)

Ventricular septal defects (VSDs) can occur in isolation or as part of complex lesions and are classified by location into four major groups: perimembranous, muscular, doubly committed outlet (subarterial), and inlet defects (Fig. 18.4). An isolated VSD is the most common congenital heart defect diagnosed in infants. Because larger defects usually are repaired in infancy and up to 60% of smaller defects close spontaneously, VSDs account for only 10% to 15% of defects observed in adults with CHD.

Perimembranous defects: These account for approximately 70% of VSDs, involve most or all of the membranous septum, and may have a muscular extension. Associated findings include an aneurysm involving the membranous septum that is composed of tricuspid valve tissue and appears as a tissue pouch. Aortic valve cusp herniation with resulting aortic regurgitation is another associated finding.

Muscular defects: These are defined by their location in the trabecular portion of the ventricular septum. They account for 20% of VSDs, can be isolated or multiple, and often are located in the central or apical portion of the trabecular septum.

Doubly committed outlet defects (subarterial): These are identified immediately below the semilunar valves. They account for 5% of VSDs and frequently are associated with aortic valve cusp prolapse that results in aortic regurgitation.

Inlet or atrioventricular canal-type defects: These account for about 5% of VSDs and are located close to the AV valves in the posterior or inlet portion of the septum. An associated primum ASD can be part of a complex defect known as an *AV septal defect,* or *AV canal defect*. This defect is common in individuals with Down syndrome.

Physiology. The physiologic consequences of a VSD are determined by the size of the defect and the pulmonary vascular resistance. Moderate-to-large defects are associated with significant left-to-right shunting and symptoms of heart failure. Severe pulmonary hypertension can develop in patients with large, long-standing VSDs and substantial pulmonary overcirculation. This in turn can lead to a reversal in the direction (right-to-left) of blood flow through the defect and cyanosis. Increased pulmonary vascular resistance secondary to irreversible vascular changes leads to pulmonary hypertension, a condition known as *Eisenmenger syndrome.* Adults in whom Eisenmenger syndrome develops have a decreased survival rate and generally are not considered candidates for surgery. Patients with unrepaired VSDs are at increased risk for infective endocarditis.

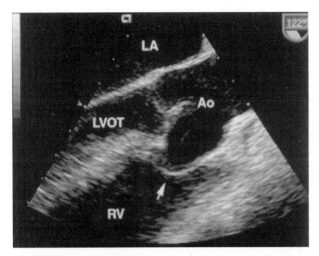

FIG. 18.5. Doubly committed subarterial ventricular septal defect. Two-dimensional transesophageal echocardiographic midesophageal aortic valve long-axis view demonstrates a subarterial ventricular septal defect and herniation of the aortic valve cusp through the defect (*arrow*). LA, left atrium; LVOT, left ventricular outflow tract; Ao, proximal ascending aorta; RV, right ventricle.

Intraoperative transesophageal echocardiographic evaluation
Two-dimensional examination: The examination should include the following:

1. Assessing defect location, size, and borders
2. Determining chamber sizes and PA dimensions
3. Inspecting for associated abnormalities
4. Identifying ventricular septal aneurysm, if present
5. Evaluating the aortic valve for herniation and prolapse (Fig. 18.5)
6. Inspecting for findings suggestive of pulmonary hypertension.

Color flow Doppler examination: Color flow Doppler is used for the following:

1. Detecting tricuspid and aortic regurgitation
2. Enhancing or confirming the presence of a defect or additional defects
3. Determining the magnitude and direction of shunt flow
4. Optimizing the alignment of the Doppler beam within the defect jet.

Hemodynamic assessment: The hemodynamic assessment includes the use of spectral Doppler to measure the tricuspid regurgitant velocity for an estimate of the PA systolic pressure. Spectral Doppler analysis helps differentiate between the high-velocity flow of a restrictive VSD and the low-velocity flow of a nonrestrictive lesion with little or no difference in ventricular pressures. Spectral Doppler is useful for measuring the peak velocity across the VSD to estimate the RV systolic pressure, which is equal to the PA systolic pressure in the absence of outflow obstruction, as follows:

$$\text{RV Systolic Pressure} = \text{Systolic Blood Pressure} - 4(v_{VSD})^2$$

where v_{VSD} is the peak velocity of the VSD jet.

Examination after repair: Intraoperative TEE immediately following surgical repair is used to detect residual shunts, determine changes in tricuspid or aortic valve regurgitation, and assess ventricular function.

Patent Ductus Arteriosus

Anatomy. Patent ductus arteriosus accounts for about 10% of cases of CHD. Normally, the patent ductus connects the junction of the main and left PAs to the descending aorta adjacent to the origin of the left subclavian artery. A ductus that remains patent 3 months after birth can be isolated or associated with other cardiac defects.

Physiology. The physiologic consequences of a patent ductus arteriosus are determined by the size of the duct and the difference between the systemic and pulmonary vascular resistances. Although a small patent ductus may have little or no physiologic effect, left-to-right shunting through a moderate-to-large ductus leads to pulmonary overcirculation and may result in an increased pulmonary vascular resistance. Most individuals with a large ductus do not survive to late adulthood unless the left-to-right flow and left ventricular (LV) volume load are limited by an increased pulmonary vascular resistance, a finding associated with the development of Eisenmenger syndrome. In many cases, symptoms of heart failure, atrial fibrillation, and cardiomegaly develop. Surgical closure of a patent ductus arteriosus in adults may require cardiopulmonary bypass and is contraindicated in adult patients with Eisenmenger syndrome. Patients with a patent ductus arteriosus are at risk for the development of infective endocarditis.

Intraoperative transesophageal echocardiographic evaluation. Examination of a patent ductus arteriosus by two-dimensional TEE can be difficult because views of the descending aorta are limited. The TEE examination includes the following:

1. Identification of associated cardiac malformations.
2. Detection of left atrial or ventricular dilation and LV dysfunction.
3. Color flow mapping to detect ductal flow into the main PA. This increases the diagnostic accuracy but requires the presence of a left-to-right shunt. Color flow Doppler contributes to the evaluation of tricuspid regurgitation and mitral regurgitation.
4. Spectral Doppler to estimate the PA systolic pressure and document retrograde flow in the descending aorta during diastole.

Examination after repair: After surgical or device closure, TEE may detect residual ductal flow that necessitates further intervention.

Coarctation of the Aorta

Anatomy. *Coarctation of the aorta* is a narrowing of the aorta that typically occurs immediately beyond the takeoff of the left subclavian artery or just beyond the insertion of the ligamentum arteriosum (juxtaductal) (Fig 18.6). The location in adults tends to be juxtaductal; a discrete, obstructing shelf project into the aortic lumen. Associated defects may include patent ductus arteriosus, VSD, and bicuspid aortic valve. Coarctation of the aorta accounts for approximately 8% of all cases of CHD, and 20% of cases of coarctation of the aorta are diagnosed in adolescents or adults

Physiology. The main physiologic consequence of coarctation of the aorta is an increased LV afterload. The systolic arterial blood pressure is increased proximal to the coarctation site and decreased distal to it, and diastolic hypertension develops subsequently. Most adults with coarctation of the aorta are asymptomatic, although recurrent epistaxis, headache, claudication, dizziness, and palpitations may develop. Major complications include dissection, rupture, or endarteritis of the aorta, cerebral hemorrhage, infective endocarditis, and LV failure. Patients with prolonged preoperative hypertension who undergo surgical repair after the age of 25 years are at increased risk for death from cardiovascular causes. Selected patients may undergo balloon angioplasty of the coarctation site.

Intraoperative transesophageal echocardiographic evaluation. The TEE evaluation of coarctation should include the following:

1. Identification of associated lesions and evaluation of the aortic arch. *The anterior position of the air-filled trachea relative to the esophagus limits the TEE examination of the distal ascending aorta and proximal aortic arch, so that this a difficult lesion to examine by TEE.*

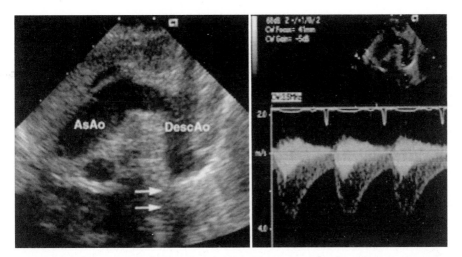

FIG. 18.6. Coarctation of the aorta. **Left:** Two-dimensional transthoracic image of aortic coarctation. The tight area of obstruction is indicated by the *arrows*. AsAo, ascending aorta; Desc Ao, descending aorta. **Right:** Typical spectral Doppler flow pattern across the coarctation site. The lighter and darker velocities correspond to the dual population of blood elements across the region. The peak Doppler velocity allows the degree obstruction to be quantified.

2. Color flow Doppler examination to detect turbulent, eccentric jets or flow acceleration in the descending aorta.
3. Spectral Doppler determination of flow velocities across the lesion. This examination is complicated by the limited ability to align the Doppler beam parallel to the direction of flow.

TEE in surgical repair of coarctation of the aorta can be used to monitor LV function during aortic clamp application and to detect residual obstruction.

Aortic Valve Stenosis

Anatomy. *Bicuspid aortic valve* is the most frequent malformation of the normally tricuspid aortic valve and frequently results from commissural fusion. After cusp fusion, a raphe or false commissure may remain, and the resultant cusps may be equal or markedly different in size with an eccentric line of closure (Fig. 18.7). *Aortic stenosis* accounts for 5% of all CHD lesions. Bicuspid aortic valve is the most common defect in patients with symptomatic aortic stenosis who are younger than 65 years of age. In some patients, a weakness in the media of the ascending and transverse aorta predisposes to aneurysm formation. Other associated defects include VSD and coarctation of the aorta. Patients are at risk for infective endocarditis.

Physiology. Gradually, the bicuspid aortic valve can thicken, calcify, and become immobile. As valve stenosis develops, the LV systolic pressure increases and the LV becomes hypertrophic. As the area of the valve orifice becomes critical, LV systolic function decreases and heart failure occurs. Aortic regurgitation may develop and lead to an increase in LV preload and dilation.

Intraoperative transesophageal echocardiographic evaluation. Methods to determine the aortic valve area are discussed elsewhere in this text. In particular, the use of planimetry of two-dimensional images to estimate the aortic valve area is unreliable in patients with a bicuspid aortic valve.

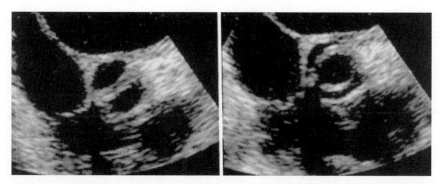

FIG. 18.7. Bicuspid aortic valve. Two-dimensional transesophageal echocardiographic midesophageal aortic valve short-axis view of a bicuspid aortic valve demonstrates the single closure line in diastole (**left**) and the abnormal valve opening during systole (**right**).

Two-dimensional evaluation: The two-dimensional evaluation of aortic stenosis should include the following:

1. Determination of aortic valve morphology and mobility
2. Measurement of annulus size
3. Identification of post-stenotic dilation of the ascending aorta
4. Detection of concentric LV hypertrophy or dilation
5. Assessment of global and segmental LV function
6. Identification of concurrent pathology.

Doppler examination
1. Color flow Doppler is used to identify turbulence of forward flow or aortic regurgitation.
2. Spectral Doppler can be used to estimate the peak instantaneous gradient across the aortic valve with the transgastric (TG) or deep TG long-axis view. Residual defects depend on the type of surgical intervention. Aortic regurgitation may be present after valvuloplasty, surgical valvotomy, or aortic valve replacement with a pulmonary autograft (Ross procedure). Following pulmonary autograft placement, a homograft is placed in the pulmonary valve position, and assessment for pulmonary homograft stenosis or regurgitation and biventricular function is also important. Paravalvular leaks can occur following placement of a prosthetic valve.

COMPLEX LESIONS

Tetralogy of Fallot

Anatomy. The initial description of *tetralogy of Fallot* consisted of a VSD, RV outflow tract (RVOT) obstruction, aortic override, and RV hypertrophy. In approximately a third of the cases, an ASD is present. This is one of the most common complex malformations seen in adults. Associated lesions include a right aortic arch, additional VSDs, absence of the pulmonic valve, coronary artery anomalies, systemic venous anomalies, aortopulmonary window, and LV outflow tract obstruction.

Physiology. The clinical findings in patients with tetralogy of Fallot are related mainly to the RVOT obstruction and the large, nonrestrictive perimembranous VSD. The degree of ventricular right-to-left shunting accounts for the degree of cyanosis. The enlarged aortic root in dextroposition and RV hypertrophy are secondary features of this anomaly.

Intraoperative transesophageal echocardiographic evaluation. The goals of the echocardiographic examination are to confirm the diagnosis, define the RVOT obstruction, estimate the size and direction of the ventricular shunt, and exclude associated pathology.

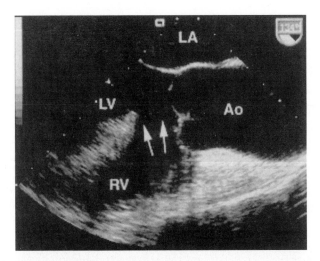

FIG. 18.8. Tetralogy of Fallot. Two-dimensional transesophageal echocardiographic midesophageal aortic valve long-axis view demonstrates two features of tetralogy of Fallot: a large ventricular septal defect (*arrows*) and an overriding aorta. LA, left atrium; LV, left ventricle; RV, right ventricle; Ao, proximal ascending aorta.

Two-dimensional examination: The perimembranous VSD is frequently demonstrated as a large subaortic defect between the right and noncoronary cusps in the midesophageal (ME) aortic valve short- and long-axis views (Fig. 18.8). Additional communications at the atrial and ventricular levels should be considered. Aortic override is best appreciated in the ME aortic valve long-axis view (Fig. 18.8). Evaluation of the RVOT and PAs requires a combination of scanning planes that define the subvalvular, valvular, and supravalvular regions.

Spectral and color flow Doppler examination: This is essential to interrogate the direction and velocity of the ventricular shunt. Determination of the severity of the RVOT obstruction is assisted by spectral Doppler measurements. The TEE examination should also include an assessment of aortic valve competence. The TEE evaluation of the distal pulmonary bed and aortopulmonary collaterals, if suspected or present, is suboptimal at best because of limited views of the structures.

Examination after repair: Patients who undergo surgical intervention may be at risk for residual RVOT obstruction and intracardiac shunts. The important TEE evaluation after bypass includes an evaluation for possible tricuspid, pulmonary, and aortic regurgitation and an estimation of RV and LV size, thickness, and function. In patients who require placement of a conduit from the RV to the PA, conduit stenosis or regurgitation may eventually develop.

Dextro-transposition of the Great Arteries

Anatomy. *Dextro-transposition of the great vessels* is characterized by concordance of the AV connection and discordance of the ventriculoarterial connection. A morphologic right atrium is connected to a morphologic RV, but the RV-arterial connection is to the aorta. Furthermore, a morphologic left atrium drains into a morphologic LV that gives rise to the PA. Transposition is a relatively frequent cardiac malformation, accounting for 5% to 7% of all cases of CHD. Associated pathology may include ASD, VSD, patent ductus arteriosus, obstruction of the pulmonary blood flow, aortic valve abnormalities, variation in the origin and course of the coronary arteries, and aortic arch anomalies.

Physiology. In this condition, the systemic and pulmonary circulations function in parallel rather than in series, so that cyanosis results. Some communication at the level of the atria, ventricles, or great arteries is essential for survival.

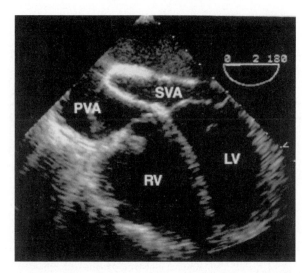

FIG. 18.9. Dextro-transposition of the great arteries. Two-dimensional transesophageal echocardiographic midesophageal four-chamber view demonstrates the features of an atrial redirection procedure for dextro-transposition. In this procedure, the systemic and pulmonary venous returns are rerouted by creating a baffle or pathway. The desaturated blood from the superior and inferior venae cavae drains into the systemic venous atrium (SVA), left ventricle, and pulmonary artery. The pulmonary venous atrium (PVA) receives oxygenated blood from the pulmonary veins, which then empties into the right ventricle and aorta. LV, left ventricle; RV, right ventricle; PA, pulmonary artery; AO, aorta.

Intraoperative transesophageal echocardiographic evaluation (systemic-pulmonary atrial baffle or redirection procedure). The surgical management of this lesion has changed dramatically through the years. Currently, the favored approach for infants with dextro-transposition is anatomic correction, or the Jatene procedure (arterial switch operation). In this operation, the great arteries are transected and anastomosed to their appropriate ventricular outflows, and the coronary arteries are translocated to the systemic outflow.

Adults with dextro-transposition are most likely to have undergone palliation or an atrial baffle procedure (Fig 18.9). The echocardiographic evaluation of such patients should include a pulsed wave Doppler examination, color flow mapping, and contrast echocardiography. The use of multiple imaging planes allows visualization of the caval junctions, the entrance of the pulmonary veins, and the mid aspect of the baffle. The administration of agitated saline solution via a peripheral or central vein may assist in the identification of baffle leaks and systemic or pulmonary obstruction.

In these patients, the RV functions as the systemic pump, and late dysfunction is not an uncommon occurrence. The tricuspid valve, which remains as the systemic atrioventricular valve, should be evaluated for regurgitation.

Congenitally Corrected Transposition (Levo-transposition)

Anatomy. Congenitally corrected transposition is also known as *levo-transposition of the great arteries,* a term that refers to the abnormal *l*-looping pattern of the heart tube during development that results in discordance between the AV and ventriculoarterial connections. The morphologic LV lies to the right and the morphologic RV to the left in a side-by-side arrangement (Fig. 18.10). Corrected transposition is frequently associated with other cardiac

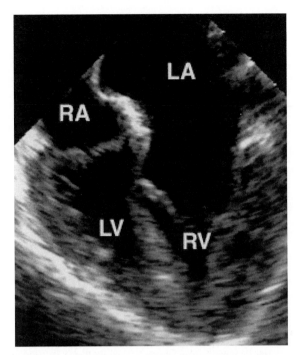

FIG. 18.10. Congenitally corrected transposition. Two-dimensional transesophageal echocardiographic midesophageal four-chamber view displays the abnormal (discordant) atrioventricular connection of this lesion. The right atrium empties into the morphologic left ventricle through a mitral valve, and the left atrium empties into the morphologic right ventricle through a tricuspid valve. Note the apical displacement of the tricuspid valve, common in this lesion. RA, right atrium; LA, left atrium; LV, left ventricle; RV, right ventricle.

anomalies, such as VSD, obstruction to pulmonary blood flow, and left AV valve (tricuspid valve) anomalies.

Physiology. In this lesion, the systemic veins drain into the anatomic right atrium, which is connected to the morphologic LV and PA. The pulmonary venous return is into the anatomic left atrium and then the morphologic RV, which is connected to the aorta. Thus, the systemic and pulmonary circulations are in series and the physiology is normal—hence the term *corrected*.

Intraoperative transesophageal echocardiographic evaluation. Definition of the AV connections by echocardiography requires identification of the characteristic features that establish ventricular morphology. The AV valves are associated with their corresponding ventricles, so that the morphologic tricuspid valve will identify the RV and the morphologic mitral valve will identify the LV. In the ME four-chamber view, the morphologic RV is characterized by inferior insertion of the septal leaflet of the tricuspid valve to the ventricular septum and by the moderator band (Fig. 18.10). The LV is identified by two distinct papillary muscles in the TG mid short-axis view. Typically, an aorta that is anterior and to the left relative to the PA is also present. A comprehensive TEE examination should focus on associated defects, such as interventricular communications, pulmonary outflow obstruction, tricuspid valve morphology and competence, and ventricular function.

The main issues of concern following surgical intervention are residual shunts, outflow obstruction, left AV valve regurgitation, and progressively decreased function of a morphologic RV in the systemic circulation.

Single-Ventricle Lesions or Univentricular Heart

Anatomy. The spectrum of single-ventricle, or univentricular, heart encompasses a wide variety of anatomic arrangements. In some patients with a biventricular heart, a two-ventricle repair may not be feasible, so that single-ventricle management is required. This group of patients may also be considered functionally to be in the univentricular group.

Physiology. The major anatomic variants of the single ventricle include double-inlet LV, tricuspid atresia, and hypoplastic left heart syndrome. A common feature of these lesions is complete mixing of the systemic and pulmonary venous blood at the atrial or ventricular level. Another frequent finding is systemic or pulmonary outflow tract obstruction.

Intraoperative transesophageal echocardiographic evaluation. Diagnostic assessment of the functional single ventricle requires a combination of multiple imaging planes. The ME four-chamber view is particularly helpful in demonstrating the crux of the heart and characterizing the AV connections. Additional views contribute to the segmental analysis by defining the ventriculoarterial connections, ventricular morphology, and location of hypoplastic or rudimentary chambers. Color flow and spectral Doppler interrogation is essential to determine AV and semilunar valve competence and inflow/outflow tract obstruction.

Surgical procedures attempt initially to protect the integrity of the pulmonary vascular bed and myocardium. Specific goals are to prevent pulmonary overcirculation, which may lead to elevation of the PA pressure, ventricular overload, and ventricular dysfunction.

Norwood procedure: In infants with LV hypoplasia (hypoplastic left heart syndrome), the initial surgical intervention is a Norwood procedure. This consists of enlargement of the hypoplastic aorta, creation of an aortopulmonary connection to provide a source of pulmonary blood flow, and atrial septectomy to ensure the unrestricted return of pulmonary venous blood into the systemic RV.

Modified Blalock-Taussig shunt: In other patients whose anatomy is associated with restricted pulmonary blood flow, a systemic-to-pulmonary connection is created (Gore-Tex tube graft) in the form of a *modified Blalock-Taussig shunt.* Two-dimensional imaging of this connection may not be feasible by TEE because of its distal location on the subclavian artery.

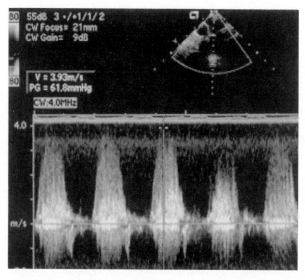

FIG. 18.11. Pulmonary artery band. Spectral Doppler interrogation across a pulmonary artery band. The peak velocity obtained by continuous wave Doppler can be used to estimate the right ventricular outflow tract systolic gradient with the modified Bernoulli equation.

Pulmonary artery band: Alternatively, in patients with excessive pulmonary blood flow, a *PA band* is created to limit overcirculation and prevent pulmonary hypertension. The peak systolic pressure gradient across the PA band can be predicted by spectral Doppler with use of the simplified Bernoulli equation (pressure gradient $= 4v^2$; Fig. 18.11). Ideally, the gradient across the PA band limits the PA systolic pressure to approximately one-third the systemic arterial blood pressure.

Glenn anastomosis and Fontan procedure: The eventual goal of surgical management is to separate the pulmonary and systemic circulations. At present, the favored approach is sequential diversion of the systemic venous blood directly into the pulmonary vascular bed via the *Glenn anastomosis* and *Fontan procedure.* In the *bidirectional Glenn procedure* (cavopulmonary anastomosis), the superior vena cava is connected to the PA. Imaging of the Glenn connection is not always possible by TEE because of limited imaging planes. The eventual separation of the pulmonary and systemic circulations in patients with single-ventricle physiology requires a *Fontan procedure* to direct blood from the inferior vena cava into the PAs. TEE is essential in the intraoperative and postoperative evaluation of valvular competence, ventricular function, and thrombosis in venous pathways.

TRANSESOPHAGEAL ECHOCARDIOGRAPHY IN THE CARDIAC CATHETERIZATION LABORATORY FOR ADULTS WITH CONGENITAL HEART DISEASE

The use of TEE in the cardiac catheterization laboratory to acquire detailed anatomic and hemodynamic data before and during interventions is increasing. TEE provides a real-time evaluation of catheter placement across valves and vessels and an immediate assessment of procedures in which closure devices are placed. It is also valuable in monitoring for catheter-induced complications, such as cardiac tamponade.

TRANSESOPHAGEAL ECHOCARDIOGRAPHY FOR NONCARDIAC SURGERY IN ADULTS WITH CONGENITAL HEART DISEASE

TEE can be used in this setting to evaluate ventricular volume and function, detect intracardiac shunts and air, identify valvular disease, and assess RV or PA systolic pressures. Adults with CHD may have concurrent acquired heart disease that puts them at increased risk for additional hemodynamic disturbances. Intraoperative TEE should be considered for patients with poor exercise tolerance.

LIMITATIONS OF TRANSESOPHAGEAL ECHOCARDIOGRAPHY IN CONGENITAL HEART DISEASE

Despite the significant contributions of TEE to perioperative care some limitations are identified. A variety of perioperative factors (level of inotropic support, high level of catecholamines immediately after bypass, loading conditions, functional state of the myocardium) may influence the echocardiographic findings and lead to an underestimate or overestimate of the hemodynamic severity of the condition in question. Thus, decisions regarding a return to bypass to address significant residual lesions must be made in the context of the hemodynamic state, with the understanding that for an optimal hemodynamic assessment, conditions that reflect the patient's baseline state are required.

SUMMARY

Intraoperative TEE is known to provide anatomic information beyond that acquired with conventional transthoracic imaging, and the opportunity to confirm preoperative diagnoses and modify the surgical approach as appropriate. TEE assists in the formulation of anesthetic plans by guiding the management of fluids, inotropes, and vasodilators, and allows the continuous monitoring of myocardial function and the detection of intracavitary/intravascular air and myocardial ischemia. Suboptimal surgical repairs and significant postoperative residua can be identified immediately with this technology. TEE can also be of benefit in evaluating factors that may contribute to difficulties in weaning from cardiopulmonary bypass. In several series, the reinstitution of cardiopulmonary bypass and reoperation were prompted by TEE in as many as 5% to 7% of congenital repairs. In operative situations such as these, TEE can provide substantial cost-saving benefits.

SUGGESTED READINGS

Brickner ME, Hillis LD, Lange RA. Congenital heart disease in adults, part I. *N Engl J Med* 2000;342:256–263.

Brickner ME, Hillis LD, Lange RA. Congenital heart disease in adults, part II. *N Engl J Med* 2000;342:334–342.

Child JS, Perloff JK. *Congenital heart disease in adults.* Philadelphia: Harcourt Health Sciences, 1998.

Garson A Jr, Bricker JT, Fisher DJ, et al. *The science and practice of pediatric cardiology.* Baltimore: Williams & Wilkins, 1998.

Miller-Hance WC, Silverman NH. Transesophageal echocardiography in congenital heart disease with focus on the adult. *Cardiol Clin* 2000:861–892.

Shanewise JS, Cheung AT, Aronson S, et al. ASE/SCA guidelines for performing a comprehensive intraoperative multiplane echocardiography examination: recommendations of the American Society of Echocardiography Council for Intraoperative Echocardiography and the Society of Cardiovascular Anesthesiologists Task Force for Certification in Perioperative Transesophageal Echocardiography. *Anesth Analg* 1999;89:870–884.

Silverman NH. *Pediatric echocardiography.* Baltimore: Williams & Wilkins, 1992.

Stumper O, Sutherland R. *Transesophageal echocardiography in congenital heart disease.* London: Hodder Headline Group, 1994.

Therrien J, Dore A, Gersony W, et al. CCS Consensus Conference 2001 update: recommendations for the management of adults with congenital heart disease, part I. *Can J Cardiol* 2001;17:943–959.

Therrien J, Dore A, Gersony W, et al. CCS Consensus Conference 2001 update: recommendations for the management of adults with congenital heart disease, part II. *Can J Cardiol* 2001;17:1029–1050.

Therrien J, Dore A, Gersony W, et al. CCS Consensus Conference 2001 update: recommendations for the management of adults with congenital heart disease, part III. *Can J Cardiol* 2001;17:1135–1158.

Warnes CA, Liberthson R, Danielson GK, et al. Task force 1: the changing profile of congenital heart disease in adult Life. *J Am Coll Cardiol* 2001;37:1170–1175.

Webb GD, Harrison DA, Connelly MS. Challenges posed by the adult with congenital heart disease. *Adv Intern Med* 1996;41:437–495.

Webb GD, Williams RG. Care of the adult with congenital heart disease: introduction. *J Am Coll Cardiol* 2001;37:1166.

QUESTIONS

1. A common TEE finding in an adult with a substantial shunt from a large secundum ASD is
   a. Bicuspid aortic valve
   b. Mitral valve stenosis
   c. Abnormal pulmonary venous connections
   d. Dilation of the RV
2. Eisenmenger syndrome
   a. Is common in adults with tetralogy of Fallot
   b. Is associated with coarctation of the aorta
   c. Does not alter patient survival
   d. Can occur in adults with a large patent ductus arteriosus

3. A previously undiagnosed perimembranous VSD in an adult is likely to be associated with
   a. Tricuspid valve stenosis
   b. Mitral valve regurgitation
   c. Aortic valve cusp herniation
   d. Doubly committed outlet VSD
4. TEE evaluation of an adult with a large patent ductus arteriosus is likely to
   a. Define the size, length, and position of the patent ductus arteriosus
   b. Detect LV hypertrophy
   c. Estimate PA pressure within the normal range
   d. Document retrograde flow in the descending aorta during diastole
5. Adults with a bicuspid aortic valve
   a. Often have a primum ASD
   b. Are at risk for aneurysm formation in the ascending aorta
   c. Also have a patent ductus arteriosus in about 40% of cases
   d. Have a central line of valve closure detected by TEE
6. Preoperative TEE assessment in tetralogy of Fallot includes all the following **except**
   a. Evaluation of the size of the VSD
   b. Doppler interrogation of the RVOT
   c. Functional evaluation of the aortic valve
   d. Two-dimensional definition of the transverse aorta
7. Classic anatomic findings in dextro-transposition of the great arteries include
   a. Bicuspid aortic valve
   b. Discordance of the AV connections
   c. Aorta originating from the RV
   d. Single-chamber heart
8. Contributions of TEE in patients with a univentricular heart include all of the following **except**
   a. Evaluation of ventricular function
   b. Assessment of valvular regurgitation
   c. Detailed inspection of the distal pulmonary bed
   d. Exclusion of venous pathway pathology
9. Which of the following statements regarding the use of TEE in CHD is true?
   a. It may modify the intraoperative surgical plan.
   b. It plays no role in the catheterization laboratory.
   c. It may document pathology after surgery, in which case a return to bypass is always required.
   d. It is too expensive for its use in selective noncardiac surgery to be justified.
10. A 19-year-old patient is undergoing closure of a VSD. A TEE probe is placed for the procedure. In the post-bypass views, a residual defect is noted with left-to-right shunting. The following hemodynamic and echocardiographic data are obtained:

Heart rate, 90 beats/min
Blood pressure (BP), 112/76 mm Hg
Body surface area (BSA), 1.8 m^2
Main PA (MPA) diameter, 2.1 cm
MPA time-velocity integral (TVI), 15.3 cm/s
LV outflow tract (LVOT) diameter, 1.9 cm
LVOT TVI, 14.8 cm/s
Peak Doppler velocity across the VSD, 4.6 m/s.

Calculate the following: LV stroke volume (SV), RV SV, cardiac output (CO), cardiac index (CI), Q_p/Q_s, and RV systolic pressure (RVSP).

PART V

MAN AND MACHINE

Common Artifacts and Pitfalls of Clinical Echocardiography

Joseph P. Miller, Albert C. Perrino, Jr., and Zak Hillel

Clinically important imaging artifacts result from the interplay of the ultrasound system, the patient, and the interpreting echocardiographer. The most common artifacts seen in clinical practice are the result of (a) normal or variant anatomic structures that are misdiagnosed, (b) the physical limitations of ultrasound imaging, and (c) undesirable interactions of ultrasound with tissues or medical devices. Accordingly, this chapter is organized into three sections. First, we review common false interpretations of normal anatomy. Second, we discuss the artifacts commonly encountered in two-dimensional imaging, and finally, we discuss the artifacts commonly encountered in Doppler examinations.

NORMAL ANATOMIC VARIANTS IN TWO-DIMENSIONAL IMAGING

Both novice and experienced echocardiographers may call normal structures abnormal. These normal variants can affect the intraoperative diagnosis and lead to inappropriate surgery, which can have a devastating impact on outcome. Careful evaluation and a consideration of the common variants discussed below can help limit problems related to misdiagnosis.

Crista Terminalis

The crista terminalis has been misinterpreted as a right atrial tumor or thrombus. This prominent muscular ridge can be differentiated from an anomaly by its characteristic appearance and position. The crista terminalis originates at the junction of the right atrium and superior vena cava junction and runs longitudinally toward the inferior vena cava. The trabeculations of the appendage originate from the crista terminalis. The crista terminalis separates the trabeculated appendage of the atrium from the smooth tubular portion. The structure is best visualized in the midesophageal (ME) bicaval view (Fig. 19.1).

Eustachian Valve or Chiari Network

The eustachian valve is often misdiagnosed as an intraatrial thrombus. The eustachian valve (called a *Chiari network* when fenestrated) is the remnant of the embryologic right venous valve, which is important in utero to direct inferior vena cava blood flow across the fossa ovalis. The filamentous structures can be differentiated from thrombus by their characteristic "insertion" into the atrial wall. They are best visualized in the ME bicaval view, in which they can be seen originating from the junction of the right atrium and inferior vena cava (Fig. 19.1).

Lipomatous Hypertrophy of the Atrial Septum

Myxomas, the most common cardiac tumors, often originate from the interatrial septum and typically involve the fossa ovalis. Lipomatous hypertrophy of the atrial septum can mimic atrial masses such as myxomas. The characteristic "dumbbell" shape seen in the ME four-chamber or ME bicaval view differentiates lipomatous hypertrophy from other structures.

The opinions or assertions contained herein are the private views of the author(s) and are not to be construed as official or as reflecting the views of the Department of Defense.

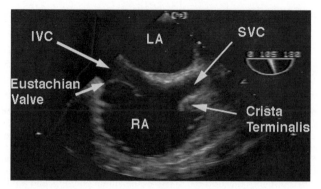

FIG. 19.1. The **crista terminalis** and **eustachian valve** are easily seen in this midesophageal bicaval view.

The appearance is caused by fatty infiltration of the atrial septum with *sparing* of the fossa ovalis (Fig. 19.2).

Coumadin Ridge

A prominent muscle ridge is formed between the left atrial appendage and the atrial insertion of the left upper pulmonary vein. This prominence is often misdiagnosed as thrombus and is referred to as the *coumadin ridge* or *"Q-tip" sign*. The lack of mobility and characteristic location, best seen in the ME two-chamber view, help distinguish it from an abnormal structure (Fig. 19.3).

Pericardial Sinuses

Pericardial sinuses (or folds) between the atria and great vessels can give rise to echo-lucent spaces despite only minimal amounts of pericardial fluid. The transverse and oblique sinuses

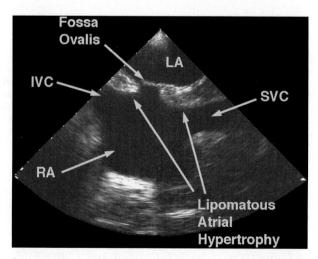

FIG. 19.2. The characteristic dumbbell shape of a **lipomatous atrial septum** with sparing of the fossa ovalis is seen in this midesophageal bicaval view.

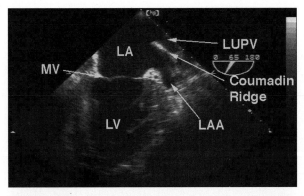

FIG. 19.3. A **Coumadin ridge** is seen between the left atrial appendage and the left upper pulmonary vein. Notably, the parallel arcs of electrocautery interference are also seen in this midesophageal two-chamber view.

of the pericardium can easily mimic pericardial cysts or abscesses. Pericardial fat seen in these extracardiac structures can also mimic intracardiac thrombus (Fig. 19.4).

Lambl Excrescences

Fine filamentous strands, Lambl excrescences, can be seen originating from the aortic valve of elderly patients. These structures can be differentiated from valvular vegetations by their characteristic "delicate" appearance in the absence of any clinical evidence of endocarditis (Fig. 19.5).

Moderator Band

The moderator band of the right ventricle has been misinterpreted as an intracardiac mass. This specialized cardiac trabeculation runs from the right ventricular free wall to the interventricular septum. It is often best seen in the ME four-chamber view (Fig. 19.6).

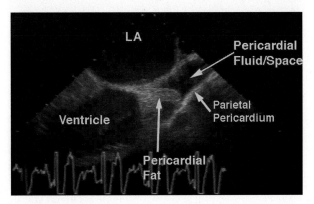

FIG. 19.4. **Pericardial fat** can be seen floating in the pericardial space.

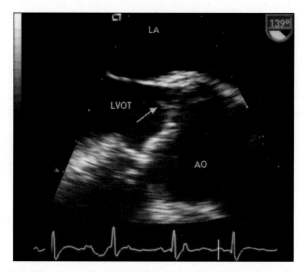

FIG. 19.5. A **Lambl excrescence** is seen on the ventricular surface of the aortic valve (*arrow*) in this midesophageal aortic valve long-axis view.

Pleural Effusion

Pleural effusions of the left side of the chest can mimic aortic dissection. In the descending aorta long-axis view, a pleural effusion will parallel the course of the aorta and have the appearance of a true lumen–false lumen dissection. Changing to the descending aorta short-axis view and identifying the characteristic triangular shape of a left-sided pleural effusion easily confirms the diagnosis of effusion versus dissection (Fig. 19.7A,B).

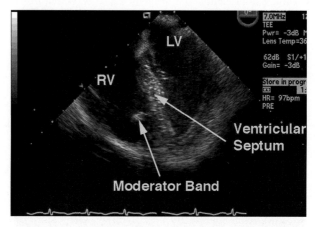

FIG. 19.6. The **moderator band** of the right ventricle is seen in this midesophageal four-chamber view.

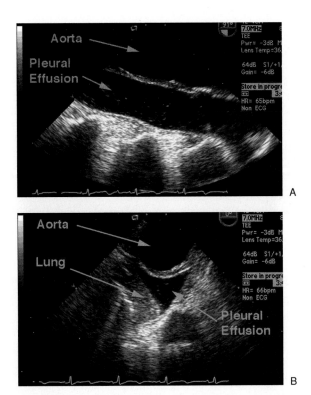

FIG. 19.7. A **pleural effusion** is seen abutting the descending aorta in the longitudinal (**A**) and transverse (**B**) planes.

TWO-DIMENSIONAL ECHOCARDIOGRAPHIC IMAGING ARTIFACTS

Suboptimal Image Quality

The inability to visualize cardiac structures because of suboptimal image quality remains a challenge in transesophageal echocardiographic diagnosis. Most commonly, improper settings of the ultrasound unit are to blame, but patient anatomy, acoustic interfaces (e.g., air between the probe and the stomach or esophageal wall, hiatal hernia), and sonographer skill play a definite role. Surprisingly, adjustments in machine settings coupled with minor manipulations of the ultrasound probe can lead to substantial improvement in the quality of images that are difficult to obtain. This topic is discussed further in Chapter 20.

Air between the transducer surface and tissue, encountered in transesophageal views more often than in transgastric (TG) views, causes severe image degradation to the point of complete inability to image. *Gastric suctioning before the transesophageal echocardiographic examination can reduce the poor acoustic contact caused by an air-tissue interface.*

Imaging is also frequently suboptimal when the cardiac structure of interest is parallel to the ultrasound beam. A common example of this artifact is "dropout" of the lateral and septal walls in the TG mid short-axis and ME four-chamber views (Fig. 19.8). Specular reflections are maximized when tissue interfaces lie perpendicular to the ultrasound beam, and this artifact is overcome by repositioning the ultrasound probe to a more favorable vantage point. An example of this phenomenon is the impaired ability to visualize thin linear structures, such as the chordae tendineae of the mitral valve, when they are parallel to the

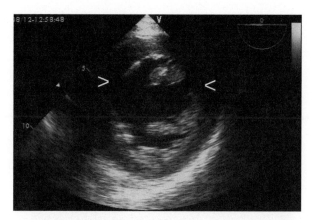

FIG. 19.8. Transgastric midesophageal short-axis view demonstrating septal and lateral wall dropout (*arrowheads*).

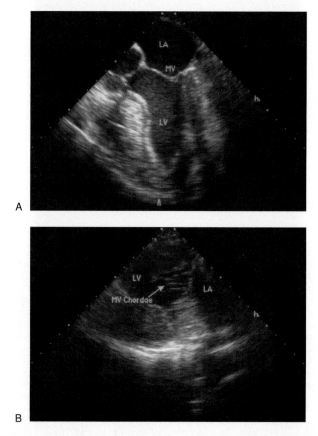

FIG. 19.9. A: Mitral valve and apparatus imaged with chordae tendineae parallel to the ultrasound beam (midesophageal five-chamber view). **B:** Markedly improved delineation of the chordae tendineae with the ultrasound beam perpendicular to the chordae tendineae (transgastric long-axis view).

ultrasound beam (ME five-chamber view) (Fig. 19.9A). However, when these structures are perpendicular to the beam (TG long-axis view), they are easily visualized (Fig. 19.9B).

Acoustic Shadowing

Acoustic shadowing occurs when the ultrasound beam meets an interface of two structures with marked differences in acoustic impedance. Common examples include structures with a high level of acoustic impedance, such as calcific aortic or mitral valves. These strongly reflect and scatter the ultrasound signal, thus limiting distal penetration of the sound waves. Similarly, mechanical prostheses and the struts of bioprosthetic valves produce shadowing. The resultant image reveals an echo-dense structure with a lack of signal in the sector beyond the structure (Fig. 19.10).

Lateral Resolution

The two-dimensional image is created from a series of individual ultrasound beams. Because structures lying between any two beams are not interrogated, the machine creates their display by averaging information received from the adjacent beams. This causes two problems. First, determinations of the size of a structure between beams (lateral resolution) are never as good as measurements made down a single beam (axial resolution). In most systems, axial resolution is at least twice lateral resolution. Second, the ultrasound beam fans out as it travels farther from the transducer, so that the distance between individual scan lines increases. This differential resolution of two-dimensional echocardiography can produce shape distortion. Lateral stretching of small but strongly echogenic objects, such as intracardiac catheters or wires, may occur. The images may show a markedly elongated shape instead of the true round cross-sectional shape. Similarly, intracardiac contrast (very small air bubbles at times) may incorrectly appear elongated laterally instead of round (Fig. 19.11).

Side Lobe and Beam Width

Side lobes are weak "beam leaks" outside the path of the main ultrasound beam. Although weak, when they encounter an echo-dense structure, such as a calcified aorta, mitral valve ring, any prosthetic material, or a catheter (Fig. 19.12), they cause reflections strong enough to be detected. The scanner misplaces these echoes in the image, incorrectly assuming that

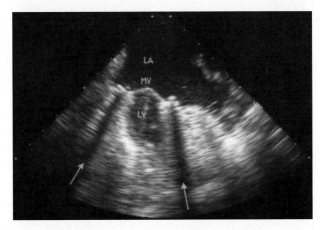

FIG. 19.10. Acoustic shadowing caused by a prosthetic mitral valve ring imaged in the midesophageal mitral commissural view. The *arrow* points to the long axial shadows.

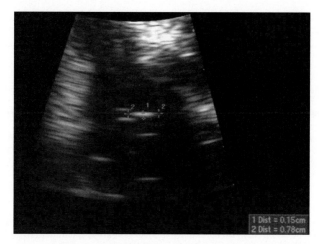

FIG. 19.11. Discrepancy between **axial** and **lateral** sizes of microbubbles as a consequence of resolution artifact. *1Dist* and *2Dist* indicate axial and lateral sizes, respectively.

they have been generated by structures lying in the path of the main beam. The artifact is displayed at the appropriate distance from the transducer but at the wrong lateral position. Some dramatic artifacts are produced when the examiner sees the image of a structure that is physically outside the scan sector overlying the two-dimensional image from the main beam! Because the main beam sweeps the entire scan sector, side lobe artifacts may appear as narrow, curvilinear densities smeared over its entire width.

Beam width artifacts occur because ultrasound waves are three-dimensional, cone-shaped structures, not just two-dimensional planar structures. Structures adjacent to the imaging plane but still within the imaging cone can be displayed in the imaging plane. The result varies depending on the location of the structures outside the imaging plane. They can appear as flaps in the aorta, structures or catheters in the wrong position (Fig. 19.12), or elongated structures. Beam width artifacts also occur with spectral Doppler and are discussed later.

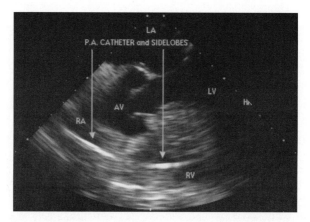

FIG. 19.12. Side lobe artifact of a pulmonary artery catheter imaged in the right atrium and right ventricle demonstrated in the midesophageal five-chamber view.

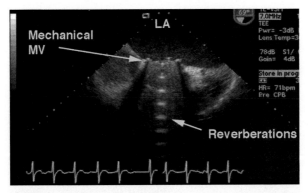

FIG. 19.13. Reverberation artifact resulting from a mechanical mitral valve is easily seen distal to the valve.

Reverberation

Reverberations are caused by the repeated back-and-forth reflection of an ultrasound wave between two strong specular reflectors. This phenomenon leads to two types of imaging artifacts. In the first, multiple linear densities are produced in the area of the imaging sector distal to the reflecting structures (Fig. 19.13). The second type of artifact occurs when the strong echoes are reflected from the transducer itself. The reflection then travels back to the same target, where it is echoed a second time toward the detecting transducer. As a result, an artifact is produced that appears as a duplication of the structure in the far field. Because this second trip doubles the travel distance and hence the travel time, the target structure is imaged once at the correct distance and a second time at twice the distance from the transducer. The descending thoracic aorta in both the transverse and longitudinal scans is a common source of this type of reverberation artifact. The vessel is imaged correctly in the near field and falsely duplicated immediately below. The duplicating reverberation artifact also extends in this case to color flow imaging (Fig. 19.14; see Color Plate 32 following page 212).

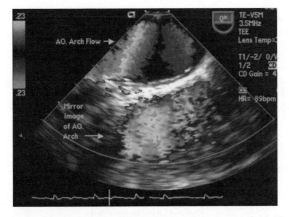

FIG. 19.14. A **mirror image** of the true aortic arch is seen in the far field. Note that the false arch is the same size as the true structure. The color flow Doppler signals are also duplicated. (See Color Plate 32 following page 212.)

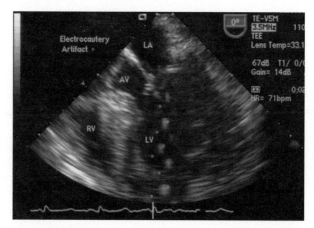

FIG. 19.15. Electrocautery artifacts are indicated by the *asterisk* in the midesophageal five-chamber view.

Electronic Noise

Electronic noise, of which electrocautery is the major source, cause an imaging artifact that resembles a "snowed image" pattern. Viewing cardiac anatomy through this snowstorm is an annoying reality of working with surgeons who use this technology (Fig. 19.15).

ARTIFACTS IN SPECTRAL AND COLOR FLOW DOPPLER

Spectral and color flow Doppler are susceptible to several of the mechanisms of artifact production that occur in two-dimensional imaging; however, the appearance of the artifacts is quite different. In addition, the Doppler examinations are susceptible to a number of artifacts unique to this method.

Aliasing

A shortcoming of pulsed wave Doppler systems, which includes color flow Doppler, is that the maximal blood velocities that can be accurately quantified are limited by the pulse repetition frequency. Specifically, any Doppler frequency shift greater than one-half the pulse repetition frequency, known as the *Nyquist limit,* results in a distorted spectral signal. The distortion in the Doppler signal, called *aliasing,* causes several types of artifacts in the pulse wave spectral signal or color flow map. Common examples include "wraparound" of the spectral signal (see Fig. 5.10) and red-blue stippling on the color flow map (see Fig. 5.14; see Color Plate 5 following page 212).

Acoustic Shadowing in Color Flow

Strong specular reflectors result in acoustic shadowing not only with two-dimensional imaging but also with Doppler modes. This artifact can be misinterpreted as a lack of blood flow in the shadowed region and is commonly seen during interrogation of prosthetic or heavily calcified valves (Fig. 19.16; see Color Plate 33 following page 212).

Nonparallel Beam Angle

Because the Doppler shift is proportional to the cosine of the angle between the path of the ultrasound beam and that of the blood flow, blood flow velocities are underestimated when the orientation of the ultrasound beam is not parallel to blood flow. With color flow Doppler,

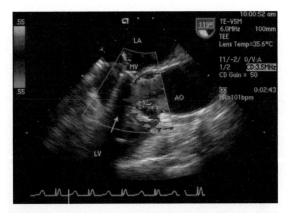

FIG. 19.16. Acoustic shadowing in color flow Doppler caused by a prosthetic mitral valve ring in the midesophageal aortic valve long-axis view. The *arrow* points to the long axial shadow. (See Color Plate 33 following page 212.)

this artifact typically occurs when the course of a vessel is oblique to the ultrasound beam. The blood flow perpendicular to the path of the Doppler beam is color-coded black (i.e., no flow). Also, as the Doppler beam sweeps across the imaging sector, it intersects the blood path at varying angles, causing a peculiar artifact in the color flow map. For example, if the blood flow in an artery is directed from left to right across the ultrasound sector, the color mapper will characterize the flow in the left side of the sector red (i.e., directed toward the transducer) and the blood flow in the right side of the sector blue (i.e., moving away from the transducer). Thus, an image is created in which it appears as if the blood were colliding in the middle portion of the vessel (Fig. 19.17; see Color Plate 34 following page 212).

Mirroring

This artifact appears in the spectral display as a symmetric duplication of the actual flow signal, but in the opposite direction (Fig. 19.18). It is related to a process known as *quadrature phase demodulation,* which allows the echo system to separate the Doppler-shifted signal

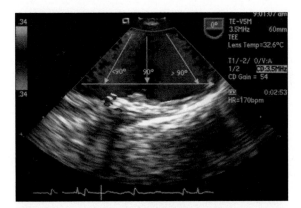

FIG. 19.17. Nonparallel beam angle color flow Doppler artifact in the aortic arch. The direction of blood flow is indicated by the *horizontal arrow*. The *angled arrows* indicate the direction of the Doppler ultrasound interrogating beam. (See Color Plate 34 following page 212.)

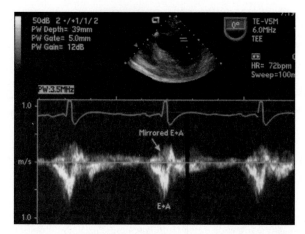

FIG. 19.18. Pulsed wave Doppler mirroring artifact. Transmitral flow and its weaker mirrored signal.

from the complex returning signal. The demodulation procedure uses a weaker signal that is generated out of phase with the broadcast signal. Excessive gain in the system causes the weak but incompletely canceled signal to be displayed as a mirror image of the actual flow signal.

Color Flow Reverberation and Gain-Related Anomalies

Reverberations are secondary reflections that occur when ultrasound is reflected a second time, typically from the transducer, highly reflective tissue, or intracardiac materials (e.g., a pulmonary artery catheter). The secondary reflection creates a ghost of the primary image that often appears at twice the distance of the actual target from the transducer. With Doppler reverberation, the reflected signal from a moving target is stronger than the original signal, so that the color intensity of the ghost is increased in comparison with that of the primary target (Figs. 19.14 and 19.19; see Color Plates 32 and 35 following page 212).

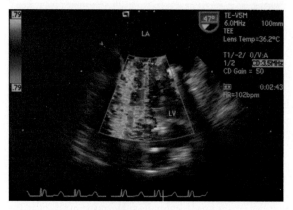

FIG. 19.19. Color flow Doppler **reverberations** are seen distal to a mechanical mitral valve in this midesophageal commissural view. (See Color Plate 35 following page 212.)

Beam Width Flow Artifacts

Although we view the heart with echocardiography as a two-dimensional image, the image is actually created by three-dimensional ultrasound signals. Because the width of the ultrasound signal increases with the distance from the transducer, it becomes possible to detect structures or blood flow outside the displayed two-dimensional image. An example of this phenomenon is shown in Figure 19.20A, in which interrogation of the interventricular septum reveals high-velocity flow. This is not the result of a ventricular septal defect but an

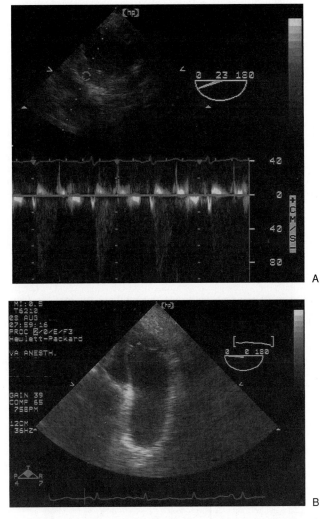

A

B

FIG. 19.20. **A:** From the transgastric short-axis view, the pulsed wave sample volume is shown placed on the interventricular septum. Spectral signals show high-velocity flow during systole. This is not caused by an interventricular septal defect; rather, it is an artifact of blood flow from the adjacent left ventricular outflow tract (LVOT), which lies just anterior to the imaged plane. With slight anteroflexion of the probe, the LVOT is visualized in the deep transgastric view (**B**).

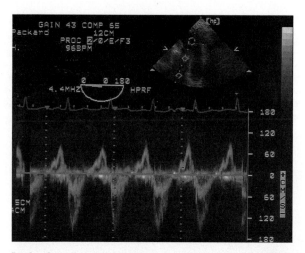

FIG. 19.21. Top: In the deep transgastric view, the pulsed wave Doppler sample volume is positioned at the tips of the mitral valve leaflets. Note that the left ventricular outflow tract and ascending aorta lie in the path of the beam in the far field. **Bottom:** The displayed pulsed wave spectral signal shows not only diastolic flow through the mitral valve but also the left ventricular outflow tract and aortic blood flow velocities during systole. These measurements of the far field velocities are at exactly two and three times the distance to the primary measurement.

artifact caused by blood flow in the left ventricular outflow tract, which lies in a plane just anterior to the TG short-axis view seen in Figure 19.20B.

Range Ambiguity with Pulsed Wave Doppler

One of the main advantages of pulsed wave Doppler is the ability to range-gate a sample volume. However, strong reflected signals originating from blood flow at two or three times the depth of the pulsed wave sample volume arrive at the transducer simultaneously with those from the target. These signals are displayed and can be misinterpreted as blood flow within the target volume (Fig. 19.21). Range ambiguity is particularly problematic with high pulse repetition frequency Doppler.

SUMMARY

An appreciation of cardiac embryology and anatomy will enable the echocardiographer to interpret cardiac structures with an unusual appearance accurately, so that unnecessary surgical intervention is prevented. A thorough understanding of two-dimensional and Doppler technologies is required to minimize misinterpretation.

SUGGESTED READINGS

Appelbe AF, Walker PG, Yeoh JK, et al. Clinical significance and origin of artifacts in transesophageal echocardiography of the thoracic aorta. *J Am Coll Cardiol* 1993;21:754–760.

Blanchard DG, Dittrich HC, Mitchell M, et al. Diagnostic pitfalls in transesophageal echocardiography. *J Am Soc Echocardiogr* 1992;5:525–540.

Cahalan MK. *Intraoperative transesophageal echocardiography. An interactive text and atlas.* New York: Churchill Livingstone, 1997.

Ducart AR, Broka SM, Collard EL. Linear reverberation in the ascending aorta: a cause of multiplane transesophageal echocardiographic artifact. *Anesthesiology* 1996;85:1497–1498.

Freeman WK, Seward JB, Khandheria BJ, et al. *Transesophageal echocardiography.* Boston: Little, Brown and Company, 1994.

Otto CM, Pearlman AS. *Textbook of clinical echocardiography.* Philadelphia: WB Saunders, 1995.

Seward JB, Khandheria BJ, Oh JK, et al. Critical appraisal of transesophageal echocardiography: limitations, pitfalls and complications. *J Am Soc Echocardiogr* 1992;5:288–305.

St. John Sutton MG, Oldershaw PJ, Kotler MN. *Textbook of echocardiography and Doppler in adults and children,* 2nd ed. Boston: Blackwell Science, 1996.

Stoddard MF, Liddell NE, Longaker RA, et al. Transesophageal echocardiography: normal variants and mimickers. *Am Heart J* 1992;124:1587–1598.

Weyman AE. *Principles and practice of echocardiography,* 2nd ed. Philadelphia: Lea & Febiger, 1994.

QUESTIONS

1. What is the most common type of imaging artifact?
   a. Acoustic shadowing
   b. Reverberation
   c. Suboptimal image quality
   d. Mirroring
2. Acoustic shadowing will produce a dark area
   a. Proximal to the strong reflector
   b. Distal to the strong reflector
   c. Left of the strong reflector
   d. Right of the strong reflector
3. In most imaging systems, axial resolution is at least
   a. Equal to lateral resolution
   b. Twice lateral resolution
   c. Ten times lateral resolution
   d. Half of lateral resolution
4. Which of the following factors is not related to aliasing in spectral Doppler imaging?
   a. Pulse repetition frequency
   b. Nyquist limit
   c. "Wraparound"
   d. Lateral resolution
5. The crista terminalis is located in the
   a. Right atrium
   b. Left atrium
   c. Right ventricle
   d. Left ventricle
6. The moderator band is in the
   a. Right atrium
   b. Left atrium
   c. Right ventricle
   d. Left ventricle
7. Which of the following statements is NOT true of a lipomatous atrial septum?
   a. It has a dumbbell shape.
   b. The fatty infiltration is echo-dense.
   c. The fossa ovalis is thickened.
   d. The fossa ovalis is spared.

8. In an interrogation of flow with spectral Doppler, a nonparallel beam angle will
   a. Overestimate the true velocity
   b. Underestimate the true velocity
   c. Correctly measure the velocity
   d. Spectral Doppler does not measure velocities.
9. Side lobe artifacts
   a. Are true structures outside the path of the main beam
   b. Are incorrectly displayed in the two-dimensional sector
   c. Are true structures in the path of the main beam
   d. **a** and **b**
10. Reverberation artifacts will not produce
   a. Multiple linear densities
   b. Dual structures in an axial orientation
   c. Dual structures in a left-right orientation
   d. A duplication that is the same size as the original

20

Techniques and Tricks for Optimizing Transesophageal Images

Herbert W. Dyal II, Michael D. Frith, and Scott T. Reeves

The accuracy and diagnostic confidence of a transesophageal echocardiographic (TEE) study depend greatly on the quality of the ultrasound image. Image quality is affected by several factors, including patient anatomy, the quality of the ultrasound system, and the skill of the echocardiographer. This chapter discusses the controls on the echocardiography machine and the process of optimizing their settings to obtain images of the highest quality.

TWO-DIMENSIONAL CONTROLS

Preprocessing versus Postprocessing Controls

Preprocessing controls adjust the transmission and acquisition of the ultrasound signals. Preprocessing settings control the formatting of the ultrasound signal for conversion into an electric signal. Changes in the preprocessing controls affect the information that the scanner will access to create an image (1), and this formatted information is the basis on which an image is created. Postprocessing settings affect the manner in which the formatted information is displayed on the monitor. Simply put, postprocessing defines the "cosmetic appearance" of the ultrasound data displayed on the monitor

Transmit Power

Transmit power controls the amplitude (acoustic power) of the transmitted ultrasound signal. Modern echocardiography systems default to a high-power setting to maximize the signal-to-noise ratio. A theoretic concern is that high-power ultrasound can have deleterious effects on tissue, particularly in fetal echocardiography. Federal standards restrict the maximal intensities allowed for transmit power settings on commercially available ultrasound systems. Typically, echocardiography systems default to the maximum transmit power, however, proper adjustment of transmit power becomes critical when echo contrast studies are performed.

Gain

Increasing the gain increases the amplitude of the electric signal generated by returning ultrasound signals received at all depths. Unfortunately, any noise present is also amplified. Setting the gain too high or too low affects the ability to read the image correctly. When the gain is set too high, the image appears quite bright, and linear structures, such as the mitral valve, appear thickened. Increases in the gain also increase the amount of visible noise. For instance, with moderately excessive gain settings, the left ventricular (LV) cavity acquires a speckled appearance, which can make it difficult to differentiate the LV cavity from the myocardium. With further increases in the gain, the entire LV takes on a whitened appearance, and the ability to differentiate structures is lost.

When the gain is set too low, only bright signals, such as those from the pericardium, are visible, and very low-amplitude signals, such as the signal from an LV thrombus or "smoke" in the LV, are lost (2). Therefore, the gain should be adjusted to obtain an image with a gray scale ranging from low-amplitude (dark gray) to high-amplitude (white) signals. The gray scale, displayed as a bar graph on the right side of the image, is useful for guiding adjustments. Figure 20.1 demonstrates the effect of three separate gain settings on the same midesophageal (ME) four-chamber view.

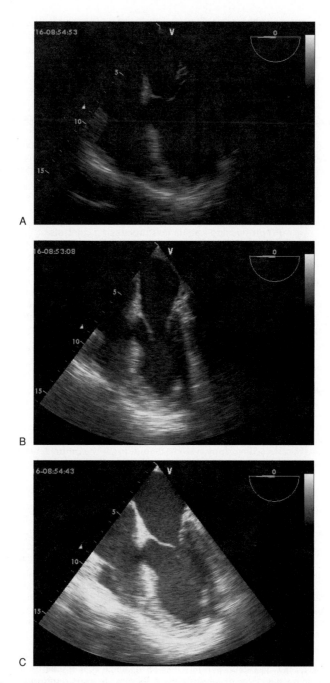

FIG. 20.1. The midesophageal four-chamber view with the gain setting too low (**A**), normal (**B**), and too high (**C**).

Clinical pearl. *The bright ambient lighting of the operating room often misleads the echocardiographer to use excessive gain settings. This problem can be overcome by eliminating the operating room lights briefly during the examination or shielding the screen with a hood.*

Time Gain Compensation

Because the amplitude of the reflected ultrasound depends on the distance traveled (depth) and the echogenicity of the tissue, the ability to adjust the gain setting selectively at each depth is essential to optimize the image. Time gain compensation allows the operator to adjust the gain at specific depths (3). For example, the echocardiographer can use the time gain compensation to amplify the weaker signals returning from the far field more than the signals returning from shallower depths (near field). The echocardiographer should be careful when adjusting the time gain compensation. If it is set too low, the elimination of true tissue signals is a risk. The time gain compensation should be used to eliminate gain-related artifacts and optimize far field structures. The effects of time gain compensation settings on image quality are shown in Figure 20.2.

Clinical pearl. *In a normal examination, the time gain compensation controls are set lower in the near field and higher in the far field. However, for imaging pathology in the near field with low echogenicity (e.g., thrombus in the aorta or left atrium), the near field time gain compensation should be increased.*

Depth

This control selects the maximal distance to be displayed. Increasing depth beyond the structure of interest has several negative consequences.

1. *The image size is reduced.* The most obvious consequence is that the image size is reduced because a larger area of the cardiac anatomy must be displayed on a screen of fixed size. The display of the cardiac structure of interest will be smaller and thus more difficult to evaluate.

2. *The frame rate is lower.* In addition, as the depth is increased, the frame rate of the two-dimensional ultrasound is slowed because the system must wait longer for signals to be received. Doubling the depth of penetration doubles the wait time before another pulse can be sent, so that the pulse repetition frequency and subsequently the frame rate are decreased (4).

Thus, to optimize image display and temporal resolution, the depth should be set just beyond the structure of interest, as shown in Figure 20.3.

It also must be appreciated that the lateral resolution of the ultrasound system is inversely proportional to the depth. Therefore, it is practical to have the position of the probe as close as possible to the structure of interest. For example, when the leaflets of the aortic valve are being evaluated, the ME aortic valve short-axis view is preferable to the deep transgastric (TG) long-axis view because the probe is closer to the aortic valve and lateral resolution is improved.

Clinical pearl. *Resist increasing the depth beyond the setting that displays the structure of interest.*

Focus

The focus control enables the operator to focus the ultrasound beam at a selected distance from the transducer. This is achieved by altering the sequences of electric impulses sent to the transducer elements. The goal of focusing is to have the beam narrowest at the location of the structure being evaluated because a thinner beam improves lateral resolution (5). The user must be cognizant of the focus depth of the system, which is typically marked

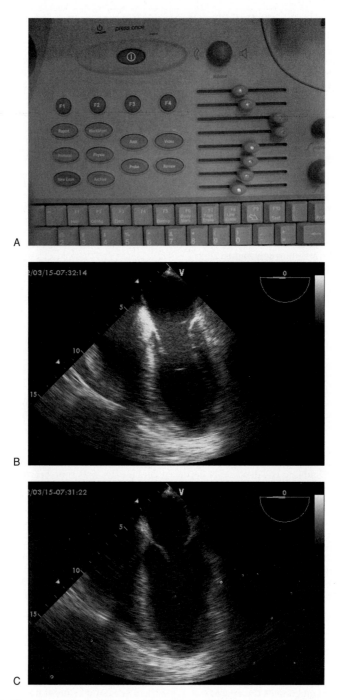

FIG. 20.2. A: The time gain compensation is determined by a series of sliding controls. The upper controls affect the near field and the lower controls the far field. Note the high settings of the third and fourth controls and their effects on the midfield in **B**. **B:** The mitral valve apparatus is obscured by specular noise. **C:** The time gain compensation controls were subsequently reduced, after which the image quality improved markedly.

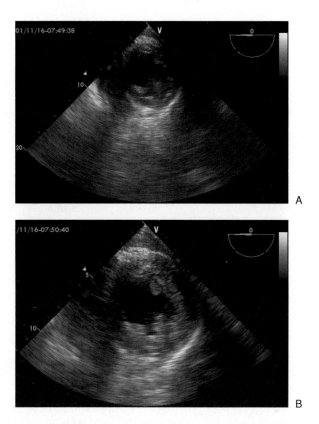

FIG. 20.3. The transgastric mid short-axis view with too much depth (**A**) and with the depth correctly set (**B**). Note that the focal point in image **B** is located at 5 cm, exactly in the center of the left ventricle. The focal point is marked with a *solid arrow head*.

on the edge of the sector (Fig. 20.3). If the focal zone is located too far from the area of interest, the image resolution may not be sufficient for proper evaluation. When the atrial septum is being evaluated for a patent foramen ovale, the focus should be placed at this level. Remember that structures distal to the focal point lie in the far field and may appear "fuzzy" or abnormally thick. Avoid evaluating small structures distal to the focal point until the focal point is moved to that level.

Clinical pearl. Adjust the focus point to the level of the structure of interest for high-resolution imaging.

Frequency

A feature of modern TEE systems is that they are capable of multiple frequencies, so that the transmitted ultrasound frequency can be adjusted. This can be especially important in TEE applications. When the structures being evaluated are in close proximity to the transducer (atria, aorta), higher frequencies are used to optimize resolution (6). When the structures being evaluated are farther from the transducer (deep TG views), higher frequencies may not be adequate because penetration is poor. In these situations, the frequency should be reduced until a satisfactory image is produced.

Clinical pearl. Use higher frequencies when evaluating shallow structures and lower frequencies when evaluating deep structures (i.e., TG views).

Dynamic Range

Modern ultrasound transducers are capable of detecting reflected ultrasound signals with amplitudes over a range of approximately 100 dB (7). Unfortunately, the monitors used in these systems are capable of displaying only a much smaller range (~30 dB). Therefore, to display the range of ultrasound signals detected by the transducer, the dynamic range control allows the wide spectrum of ultrasound amplitudes to be compressed. The compressed signals are then displayed on the monitor as varying shades of gray.

Ultrasound systems have both a fixed dynamic range, which is limited by the hardware of the system, and a selectable dynamic range, which can be changed according to the echocardiographer's preference. Increasing the dynamic range of the system increases the number of shades of gray between black and white within the image and therefore increases image detail, so that a smoother image appears on the display screen. Decreasing the dynamic range of the system increases the contrast of the image, with more black and white areas than shades of gray. The effect of dynamic range on image quality is shown in Figure 20.4.

Compression

Compression is a postprocessing tool that in conjunction with the preprocessing dynamic range control setting alters the range of the displayed gray scale (8). The compression control changes how the given dynamic range of ultrasound data is displayed. When the compression control is reduced, the given dynamic range is displayed with the largest range of allowable shades of gray. The lowest-intensity signal is displayed as black, and the highest-intensity signal is displayed as white. As the compression control is increased, the range of shades of gray used to produce the image is reduced to produce a softer, smoother image. The gray scale is therefore compressed by eliminating the display of shades of gray at each end of the spectrum. Compression settings are a personal preference of the echocardiographer.

Reject

In the early stages of ultrasound development, it was discovered that ultrasound transducers detect many sources of low-level interference from within the body. Examples include movement artifacts, the electronic noise of equipment, such as ventilators, and aberrant ultrasound resulting from refraction of the ultrasound signal. These low-level signals are detected by the scanner and displayed in the image as "noise." To eliminate such signals, all ultrasound systems have a fixed or default "filter" that removes any signal below a certain amplitude threshold (the lower limit of the displayed dynamic range) (9). Sometimes, the default filter is not enough to remove the noise in an image. The reject control is an adjustable control that enables the user to eliminate a greater number of low-intensity signals. The reject control is used to eliminate signals that are usually located in blood pools and are a result of artifacts. When the reject control is adjusted, care must be taken not to eliminate important low-intensity echoes from certain pathologic conditions. Specifically, fresh thrombi within a cardiac chamber or vessel have a low-intensity (dark) signal that may be eliminated from the image if the reject is set too high.

Clinical pearl. Increase the reject control to eliminate noise (random echoes often found in blood pools and other low-intensity areas). Do not use excessive reject because low-intensity echoes such as thrombi may be removed from the image.

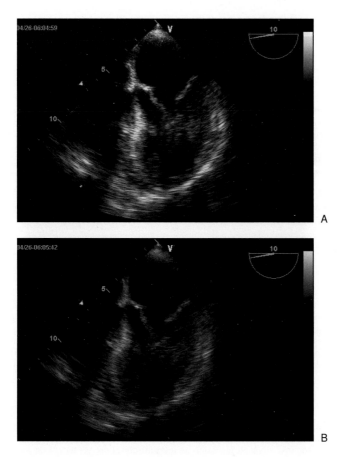

FIG. 20.4. A partial midesophageal four-chamber view concentrating on the left atrium and left ventricle. **A:** The dynamic range is set too low. Note the increased contrast in the image, with more black and white than shades of gray. **B:** The same image with the proper dynamic range setting.

Persistence

Persistence is a postprocessing control that can best be described as signal averaging or image blending. The term is derived from earlier ultrasound systems that used cathode ray tubes for display. After the phosphor elements in the tube were illuminated to form an image, rather than disappearing instantly, the luminescence faded gradually (or persisted). As a result, new images were displayed while the old, dimmer image was still on the screen (10). With the advent of digital scan converters and the replacement of cathode ray tubes with modern monitors, the term *persistence* is now used for frame averaging in the digital scan converter. As incoming signals are processed by the system, images are displayed as they are created in their purest form (no persistence), or the system can average one image with the next and display the averaged image. Persistence is used to smooth the appearance of the heart in motion. As the persistence control is increased, more images are used to create the averaged image, and temporal and spatial resolution is decreased. If the persistence is set too high, the image is often described as appearing to be in "slow motion." Because valvular structures move rapidly, persistence is usually set low in echocardiographic applications to retain temporal resolution and a real-time appearance.

Sector Size

Sector size controls the angle of the sector displayed on the monitor. Most ultrasound scanners can display sectors with angles ranging from 15 to 90 degrees. Wide angles allow the operator to survey a broad array of cardiac structures in a single view. The most important effect of the sector size is on the frame rate. The wider the sector size, the lower the frame rate and the temporal resolution. For a proper evaluation of fast-moving structures, the sector size should be kept small to allow for higher frame rates. Some scanning systems do not depend on sector size for high frame rates and can achieve adequate frame rates with a full 90-degree sector.

Clinical pearl. *Larger sector sizes result in lower frame rates and a lower level of temporal resolution. When valvular structures are evaluated, it is helpful to decrease the sector size (or use M-mode) to improve the frame rates.*

COLOR CONTROLS

Region of Interest

The region of interest is the area that defines where the color will be displayed. There are certain limitations to setting the size of the region of interest. As the width of the region of interest increases, the frame rate decreases (11). The goal is to optimize the frame rate to improve temporal resolution and the assessment of blood flow. The depth also affects the color frame rate. As the depth increases, the system must wait longer for the returning signal; therefore, the frame rate is slower.

Color Gain

Color gain is similar to two-dimensional gain in that it increases or amplifies the signal generated by the returning echoes. It is very important to have the color gain set properly. If the gain is set too low, a small jet, such as a small atrial septal defect or patent foramen ovale, can be missed. If the gain is set too high, the size of a regurgitant jet is frequently overestimated. The color gain is adjusted simply by increasing the color gain control until speckles of color lay outside the blood pools and then decreasing the gain one to two settings until the speckles go away. Figure 20.5 (see also Color Plate 36 following page 212) shows different color gain settings.

Color Scale

The color scale is the range of color velocities displayed. To optimize the color scale, one must be cognizant of the general velocities of the blood flow being evaluated. For example, when lower-flow velocities in the pulmonary veins are evaluated, one must decrease the color scale. Adjusting the scale will affect the Nyquist limit. Velocities sampled outside this range cause aliasing within the color display. In certain applications, such as when the proximal isovelocity surface area (PISA) is calculated, adjusting the color scale to produce aliasing is required to create an adequate flow convergence hemisphere for measurement.

Variance

The variance color flow map displays the range of velocities in any given sample volume. The variance in flow is displayed as shades of green, whereas normal flows are displayed

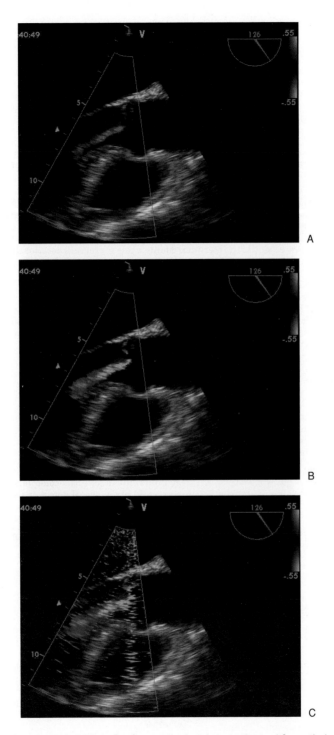

FIG. 20.5. Midesophageal aortic valve long-axis view in a patient with aortic insufficiency. **A:** The color gain is set too low, so that the width of the aortic insufficiency jet is underestimated. **B:** The color gain is correctly set. **C:** The color gain is too high. (See Color Plate 36 following page 212.)

with the standard red-blue color flow map. In laminar flow, the range of velocities in a given sample volume is relatively small, and laminar flow appears color-coded as red or blue. In turbulent flow, the number of velocities is increased (i.e., increased variance) such that turbulent flow is color-coded as green (12). A variance map may help to identify a small turbulent jet by tagging it with a different (i.e., green) color.

STORAGE SYSTEMS: ANALOG VIDEOTAPE VERSUS DIGITAL STORAGE

The advantages of videotape storage are its availability and reasonable cost. It is the most common storage format used today. A patient's study can be reviewed anywhere a videocassette recorder is available. A shortcoming is that it is difficult to archive and retrieve studies, and to directly compare different studies of the same patient. For example, if a patient has an LV ejection fraction of 40% on one examination and on a subsequent examination a value of 30% is reported, it is essential to determine whether this represents deterioration in function or differences in interpretation. With digital technology, a direct side-by-side comparison can be performed.

Current digital technology also allows the study data to be manipulated. The reviewer can adjust the *postprocessing* controls, including contrast, brightness, and two-dimensional and Doppler gain. It is also possible to make measurements from stored images without having to recalibrate the system. Finally, optical storage media make it practical to house large databases in minimal space. In sum, digital storage offers major advantages for archiving, retrieving, and sharing echocardiographic studies.

SUMMARY

The extensive control options of modern full-platform echocardiography systems provide the echocardiographer with tools for reliably obtaining high-quality images under a broad range of conditions. With a firm understanding of the control settings available, the examiner can optimize image acquisition and display and detect pathology that might otherwise be missed.

REFERENCES

1. Marcus ML, Schelbert HR, Skorton DJ, et al. *Cardiac imaging—a companion to Braunwald's "heart disease."* Philadelphia: WB Saunders, 1991:363.
2. Feigenbaum H. *Echocardiography.* Philadelphia: Lea & Febiger, 1986:57.
3. Weyman AE. *Cross-sectional echocardiography.* Philadelphia: Lea & Febiger, 1982:26.
4. Weyman AE. *Principles and practice of echocardiography.* Philadelphia: Lea & Febiger, 1994:219.
5. Thrush A, Hartshorne T. *Peripheral vascular ultrasound how, why, and when.* London: Churchill Livingstone, 1999:17–18.
6. Weyman AE. *Cross-sectional echocardiography.* Philadelphia: Lea & Febiger, 1982:17.
7. Weyman AE. *Principles and practice of echocardiography.* Philadelphia: Lea & Febiger, 1994:49–50.
8. Hagen-Ansert SL. *Textbook of diagnostic ultrasonography.* St. Louis: Mosby, 1989:38–39.
9. Feigenbaum H. *Echocardiography.* Philadelphia: Lea & Febiger, 1986:23.
10. Weyman AE. *Cross-sectional echocardiography.* Philadelphia: Lea & Febiger, 1982:55.
11. Thrush A, Hartshorne T. *Peripheral vascular ultrasound how, why, and when.* London: Churchill Livingstone, 1999:42.
12. Weyman AE. *Principles and practice of echocardiography.* Philadelphia: Lea & Febiger, 1994:225–226.

QUESTIONS

1. The LV appears very small on the screen. Which control would you adjust to make it appear larger on the screen?
   a. Increase frequency
   b. Decrease frequency
   c. Increase depth
   d. Decrease depth
2. When obtaining a deep TG long-axis view, how would you adjust the frequency of the transducer to increase the penetration?
   a. Increase frequency
   b. Decrease frequency
   c. The frequency does not affect penetration
3. What effect does increasing the sector size have on an image?
   a. Increases the resolution
   b. Increases the frame rate
   c. Decreases the frame rate
   d. Has no effect
4. There is too much aliasing in the color Doppler display. Which control would you adjust to decrease the amount of aliasing in the display?
   a. Increase depth
   b. Decrease depth
   c. Increase the scale/pulse repetition frequency
   d. Decrease the scale/pulse repetition frequency
5. Which control is best used to adjust the brightness of the image at a specific depth?
   a. Time gain compensation
   b. Gain
   c. Depth
   d. Power
6. Which color map will help to identify a turbulent flow pattern?
   a. Red-blue
   b. Low flow
   c. Mosaic
   d. Variance
7. Which control is best used to filter out low-level noise from the two-dimensional or Doppler image?
   a. Reject
   b. Gain
   c. Dynamic range
   d. Compression
8. Which method of storage best allows the user to manipulate data after the study?
   a. Videocassette recorder tape
   b. Digital storage
   c. It is not possible to manipulate an image after it has been saved
9. Which of the following is a preprocessing control?
   a. Persistence
   b. Transmit power
   c. Contrast
   d. Color gain
10. When reviewing a study obtained in the operating room, your colleagues in the echocardiography laboratory comment that the image is too bright. What can be done in the future to optimize image quality?
    a. Decrease the gain settings
    b. Turn off the operating room lights briefly while the TEE examination is performed
    c. Shield the monitor with a hood
    d. All of the above

APPENDIX 1

TRANSESOPHAGEAL ECHOCARDIOGRAPHIC ANATOMY

ME Asc Aortic SAX	Probe Adjustment: Neutral	Sector Depth: ~6 cm
	Primary Diagnostic Issues Aortic atherosclerosis Aortic dissection Pulmonary artery pathology (emboli, dilation, other)	**Required Structures** Aorta in cross section in transverse plane (0 degree) Pulmonary artery (main and proximal right)
ME Asc Aortic LAX	Probe Adjustment: Neutral	Sector Depth: ~6 cm
	Primary Diagnostic Issues Aortic atherosclerosis Aortic dissection	**Required Structures** Ascending aorta in long axis Right pulmonary artery in cross section
UE Aortic Arch SAX	Probe Adjustment: Neutral	Sector Depth: ~6 cm
	Primary Diagnostic Issues Aortic atherosclerosis Aortic dissection Pulmonic valve	**Required Structures** Aortic arch in cross section Main pulmonary artery (often not well seen)
UE Aortic Arch LAX	Probe Adjustment: Rightward	Sector Depth: ~6 cm
	Primary Diagnostic Issues Aortic atherosclerosis Aortic dissection Visualization of aortic cannulation site	**Required Structures** Distal ascending aortal/aortic arch
Desc Aortic SAX	Probe Adjustment: Neutral	Sector Depth: ~6 cm
	Primary Diagnostic Issue Aortic atherosclerosis Aortic dissection	**Required Structures** Descending aorta in cross section in transverse plane (0 degree)
Desc Aortic LAX	Probe Adjustment: Neutral	Sector Depth: ~6 cm
	Primary Diagnostic Issues Aortic atherosclerosis Aortic dissection	**Required Structures** Descending aorta in long axis in longitudinal plane (90 degrees)

(continued)

ME AV SAX	Probe Adjustment: Neutral	Sector Depth: ~10 cm

Primary Diagnostic Issue	**Required Structures**
Aortic stenosis	Three leaflets
Valvular morphology	Commissures
	Coaptation point

ME RV Inflow-Outflow	Probe Adjustment: Neutral	Sector Depth: ~10 cm

Primary Diagnostic Issues	**Required Structures**
Pulmonic valve disease	Pulmonic valve
Pulmonary artery pathology	Tricuspid valve
RVOT pathology	Main pulmonary artery (at least
Doppler evaluation of	1 cm distal to the pulmonic valve)
tricuspid valve	RVOT (at least 1 cm proximal to the
	pulmonic valve)

ME AV LAX	Probe Adjustment: Neutral	Sector Depth: ~10 cm

Primary Diagnostic Issues	**Required Structures**
Aortic valve pathology	LVOT (at least 1 cm proximal to the
Aortic pathology (ascending	aortic valve)
and root)	Aortic valve (visualized cusps
LVOT pathology	approximately equal in size)
Anterior leaflet mitral valve	Ascending aorta (at least 1 cm
	distal to the sinotubular junction)

ME Bicaval	Probe Adjustment: Neutral	Sector Depth: ~10 cm

Primary Diagnostic Issues	**Required Structures**
Atrial septal defect	RA free wall (or appendage)
Tumor	Superior vena cava (at least its
Retrograde venous cannula	entry into the RA)
positioning	Interatrial septum

ME Four-Chamber	Probe Adjustment: Neutral-Retroflex	Sector Depth: ~14 cm

Primary Diagnostic Issues	**Required Structures**
Atrial septal defect	LA
Chamber enlargement	LV
dysfunction	Mitral valve
Mitral disease	Tricuspid valve (maximal annular
Tricuspid disease	dimension)
Detection of intracardiac air	

ME Two-Chamber	Probe Adjustment: Neutral	Sector Depth: ~14 cm

Primary Diagnostic Issues	**Required Structures**
LA appendage	LA appendage
Mass/thrombus	Mitral valve
LV apex pathology	LV apex (i.e., maximal LV length)
LV systolic dysfunction	
(apical segments)	

(continued)

ME LAX	Probe Adjustment: Neutral	Sector Depth: ~12 cm
	Primary Diagnostic Issues Mitral valve pathology LVOT pathology	**Required Structures** LV Mitral valve LVOT

ME Mitral Commissural	Probe Adjustment: Neutral	Sector Depth: ~12 cm

	Primary Diagnostic Issues
	Localization of mitral valve
	    pathology
		Required Structures
		Mitral valve (P1, P3, and A2
		    scallops)
		Papillary muscles/chordae
		    tendineae
		LA
		LV

TG Mid SAX	Probe Adjustment: Neutral	Sector Depth: ~ 12 cm

	Primary Diagnostic Issues
	Hemodynamic instability
	LV enlargement
	LV hypertrophy
	LV systolic dysfunction
	    (global and regional)
		Required Structures
		LV cavity
		LV walls (at least 50% of
		    circumference with visible
		    endocardium)
		Papillary muscles (approximately
		    equal in size and distinct from
		    ventricular wall)

TG Two-Chamber	Probe Adjustment: Neutral	Sector Depth: ~12 cm

	Primary Diagnostic Issues
	LV systolic dysfunction
	    (anterior and inferior basal
	    segments)
		Required Structures
		Mitral leaflets
		Mitral subvalvular apparatus
		LV (anterior and inferior: basal plus
		    mild segments)

TG RV Inflow	Probe Adjustment: Neutral-Rightward	Sector Depth: ~12 cm
	Primary Diagnostic Issues RV systolic dysfunction Tricuspid valve pathology	**Required Structures** Tricuspid leaflets Tricuspid subvalvular apparatus RV

TG RV Inflow-Outflow	Probe Adjustment: Neutral-Rightward	Sector Depth: ~14 cm
	Primary Diagnostic Issues RV systolic dysfunction RVOT pathology Pulmonary artery pathology Pulmonic valve evaluation	**Required Structures** RA RV Main pulmonary artery Pulmonic valve

(continued)

TG Basal SAX	Probe Adjustment: Neutral	Sector Depth: ~12 cm

	Primary Diagnostic Issues	**Required Structures**
	LV systolic dysfunction (basal segments)	Mitral leaflets
		Mitral subvalvular apparatus
	Mitral valve pathology	LV (basal segments)

TG LAX	Probe Adjustment: Neutral-Leftward	Sector Depth: ~12 cm

	Primary Diagnostic Issues	**Required Structures**
	LV systolic dysfunction (anteroseptal and posterior: basal segments)	Mitral leaflets
		Mitral subvalvular apparatus
		LV (anteroseptal and posterior: basal plus mid segments)
	Doppler evaluation of aortic valve	Aortic valve

Deep TG LAX	Probe Adjustment: Neutral	Sector Depth: ~16 cm

	Primary Diagnostic Issues	**Required Structures**
	Aortic valve pathology	LV
	LVOT pathology	Aortic valve
	Doppler evaluation of aortic valve	Aorta

Abbreviations: Asc, ascending; AV, aortic valve; Desc, descending; LA, left atrium; LAX, long axis; LVOT, left ventricular outflow tract; ME, midesophageal; RA, right atrium; RVOT, right ventricular outflow tract; SAX, short axis; TG, transgastric; UE, upper esophageal.

Modified from Miller JP, Lambert SA, Shapiro WA, et al. The adequacy of basic intraoperative transesophageal echocardiography performed by experienced anesthesiologists. *Anesth Analg* 2001;92:1103–1110, with permission.

APPENDIX 2

SUMMARIES OF VALVULAR STENOSIS AND INSUFFICIENCY

A. SEVERITY OF AORTIC INSUFFICIENCY

Method of Evaluation (View)	Trivial (0–1$^+$)	Mild (1$^+$–2$^+$)	Moderate (2$^+$–3$^+$)	Severe (3$^+$–4$^+$)
AI jet height/LVOT diameter (ME AV LAX)	1%–24%	25%–46%	47%–64%	>65%
AI area/LVOT area (ME AV SAX)	<4%	4%–24%	25%–59%	>60%
Jet depth mapping (ME LAX)	LVOT	Mid anterior mitral leaflet	Tip anterior mitral leaflet	Papillary muscle head
Vena contracta mapping (ME LAX, ME AV SAX)				Width >6 mm Area >7.5 mm^2
Aortic diastolic flow reversal (UE aortic arch LAX)				Holodiastolic retrograde flow in the descending aorta
Slope of AR jet decay (TG LAX, deep TE LAX)			≥2 m/s	≥3 m/s
Pressure half-time (deep TG LAX, TG LAX)		>500 ms	200–500 ms	<200 ms

AI, aortic insufficiency; LVOT, left ventricular outflow tract; ME, midesophageal; AV, aortic valve; LAX, long axis; SAX, short axis; UE, upper esophageal; AR, aortic regurgitation; TG, transgastric.

B. SEVERITY OF AORTIC STENOSIS

Method of Evaluation	Normal	Mild	Moderate	Severe
Peak velocity (m/s)	1.0–1.7			>4.5
Mean gradient (mm Hg)		<20	20–50	>50
Maximal pressure gradient (mm Hg)		<36	>50	>80
TVI$_{LVOT}$/TVI$_{AV}$ ratio				<0.25
AVA (cm^2)	2.6–3.5	1.0–1.5	0.80–1.0	<0.80

TVI, time-velocity integral; LVOT, left ventricular outflow tract; AVA, aortic valve area.

C. SEVERITY OF MITRAL INSUFFIENCY

Method	Mild	Moderate	Severe
MR jet area/atrial area	20%–30%	30%–40%	>40%
Vena contracta width			>5.5 mm
MR jet area	<3 cm^2	3.0–6.0 cm^2	>6 cm^2
Pulmonary vein flow	Blunted S wave	S wave < D wave	Systolic reversal
MR fraction	20%–30%	30%–50%	>55%
Mitral orifice (PISA)	<10 mm^2	10–25 mm^2	>25–35 mm^2

MR, mitral regurgitant; PISA, proximal isovelocity surface area.

D. SEVERITY OF MITRAL STENOSIS

	Grade		
	Mild	**Moderate**	**Severe**
Mean gradient (mm Hg)	6	6–10	>10
PHT (ms)	100	200	>300
MVA (cm^2)	1.6–2.0	1.0–1.5	<1.0

PHT, pressure half-time; MVA, mitral valve area.

Answers to Questions

CHAPTER 1

1. d
2. e
3. d
4. d
5. b
6. b
7. e
8. b
9. c
10. c

CHAPTER 2

1. a
2. b
3. a
4. c
5. d
6. a
7. d
8. d
9. d
10. b

CHAPTER 3

1. $SV = CSA_{LVOT} \ (cm^2) \times TVI_{LVOT} \ (cm)$
   $= \pi r_{LVOT}^2 \times TVI_{LVOT}$
   $= 3.14(1.9/2)^2 \times 14.47$
   $= 2.8 \times 14.47$
   $= 40.5 \ cc$
   $CO = SV \times HR$
   $= 40.5 \times 100$
   $= 4,050 \ cc/min$
   $= 4.0 \ L/min$
   $CI = CO/BSA \ (m^2)$
   $= 4.0/1.8$
   $= 2.2 \ L/min/m^2$

2A. $5.2 - 3.1/5.2 \times 100 = 40\%$

2B. LV function is *normal* because the shortening fraction is greater than or equal to 40%.

3. e

4. Adequate preload provides for a blood pressure or cardiac output that meets a minimum acceptable value. Optimal preload maximizes cardiac output. An "empty ventricle" by TEE does not always require IV fluid administration. Only when blood pressure and/or cardiac output are inadequate should the TEE diagnosis of low preload be treated.

5. Quantitative methods for determining cardiac output or ejection fraction are often time consuming and require obtaining ideal or multiple images. Such lengthy methods of determining ejection fraction are not compatible with a rapidly changing clinical situation.

6. a
7. c
8. e
9. d
10. e

CHAPTER 4

1. d
2. a
3. c
4. b
5. c
6. d
7. d
8. b
9. e
10. b

CHAPTER 5

1. c
2. b
3. d
4. c
5. a
6. c
7. c
8. a
9. b
10. d

CHAPTER 6

1. d
2. c
3. d
4. c
5. d
6. c
7. a
8. d
9. e
10. e

CHAPTER 7

1. d
2. a
3. d
4. c
5. a
6. b
7. d
8. c
9. a
10. b

CHAPTER 8

1. b
2. c
3. a
4. d
5. d
6. b
7. a
8. c
9. a
10. b

CHAPTER 9

1. c
2. c
3. d
4. c
5. b
6. a
7. c
8. c
9. d
10. d

CHAPTER 10

1. c
2. b
3. b
4. a
5. e
6. b
7. c
8. a
9. e
10. b

CHAPTER 11

1. d
2. d
3. e
4. d
5. e
6. b
7. e
8. a
9. e
10. a

CHAPTER 12

1. c
2. c
3. d
4. b
5. a
6. f
7. b
8. d
9. a
10. d

CHAPTER 13

1. c
2. b
3. a
4. d
5. d
6. a
7. c
8. a
9. b
10. a

CHAPTER 14

1. d
2. a
3. d
4. b
5. b
6. b
7. d
8. b
9. b
10. d

CHAPTER 15

1. d
2. b
3. c
4. d
5. c
6. d
7. a
8. b
9. c
10. b

CHAPTER 16

1. c
2. d. Konstadt showed that with TEE, up to 42% of the length of the ascending aorta, a distance of 4.5 to 10.7 cm, is not visualized. In addition, manual surgical palpation detects only 50% of important atheromas identified by epiaortic ultrasonography. Therefore, for a patient with significant disease identified by TEE in zones 1, 2, 5, or 6 as moderate to severe atheroma (grade 4 or 5), epiaortic scanning of the distal ascending and proximal arch (zones 4 and 5) is indicated.
3. e. Patients with an intramural hematoma do not have evidence of an intimal tear or dissection membrane on TEE or other diagnostic imaging modalities.
4. c
5. e
6. b. Angiography, CT, and MRI are superior in detecting thrombus.
7. b. Stanford type A criteria include DeBakey types I and II. Stanford type A and DeBakey types I and II aortic dissections require emergent surgical treatment, whereas Stanford type B and DeBakey type III dissections can be managed medically.
8. e
9. e
10. d. Coronary involvement by acute aortic dissection has been estimated to occur in 10% to 20% of cases.

CHAPTER 17

1. d
2. d
3. e
4. d
5. c
6. c
7. d
8. d
9. c
10. a

CHAPTER 18

1. d
2. d
3. c
4. d
5. b
6. d
7. c
8. c
9. a
10.

$$LVOT\text{-}SV = Area_{LVOT} \times TVI_{LVOT}$$
$$= 3.14(1.9/2)^2 \times 14.8$$
$$= 41.9 \text{ cc}$$

$$\text{RV-SV} = \text{Area}_{\text{MPA}} \times \text{TVI}_{\text{MPA}}$$
$$= 3.14(2.1/2)^2 \times 15.3$$
$$= 53 \text{ mL}$$

$$\text{CO} = \text{LVOT-SV} \times \text{HR}$$
$$= 41.9 \times 90$$
$$= 3.8 \text{ L/min}$$

$$\text{CI} = \text{CO/BSA}$$
$$= 3.8/1.8$$
$$= 2.1 \text{ L/min/m}^2$$

$$Q_p/Q_s = \text{SV of the pulmonary circuit/SV of the systemic arterial circuit}$$
$$Q_p = \text{SV from RV}$$
$$Q_s = \text{SV from LVOT}$$
$$Q_p/Q_s = 53 \text{ mL/42 mL}$$
$$= 1.3 : 1$$

$$\text{RVSP} = \text{BP} - 4(v_{vsd})2$$
$$= 112 - 4(4.6)^2$$
$$= 27 \text{ mmHg}$$

CHAPTER 19	**CHAPTER 20**
1. c	1. d
2. b	2. b
3. b	3. c
4. d	4. c
5. a	5. a
6. c	6. d
7. c	7. a
8. b	8. b
9. d	9. b
10. c	10. d

Subject Index

Page numbers followed by *f* refer to figures; page numbers followed by *t* refer to tables.

A

A2 anterior leaflet prolapse
transesophageal four-chamber view of, 169*f*
Absorption, 7
Acoustic impedance, 6
Acoustic quantification-derived fractional area change
transgastric mid short-axis view, 41*f*
Acoustic shadowing, 311, 311*f*
color flow Doppler artifacts, 314, 315*f*
Acoustic windows
ICU
TEE, 275
Acute myocardial infarction
complications, 66*t*
Adult congenital heart disease
aortic valve stenosis, 293–294
coarctation of the aorta, 292–293
congenitally corrected transposition, 296–297
dextro-transposition of the great arteries, 295*f*–296
patent ductus arteriosus, 292
prevalence of, 286
survival patterns of, 286, 287*t*
TEE, 286–300
atrial septal defects, 287–289
catheterization laboratory, 299
limitations of, 299
for noncardiac surgery, 299
tetralogy of fallot, 294–295
univentricular heart, 298–299
ventricular septal defect, 289–291
Alias artifacts, 88*f*
Aliasing, 314
Allograft valves, 209–210
American Society of Anesthesiologists
perioperative TEE practice guidelines, 56
American Society of Echocardiography
16-segment system, 61–67
midesophageal four-chamber anatomic segments and perfusion, 61*f*
midesophageal long-axis anatomic segments and perfusion, 62*f*
midesophageal two-chamber anatomic segments and perfusion, 62*f*
transgastric short-axis anatomic segments and perfusion, 63*f*
A-mode (amplitude mode), 16

Amplification, 16
Amplitude, 3
Amplitude mode, 16
Analog videotape
vs. digital storage, 330
Aneurysms
aortic. *See* Aortic aneurysms
inferobasal, 66*f*
true. *See* True aneurysms
ventricular
partial midesophageal four-chamber view, 49*f*
Antegrade cardioplegia
administration of, 242–243
Anterior leaflet prolapse
transesophageal four-chamber view of, 169*f*
Anteroseptal akinesis
following cardiopulmonary bypass, 60*f*
Aorta
ascending
transesophageal echocardiography, 242
measurement of, 209*f*
ascending thoracic
examination of, 256–257
linear streak in, 257*f*
atheromatous disease
management, 242
coarctation of the, 292–293
descending thoracic
examination of, 257–258
intimal tear
entry site of, 260*f*
diastolic flow reversal, 182
examination, 33
descending aorta long-axis view, 34
descending aorta short-axis view, 33
upper esophageal aortic arch short-axis view, 34
hematoma, 251*f*
insufficiency
severity of, 337
insufficiency height
ratio to left ventricular outflow tract diameter, 179*f*
root allografts, 209
thoracic
classification systems, 251–252
examination techniques, 255–258
TEE, 251–267
transgastric long-axis view, 43*f*

Aorta (*contd.*)
 transvalvular gradients
  equations for, 191*t*
 ultrasound, 235*f*
Aortic aneurysms
 ascending
  dilation, 262*f*
 classification of, 251
 type A
  morphology of, 253*f*
Aortic dissection
 acute
  morality rate for, 252
  true and false lumina of, 258*f*
 aortic regurgitation, 263*f*
 aortography, 253–255
 characteristics of, 258–259
 classification of, 251
 CT, 255
 diagnostic modalities for, 252–255
 imaging diagnosis, 254*t*
 MRI, 255
 TEE, 255, 258–264
  aortic graft repair intraoperative
   assessment, 264
  aortic insufficiency, 261–262
  artifacts of, 264
  coronary arteries, 262–263
  false lumen thrombosis, 261
  false *vs.* true lumen, 260–261
  ICU indications for, 279–280
  intramural hematoma, 265
  left ventricular function, 263
  limitations of, 264
  location and entry sites, 259–261
  pericardial and pleural effusion, 263
  surgeons' questions, 258
  thoracic aortic plaque, 265–267
Aortic regurgitant jet
 depth
  color flow mapping of, 181
  slope of, 182
 velocity profile
  transgastric long-axis view of,
   183*f*
 volume, 183–184
Aortic regurgitation, 177–184
 quantitative assessment of, 178–184
  aortic diastolic reversal, 182
  aortic regurgitant jet decay slope, 183
  audible Doppler signal, 184
  color flow mapping, 178–181
  pressure half-time measurement, 183
  regurgitant volume calculation, 183
  vena contracta mapping, 181
 recommended views for, 178
 scoring severity of, 180*t*
 upper esophageal aortic arch long-axis
  view, 181*f*
Aortic stenosis, 188–197
 in aortic regurgitation, 196
 low cardiac output in, 195–196

 maximal instantaneous gradient, 192*f*
 midesophageal aortic valve short-axis view
  of, 194*f*
 postoperative subaortic obstruction, 196
 quantitative Doppler assessment of,
  190–193
  aortic valve gradient, 191–193
  TEE, 190–191
 severity of, 189*t*, 336
 transgastric view of, 192*f*
Aortic valve
 annulus measurement of
  TEE, 209*f*
 bicuspid, 294*f*
 calculation of area, 193–194, 193*t*
 evaluation of, 188–195
  Bernoulli equation, 191–193
  continuity equation, 193–194
  technical considerations, 194–195
  two-dimensional planimetry, 188–190
 leaflet injury
  TEE assessment of, 172
 midesophageal aortic valve long-axis view,
  29
 midesophageal aortic valve short-axis view
  of, 189*f*
 midesophageal bicaval view, 30
 midesophageal right ventricular
  inflow-outflow, 28–29
 midesophageal short-axis view, 27–28
 prostheses
  normal maximal pressure gradients for,
   213*f*
 prosthetic
  effective orifice area of, 205*t*
 pulsed wave Doppler, 195*f*
 stenosis, 293–294
  anatomy of, 293
  color flow Doppler examination of, 294
  intraoperative TEE of, 293–294
  physiology of, 293
  spectral Doppler examination of, 294
  two-dimensional evaluation of, 294
 stepwise examination, 27–29
 vegetation, 278*f*
Apical segments
 imaging, 63
Array, 17
Artifacts
 alias, 88*f*
 color flow Doppler
  acoustic shadowing, 314, 315*f*
 echocardiographic imaging
  two-dimensional, 309–314
 electrocautery, 314*f*
 lateral resolution
  two-dimensional echocardiographic
   imaging, 311
 mirroring
  pulsed wave Doppler, 316*f*
 spectral and color flow Doppler, 314–318
  aliasing, 314

mirroring, 315–316, 316*f*
nonparallel beam angle, 314–315, 315*f*
two-dimensional echocardiographic
   imaging, 309–314
   acoustic shadowing, 311, 311*f*
   electronic noise, 314
   reverberation, 313, 313*f*
   side lobe and beam width, 311–312,
      312*f*
   suboptimal image quality, 309–311
AR-wave, 124*f*
ASD. *See* Atrial septal defects (ASD)
Asymmetric septal hypertrophy (ASH)
   LVOT, 52*f*
Atherosclerotic disease
   aorta, 235*f*
Atrial appendage thrombus
   short-axis imaging of, 149*f*
Atrial filling
   left
      Doppler echocardiographic evaluation of,
         117–118
Atrial myxoma
   transesophageal echocardiographic
      midesophageal four-chamber image,
         146*f*
   transgastric basal short-axis image, 146*f*
Atrial pressure
   left
      Bernoulli equation, 104
      mitral regurgitation velocity profile, 105
Atrial septal defects (ASD), 287–289
   anatomy of, 287
   closure device, 289*f*
   color flow Doppler examination, 289
   intraoperative TEE, 289
   location of, 288*f*
   physiology of, 287–288
   repair of
      examination after, 289
   secundum, 288*f*
   two-dimensional examination, 289
Atrial septum
   lipomatous, 306*f*
   lipomatous hypertrophy of,
      305–306
Atrioventricular septal defects
   partial, 287
Attenuation, 5*f*, 7–8
Attenuation coefficient, 7
Axial resolution, 14
   pulse length, 11*f*
Azimuth resolution, 14

B
Backing, 10
Band
   moderator, 307, 308*f*
   pulmonary artery, 298*f*, 299
Beall prosthetic valves
   echocardiographic characteristics of, 205
Beam orientation, 24*f*–25*f*

Bernoulli equation, 100*f*, 101–105
   modified, 191–192
   simplified, 102
Bidirectional Glenn procedure, 299
Bileaflet prolapse
   repair of, 167
   transesophageal five-chamber view of, 169*f*
Billowing, 134, 135*f*
Bioprosthetic valves
   stentless, 208–209
Bjork-Shiley prosthetic valves
   echocardiographic characteristics of, 206
   pannus formation on, 207*f*
Blood flow
   common profiles, 96*f*
   detecting, 78*f*
   velocity
      calculating, 79*f*
Blood flow velocity
   transmitral
      determination, 114*f*
      left ventricular diastolic dysfunction,
         116*f*
Blunt profile, 95*f*
B-mode (brightness mode), 16–17
Bovine pericardial bioprosthesis
   in aortic position
      TEE, 212*f*
Brightness mode, 16–17

C
CABG. *See* Coronary artery bypass graft
   (CABG)
Caged-ball prosthetic valves
   echocardiographic characteristics of, 205
Caged-disc prosthetic valves
   echocardiographic characteristics of, 205
Carbomedic prosthetic valve
   echocardiographic characteristics of,
      203–205
Carbomedic R-series mechanical bileaflet
      prosthetic aortic valve, 202*f*
Cardiac cycle
   diastolic phase of, 111*f*
Cardiac dysfunction
   acute
      assessment and management of,
         239–241
      TEE, 239–241
Cardiac examination
   basic, 27*f*
Cardiac function
   TEE, 237*t*
Cardiac output, 42
   calculation
      aortic valve approach, 97*f*
      pulmonary artery approach, 98*f*
      right ventricular outflow tract approach,
         99*f*
   Doppler measurement, 94–97
   left ventricular function
      quantitative assessment of, 238

Cardiac output (*contd.*)
  low
    in aortic stenosis, 195–196
Cardiac tamponade
  evaluation of, 280
  indications for TEE in ICU, 282
Cardiomyopathy
  hypertrophic, 50–53
Cardiopulmonary bypass (CPB)
  anteroseptal akinesis following, 60*f*
  diastolic dysfunction following,
    110
  new regional wall motion abnormalities
    following
    management of, 239, 239*t*
Cardiopulmonary pressure
  Bernoulli equation, 103*t*
Carpentier-Edwards prosthetic valves,
    208*f*
  echocardiographic characteristics of, 207
Carpentier nomenclature,
    162, 162*f*–163*f*
  of mitral valve, 133
Carpentier technique
  for preventing systolic anterior motion,
    168*f*
Cavopulmonary anastomosis, 299
Ceramic piezoelectric crystal, 9
Chest trauma
  blunt
    indications for TEE in ICU, 282
Chiari network, 222, 305
Chordae tendineae, 310*f*
  anatomy of, 133, 145
Cine loops
  digital capture, 65–66
Classic anatomic nomenclature
  of mitral valve, 133
Clean envelope, 83
Cleansing jets, 205
Closure backflow, 210
Coarctation of the aorta, 292–293
  anatomy of, 292
  intraoperative TEE of, 292
  physiology of, 292
  two-dimensional transthoracic image of,
    293*f*
Color controls, 328–330
  color gain, 328
  color scale, 328
  region of interest, 328
  variance, 328–330
Color flow Doppler
  artifacts, 314–318
    acoustic shadowing, 314, 315*f*
    aliasing, 314
    beam width flow artifacts, 317–318
    mirroring, 315–316, 316*f*
    nonparallel beam angle, 314–315,
      315*f*
  of mitral regurgitation severity, 136–138
  reverberation, 316*f*

Color flow mapping, 89–91
Color M-mode
  transmitral
    Doppler flow propagation velocity, 122*f*
    impaired left ventricular relaxation,
      123*f*
Color M-mode transmitral propagation
    velocity, 120–123
Compression, 3, 16
Concentric hypertrophy, 47
Congenital heart disease
  adult. *See* Adult congenital heart disease
  classification of, 286–287
  incidence of, 286
Congenitally corrected transposition
    (levo-transposition), 296–297
  anatomy of, 296–297
  intraoperative TEE of, 297
  physiology of, 297
Congestive heart failure
  diastolic dysfunction, 110
Continuity equation, 100*f*, 101, 152–154,
    193–194, 193*t*
Continuous wave Doppler, 89
Continuous wave spectral signal, 90*f*
Contractility
  TEE, 237*t*
Controls
  two-dimensional, 321–328
Coronary artery
  injury
    TEE assessment of, 172
  perfusion zones, 63
Coronary artery bypass graft (CABG)
  dobutamine stress testing, 60
  primary
    with cardiopulmonary bypass, 68, 68*t*
  redo
    ischemia during, 69
  TEE, 234*t*
Coronary revascularization
  epiaortic scanning, 234–236
  epicardial scanning, 234–236
  surface scanning, 234–236
  TEE, 233–247
    approach, 236
    complications of, 233–234
    contra indications of, 233–234
    indications of, 233
    ventricular function, 236–238
Coronary sinus
  TEE, 244, 244*f*
Coumadin ridge, 306, 307*f*
CPB. *See* Cardiopulmonary bypass (CPB)
Crawford classification, 251, 252*f*
Crista terminalis, 305, 306*f*
Cross-sectional area (CSA), 94

D
DeBakey classification, 251, 254*f*
Deceleration time, 152, 153*f*
Demodulation, 81

Dextro-transposition of the great arteries, 295–296
  anatomy of, 295
  intraoperative TEE of, 296
  physiology of, 295
Diastolic dysfunction
  clinical relevance, 110
Diastolic function filling dynamics
  TEE, 237*t*
  ventricular Doppler echocardiographic indices, 113*t*
Diastolic heart failure
  prevalence, 110
Digital scan conversion, 16
Digital scan converter, 16
  postprocessing settings, 16
  preprocessing settings, 16
Dilated cardiomyopathy, 49–50
  associated findings, 50
  midesophageal four-chamber view, 51*f*
  two-dimensional characteristics, 49–50
Dimensionless index, 195–196
Dispersion, 7
Dobutamine stress testing, 60
Doppler, 78–81
  audible signal
    in aortic regurgitation assessment, 184
  beam
    cosine relationship, 80*f*
    orientation, 79–80
  blood flow velocity
    nonparallel beam orientation, 81*f*
  color display aliasing, 91*f*
  color flow. *See* Color flow Doppler
  color flow mapping, 89–91
  continuous wave, 89
  data presentation, 81–83
    audible broadcast, 81–83
    spectral display, 83, 85*f*
  effect, 77
  equation, 78–79, 79*f*
  flow measurement
    vs. two-dimensional imaging, 83*f*–84*f*
  frequency shift, 77–78
    isolating, 81
    signal frequency and blood flow, 77–78
  high-frequency pulsed, 88
  interrogation
    jet core, 85*f*
  left ventricular filing, 113–114
  pulmonary venous blood flow (PVDF)
    velocity profile, 118*f*
  pulsed wave. *See* Pulsed wave Doppler
  spectral
    of mitral valve, 138
  spectral and color flow
    beam width flow artifacts, 317–318
  techniques, 86–91
  transmitral blood flow velocity
    determination, 114*f*

left ventricular diastolic dysfunction, 116*f*
trans-tricuspid flow velocity
  normal profile, 124*f*
  right ventricular diastolic function, 123–124
Doppler flow profiles
  left atrial
    physiologic variables influence on, 119
  left ventricle (LV)
    physiologic variables influence on, 119
Duran nomenclature
  of mitral valve, 133
Dyskinesis
  M-mode (motion mode), 58*f*

E
Eccentric hypertrophy, 47
Echocardiography
  two-dimensional, 3–20
    artifacts, 309–314
Effective orifice area, 205
Eisenmenger syndrome, 290, 292
Ejection fraction, 38
Electrical processing, 16
Electric connector, 9*f*
Electrocautery artifacts, 314*f*
Electrodes, 9
Elevational resolution, 14
Endoaortic clamp, 245
Endocarditis
  indications for TEE in ICU, 278
  prosthetic valves
    clinical caveats, 213–214
  of prosthetic valves, 213–214
Epoxy filler, 9*f*
Eustachian valve, 305, 306*f*
Expiration, 125

F
Faceplate, 9*f*, 10
False rue lumen
  identification of, 280
Far fields (Fraunhofer), 10–11
Fast Fourier transform, 81
Fasting
  TEE probe insertion, 273
Femoral arterial cannulation, 243
Femoral venous cannulation, 243
Fish mouth orifice
  mitral valve, 151*f*
Flat flow profile, 95*f*
Flow velocities
  transmitral
    physiology of, 114–115
Fontan procedure, 299
Fractional shortening, 37–38
  left ventricle, 38*f*
Frame rate, 17, 19
Frank-Starling relationship, 44–47, 46*f*
  echocardiographic determination, 45–47
Fraunhofer fields, 10–11

Frequency, 3
 soft tissue, 5*f*
Fresnel fields, 10–11

G
Gag reflex
 TEE probe insertion, 274
Gain controls, 16
Giant penetrating ulcers
 classification of, 252
Glenn anastomosis, 299
Glenn procedure
 bidirectional, 299
Gorlin equation, 190
Grating lobes, 14
Great arteries
 dextro-transposition of the, 295–296

H
Half-power distance, 9
Hancock prosthetic valves
 echocardiographic characteristics of, 207
Harken prosthetic valves
 echocardiographic characteristics of, 205
Heart
 rhythm
  pulsed wave Doppler echocardiography,
   105–106
 right side
  stroke volume calculation, 96–97
Heart valves
 mechanical
  echocardiographic characteristics of, 201
Hematomas
 intramural
  classification of, 252
Hemodynamic instability
 indications for TEE in ICU, 276–277
Hemodynamics
 Doppler quantitative assessment of,
  94–106
 quantitative
  TEE, 237*t*
Hemolysis
 prosthetic valves
  clinical caveats, 213
 of prosthetic valves, 213
Hibernating myocardium
 characteristics, 57*t*
 dobutamine stress testing, 60
Hypertrophic cardiomyopathy, 50–53
 associated findings, 52–53
 classification, 50–51
 intraoperative considerations, 52–53
 two-dimensional characteristics, 51
Hypervolemia, 67
Hypotension
 conditions associated with, 277*t*
 TEE assessment
  ICU, 277–278
Hypovolemia
 TEE, 240

Hypoxemia
 unexplained
  indications for TEE in ICU, 280

I
IABP
 TEE, 241
ICU. *See* Intensive care unit (ICU)
Incidental disease
 TEE, 245*t*
Inferobasal aneurysms, 66*f*
Inspiration, 125
Insulation, 10
Intensity, 7
Intensive care unit (ICU)
 TEE, 272–282
  challenges to, 273*t*
  complications of, 274–275, 275*t*
  contraindications to, 274–275
  disadvantages and limitations of,
   275–276
  indications for, 276–282, 276*t*
  probe insertion, 273–274
  vs. pulmonary artery catheterization,
   272–273
  vs. TTE, 272, 273*t*
Interseptal infarction, 64*f*
Intimal flap
 localization of, 279–280
 with type B aortic dissection, 279*f*
Intraaortic balloon counterpulsation (IABP)
 TEE, 241
Intracardiac pressure, 101–105
 TEE, 238
Intracardiac shunts, 101
Intracavitary pressures disease
 Bernoulli equation, 102–105
Ischemia
 characteristics, 57*t*

J
Jet
 mitral insufficiency *vs.* aortic stenosis,
  195
Jet area/left ventricular outflow tract area
 method, 180*f*

K
Kay-Shiley prosthetic valves
 echocardiographic characteristics of, 205

L
Lambl excrescences, 307, 308*f*
Lateral (azimuth) resolution, 14
Lateral wall dropout, 310*f*
Leaflet prolapse
 isolated anterior
  repair of, 167
 isolated P2 posterior
  repair of, 166–167
Leakage backflow, 210
Left subclavian artery (LSUB), 241*f*

Left ventricle (LV)
 chamber compliance, 111
 diastolic dysfunction
  Doppler echocardiographic values, 126*t*
  Doppler transmitral blood flow velocity,
   116*f*
 diastolic function
  echocardiographic evaluation of,
   112–114
  newer echocardiographic assessment
   techniques, 119–123
 distention
  TEE, 241
 Doppler flow profiles
  physiologic variables influence on, 119
 filling
  Doppler echocardiography, 113–114
 fractional shortening, 38*f*
 function
  quantitative assessment of, 238
 function assessment, 37
 hypertrophy, 47
  imaging difficulties, 67
 mass
  determination, 47
 pressure
  Bernoulli equation, 104
 pressure rise
  Doppler echocardiography, 45*f*
 pseudoaneurysm, 49
  quantitative Doppler characteristics,
   49–50
  two-dimensional characteristics,
   49–50
 quantitative measurements, 38–41
 relaxation, 111, 112*f*
 stepwise examination, 32–33
 transgastric midpapillary short-axis view,
  32
 transgastric two-chamber view, 33
 true aneurysm, 47–48
  associated findings, 48
  two-dimensional characteristics, 48
 volumes, 38
  acoustic quantification, 40–41
  calculation of, 39
  fractional area change, 40–41
 wall thickness
  determination, 47
Left ventricular ejection fraction (LVEF)
 qualitative determinations, 42, 42*t*
 TEE assessment of, 276
Left ventricular end-diastolic pressure
 (LVEDP)
 aortic valve insufficiency velocity profile,
  106*f*
 aortic valve regurgitation velocity profile,
  105
 TEE assessment of
  in ICU, 276
Left ventricular internal dimension (LVID),
 39*f*

Left ventricular outflow diameter
 jet height ratio to
  in aortic regurgitation, 178, 179*f*
Left ventricular outflow tract (LVOT), 42
 ASH, 52*f*
 jet height ratio to
  in aortic regurgitation, 178–179, 180*t*,
   180*f*
 stroke volume calculation, 96
 transesophageal longitudinal view of, 172*f*
 transgastric long-axis view, 43*f*
Left ventricular outflow tract obstruction
 (LVOTO)
 following mitral valve repair, 165
 prosthetic valves
  clinical caveats, 214
 of prosthetic valves, 214
 TEE assessment of, 171–172
Levo-transposition, 296–297
Linear array, 18
Loitering, 65
LSUB, 241*f*
LV. *See* Left ventricle (LV)
LVEDP. *See* Left ventricular end-diastolic
 pressure (LVEDP)
LVEF
 qualitative determinations, 42, 42*t*
 TEE assessment of, 276
LVID, 39*f*
LVOT. *See* Left ventricular outflow tract
 (LVOT)
LVOTO. *See* Left ventricular outflow tract
 obstruction (LVOTO)

M
MAM
 Doppler tissue imaging of, 119–120, 120*f*
ME. *See* Midesophageal (ME)
Mechanical heart valves
 echocardiographic characteristics of, 201
Medtronic Hall prosthetic valves
 echocardiographic characteristics of, 206
Method of discs, 39
Midesophageal (ME)
 aortic valve long-axis view
  color gain too high, 329*f*
 commissural view, 139
 four-chamber view
  dynamic range too low, 327*f*
  gain setting too low, 322*f*
Mirroring artifacts
 pulsed wave Doppler, 316*f*
Mitral annular motion (MAM)
 Doppler tissue imaging of, 119–120, 120*f*
Mitral annular velocities
 patterns of, 121*f*
Mitral annulus
 calcified, 170
Mitral inflow
 continuous wave Doppler, 151*f*
 diastolic spectral profile of, 150*f*, 151*f*
 patterns of, 121*f*

Mitral insufficiency
  severity of, 337
Mitral leaflet
  anterior
    anatomy of, 133, 145
    doming of, 147f, 148
    hockey stick deformity of, 170f
  fish mouth view, 164f
  motion, 134–135, 135f
    excessive, 162
    normal, 162
    restricted, 162
  posterior
    anatomy of, 133, 145
  prolapse, 136f
  repair, 166–170
Mitral regurgitant jet
  eccentric, 137f
Mitral regurgitation, 133–142
  causes, 134–135, 134t
  color flow Doppler examination, 136
  dynamic
    TEE, 240
  evaluation of
    pitfalls in, 142
  functional classification of, 162
  grading, 137t
  intraoperative examination of, 135–141
  ischemic, 65
    repair of, 167–168
  lesion location, 138–139
  mechanism, 134–135
  mitral valve repair for
    history of, 159
    indications for, 159
    intervention timing, 159
    patient assessment for, 160–165
    surgery, 166–171
  P2 segment with adjacent annular
    calcium, 171f
  severity grading, 136–138
  TEE, 246
  two-dimensional examination, 136
  valve repair, 139–141
Mitral ring annuloplasty
  in cardiomyopathy, 169
Mitral stenosis, 145–155
  echocardiographic scoring system,
    148–149, 148t
  etiology of, 145–146
  mitral valve repair for
    history of, 159
    indications for, 159
    intervention timing, 159
    pressure half-time results after, 172–173
  practical evaluation, 155
  rheumatic
    midesophageal long-axis view of, 147f
  severity of, 150t, 338
  transesophageal echocardiographic
    evaluation of, 147–155
    physiologic assessments, 149–152

two-dimensional echocardiography,
    147–149
transesophageal echocardiographic
    midesophageal four-chamber image,
    146f
transesophageal five-chamber view of, 170f
Mitral valve
  anatomy of, 133, 145
  area
    determination of, 152t
  cross section of, 141f
  disease
    pathologic anatomy of, 160f
  exposure of
    in mitral regurgitation repair, 166
  fish mouth orifice, 151f
  midesophageal four-chamber view, 30–31
  midesophageal two-chamber view, 31
  nomenclature schemes, 133, 134f
  quantitative evaluation of, 141–142
  stepwise examination, 29–31
  systemic transesophageal
    echocardiographic examination of,
    140f
Mitral valve repair, 159–173
  assessment afterwards, 171–173
    surgical valve, 171
    TEE, 171–173
  for mitral regurgitation
    freedom from reoperation, 160f–161f
    history of, 159
    indications for, 159
    intervention timing, 159
    patient assessment for, 160–165
    results of, 159–160
    surgery, 166–171
  for mitral stenosis
    history of, 159
    indications for, 159
    intervention timing, 159
  reintervention decisions, 173
  in rheumatic disease, 170
M-mode (motion mode), 17
  Doppler flow propagation velocity, 122f
    impaired left ventricular relaxation,
    123f
  dyskinesis, 58f
  normal wall motion, 58f
Moderator band, 307, 308f
Modulation, 78
Monitoring
  TEE probe insertion, 273
Motion mode. *See* M-mode (motion mode)
Myocardial infarction
  acute
    complications, 66t
  complications, 65
  diagnosis
    abnormal loading conditions, 67
    abnormal wall motion, 67
    imaging pitfalls, 67
  indications for TEE in ICU, 282

Myocardial ischemia
  anatomic localization of, 61–67
  characteristics, 57*t*
  diagnosis, 56–70
    clinical applications, 68–70
    echocardiographic, 61–67
    physiologic basis, 57–61
    TEE, 56–57
  endocardial excursion *vs.* wall thickening,
    59*t*
  ischemic mitral regurgitation, 65
  monitoring, 68
  myocardial infarction complications,
    65
  right ventricular, 67
  segmental wall motion abnormalities,
    59*t*
  TEE, 238–241
  transgastric short-axis view, 237*f*
Myocardial stunning, 238
Myocardium
  hibernating
    characteristics, 57*t*
    dobutamine stress testing, 60
  preconditioned
    characteristics, 57*t*

N
Nasogastric suction
  TEE probe insertion, 274
Near fields (Fresnel), 10–11
Nomenclature
  classic anatomic
    of mitral valve, 133
  Duran
    of mitral valve, 133
Nyquist illusions, 87*f*
Nyquist limit, 89*f*

O
Occult disease
  TEE, 245–246
Off-pump CABG (OPCAB), 56
  hemodynamic compromise, 246
  ischemia during, 69
  mitral regurgitation, 247
  patent foramen ovale, 247
  RWMA, 246–247
  TEE, 246
Optimizing resolution, 14
Ostium primum defects, 287
Ostium secundum defects, 287

P
Papillary muscles
  anatomy of, 133
  rupture
    repair of, 167
Paravalvular regurgitation, 205, 211
  TEE, 211*f*
Patent ductus arteriosus, 292
  anatomy of, 292

intraoperative TEE of, 292
  physiology of, 292
  repair of
    examination after, 292
Patent foramen ovale
  across intraatrial septum, 280*f*
  TEE, 245–246
Pathologic transmitral flow velocities,
    115–123
  impaired relaxation filling patterns,
    114
  pseudonormalized filling pattern,
    117
  restrictive filling pattern, 114–115
Pathologic transvalvular regurgitation,
    210–211
Patient positioning
  TEE probe insertion, 274
Pericardial disease, 125–126
Pericardial effusion
  indications for TEE in ICU, 282
Pericardial fat, 307*f*
Pericardial sinuses, 306–307
Pericardial tamponade, 125–126
Pericarditis
  constrictive, 125–126
Perioperative TEE practice guidelines
  American Society of Anesthesiologists/
    Society of Cardiovascular
    Anesthesiologists, 56
Phased array, 18
  transducer, 12, 13*f*
Piezoelectric crystal, 10
PISA. *See* Proximal isovelocity surface area
    (PISA)
Planimetry
  LV area, 236–237
  two-dimensional
    of aortic stenosis, 188–190
  valve area, 150
Pleural effusion, 308, 309*f*
  TEE, 246
Porcine bioprosthetic valve
  transvalvular regurgitation, 210*f*
Port access surgery
  TEE, 244–245
P2 posterior leaflet prolapse
  transesophageal four-chamber view of,
    167*f*
Preload
  TEE, 237*t*
Pressure gradients, 101–105
  calculation of, 100*f*, 149–150
Pressure half-time, 151–152
  measurement of
    in aortic regurgitation, 182–183
    mitral valve area, 152
    results after mitral stenosis, 172–173
Propagation velocity, 3–4
Prosthetic aortic valves
  effective orifice area of, 205*t*
  normal effective orifice area for, 214*f*

Prosthetic valves, 200–215. *See also* specific
        valve
    bileaflet
        aortic position, 204*f*
        color Doppler flow, 203*f*
        echocardiographic characteristics of,
            203–205
        mitral position, 203*f*
        TEE, 204*f*
    biologic
        echocardiographic characteristics of,
            206–207
    echocardiographic characteristics of,
        201–210
    endocarditis, 213–214
        clinical caveats, 213–214
    hemolysis, 213
        clinical caveats, 213
    LVOTO, 214
        clinical caveats, 214
    regurgitation, 210–211
        clinical caveats, 210–211
    stenosis, 211–212
        clinical caveats, 211–212
    stented bovine pericardial
        echocardiographic characteristics of,
            207–208
    TEE evaluation of, 200–201
        clinical role of, 201*t*
    thrombosis, 212–213
        clinical caveats, 212–213
    types of, 202*t*
Proximal isovelocity surface area
        (PISA)
    method, 153–154
    midesophageal four-chamber view, 154*f*
    mitral stenosis, 155*f*
Pseudoaneurysm
    left ventricular, 49
        quantitative Doppler characteristics,
            49–50
        two-dimensional characteristics, 49–50
        transgastric view, 50*f*
Pulmonary artery
    band, 298*f*, 299
    bifurcation
        with thrombus, 281*f*
    diastolic pressure
        Bernoulli equation, 104, 104*f*
    mean pressure
        Bernoulli equation, 104, 104*f*
    systolic pressure
        Bernoulli equation, 102–103, 103*f*
Pulmonary catheters
    TEE, 244
Pulmonary embolism
    indications for TEE in ICU, 281
Pulmonary venous atrial flow reversal,
        117–118
Pulmonary venous blood flow (PVDF)
    Doppler echocardiographic evaluation of,
        117–118

    pulsed wave Doppler scan of, 139*f*
    velocity profile, 118*f*
Pulmonic valve, 226–228
    anatomy of, 226
    midesophageal aortic valve short-axis
        view, 227
    midesophageal right ventricular
        inflow-outflow view, 227
    regurgitation, 227–228
        severity, 227*f*
    stenosis, 228
        Doppler echocardiography, 228
        two-dimensional echocardiography, 228
    TEE, 227
    transesophageal echocardiography, 228*f*
    transgastric pulmonic valve view, 227
Pulsed wave Doppler, 86–88
    aliasing
        baseline setting, 90*f*
    artifacts
        range ambiguity, 317–318
    clinical caveats, 86
    echocardiography
        heart rhythm, 105–106
    limitations, 87
    mirroring artifact, 316*f*
    sample volume, 318*f*
    system processing, 86–87
Pulsed wave sample volume, 317*f*
Pulse length
    axial resolution, 11*f*
Pulse repetition frequency, 19, 86
Pulse wave velocity measurements
    maximizing, 87–88
PVDF. *See* Pulmonary venous blood flow
        (PVDF)

Q
Quadrature phase demodulation, 81, 315
Quantitative hemodynamics
    TEE, 237*t*

R
Range ambiguity
    pulsed wave Doppler artifacts, 317–318
Rarefaction, 3
Red cell motion
    effects on ultrasound frequency, 78*f*
Reflection, 5*f*, 6–7
Refraction, 5*f*, 7
    artifact, 8*f*
Regional wall motion abnormality (RWMA),
        56
    TEE assessment of, 276
Regurgitant fraction
    calculation of, 141
Regurgitant jet area
    color map of, 136–137
Regurgitant orifice area
    calculation of, 141–142
Regurgitant volume, 98–101
    calculation of, 141

Regurgitation
  prosthetic valves
    clinical caveats, 210–211
  transvalvular, 205
Resolution, 14
Retrograde cardioplegia
  administration of, 243
Reverberation, 313, 313*f*
  color flow Doppler, 316*f*
Rheumatic heart disease
  causing mitral stenosis, 146
Right atrium, 222–223
  anatomy of, 222–223
  TEE, 223
Right-dominant system, 64
Right ventricle (RV), 218–222
  anatomy, 218, 219*f*
  diastolic function, 123–125
    Doppler trans-tricuspid flow velocity,
      123–124
  dilation, 219–220, 220*f*
  dysfunction
    TEE, 240–241
  function
    TEE assessment of, 276–277
  hepatic vein flow, 221–222, 221*f*
  hypertrophy, 218–219
  infarction, 67
  interventricular septum, 222
  ischemia, 67
  midesophageal four-chamber view,
    218
  midesophageal right ventricular
    inflow-outflow view, 218
  regional right function, 222
  systolic function, 220
  systolic pressure
    Bernoulli equation, 102–103
  TEE views, 218
  transgastric midpapillary short-axis view,
    218, 219*f*
  transgastric right ventricular inflow view,
    218, 220*f*
  tricuspid annular plane systolic excursion,
    220–221
Ross procedure, 228
RV. *See* Right ventricle (RV)
RWMA, 56
  TEE assessment of, 276

S
SAM. *See* Systolic anterior motion
    (SAM)
Sample volume, 86
Scan line density, 19
Scan lines, 18*f*
Scattering, 5*f*
Scattering reflectors, 6–7
Secundum atrial septal defect,
    288*f*
Sedation
  TEE probe insertion, 273–274

Segment system
  myocardial ischemia, 61–67, 61*f*, 62*f*, 63*f*
Septal wall dropout, 310*f*
Side lobes, 14, 15*f*
  artifacts, 15
Signal
  Doppler
    extracting low-frequency, low-amplitude,
      84*f*
Simpson's rule
  modified, 40
Simpson's rule of discs, 39
  left ventricular ejection fraction
    calculation, 41*f*
Single-plane ellipsoid model, 39, 40*f*
Single-ventricle lesions, 298–299
Sinotubular junction
  measurement of
    TEE, 209*f*
Sinus of Valsalva
  measurement of
    TEE, 209*f*
16-segment system
  myocardial ischemia, 61–67, 61*f*, 62*f*, 63*f*
Society of Cardiovascular Anesthesiologists
  perioperative TEE practice guidelines, 56
Soft tissue
  frequency, 5*f*
  wavelength, 5*f*
Sound beams
  extraneous, 14–15
Sound waves
  frequency, 3
  physical properties of, 3–9
  propagation velocity, 3–4
  ultrasound, 4–5
  vibrations, 3, 4*f*
  wavelength, 3
Spectral Doppler
  artifacts, 314–318
    aliasing, 314
    beam width flow artifacts, 317–318
    mirroring, 315–316, 316*f*
    nonparallel beam angle, 314–315, 315*f*
    of mitral valve, 138
Specular reflectors, 6
St. Jude prosthetic valve
  echocardiographic characteristics of,
    203–205
Stanford B dissections
  TEE, 264–265
Stanford classification, 254*f*
Starr-Edwards prosthetic valves
  color Doppler, 206*f*
  echocardiographic characteristics of, 205
  TEE, 206*f*
Stenosis
  prosthetic valves
    clinical caveats, 211–212
Stented bovine pericardial prosthetic valves
  echocardiographic characteristics of,
    207–208

Stented porcine heterografts
echocardiographic characteristics of, 207
Stentless bioprosthetic valves, 208–209
Stepwise examination, 27–34
aortic valve level, 27–29, 33
left ventricular level, 32–33
mitral valve level, 30–31
Storage systems, 330
Stress testing
dobutamine, 60
Stroke distance, 94
Stroke volume, 42
determination, 95*f*
Doppler measurement, 94–97
echocardiographic technique for Doppler
measurement of, 95*f*
Stunned myocardium
characteristics, 57*t*
dobutamine stress testing, 60
S-wave, 124*f*
Systemic embolism
indications for TEE in ICU, 281–282
Systolic anterior motion (SAM)
cases at high risk for, 170–171
risk assessment for, 165
TEE assessment of, 166*f*, 171–172

T
TEE. *See* Transesophageal echocardiography
(TEE)
Tetralogy of fallot, 294–295, 295*f*
anatomy of, 294
color flow Doppler examination of, 295
intraoperative TEE of, 294–295
physiology of, 294
repair of
examination after, 295
spectral Doppler examination of, 295
two-dimensional examination of, 295
Thoracic aorta
ascending
examination of, 256–257
linear streak in, 257*f*
atheroma, 266*f*, 267*f*
grading, 266*t*
classification systems, 251–252
descending
examination of, 257–258
intimal tear
entry site of, 260*f*
examination techniques, 255–258
TEE, 251–267
Thoracic esophagus
esophagus and aorta relationship, 256
Three-dimensional ultrasound beam, 10–11
Thrombosis
atrial appendage
short-axis imaging of, 149*f*
prosthetic valves
clinical caveats, 212–213
of prosthetic valves, 212–213
TEE, 245

Tilting-disc prosthetic valves
echocardiographic characteristics of, 206
Time gain compensation, 16
Time gating, 86
Time-velocity integral (TVI), 42
Tissue
acoustic properties, 6*t*
Tissue interface, 6
Tracheal intubation
TEE probe insertion, 274
Transaortic valve
stroke volume calculation, 96
Transducer, 3
components, 9–10, 9*f*
ICU
TEE, 275
transmit and receive modes
cycling, 15
Transesophageal echocardiography (TEE)
anatomy, 333–336
for aortic stenosis assessment, 190–193
assessing mitral valve repair, 162–165,
171–173
adequacy, 171–172
complications, 171–172
direct surgical inspection of mitral
apparatus, 165
mitral regurgitation functional
classification, 162
nomenclature, 162
pitfalls of, 173
rationale, 162
reporting findings, 165
systolic anterior motion risk
assessment, 165
assessing prosthetic valves, 200–201
clinical role of, 201*t*
Doppler examination
clinical caveats, 80–81
measurements
normal, 48*t*
probe
advancement, 23*f*
insertion in two-dimensional
examination, 22
manipulation in two-dimensional
examination, 22
Transesophageal images
optimizing, 321–330
color controls, 321–330
storage systems, 330
two-dimensional controls, 321–328
Transmyocardial laser revascularization, 69
left ventricle laser beam penetration, 70*f*
Transthoracic echocardiography (TTE), 63
Tricuspid annulus, 222
Tricuspid regurgitation, 224–225
Doppler image, 224*f*, 226*f*
hepatic venous flow, 225*f*
Tricuspid stenosis, 225
Doppler echocardiography, 225
two-dimensional echocardiography, 225

Tricuspid valve, 223–226
  anatomy of, 223, 223*f*
  annular dilation, 225
  carcinoid syndrome, 226
  diseases
    etiology, 225–226
  Ebstein anomaly, 226
  endocarditis, 226
  midesophageal four-chamber view, 224
  midesophageal right ventricular
    inflow-outflow view, 224
  rheumatic disease, 226
  TEE, 223–224
  transgastric view, 224
True aneurysm
  left ventricular, 47–48
    associated findings, 48
    two-dimensional characteristics, 48
True aortic arch
  mirror image of, 313*f*
True lumen
  early systolic flow within, 259*f*
  flow to false lumen, 260*f*
  identification of, 280
TTE, 63
TVI, 42
Two-dimensional controls, 321–328
  compression, 326
  depth, 323
  dynamic range, 326
  focus, 323–325
  frequency, 325–326
  gain, 321–325
  persistence, 326–327
  preprocessing *vs.* postprocessing, 321
  reject, 326
  sector size, 328
  time gain compensation, 323, 324*f*
  transmit power, 321
Two-dimensional echocardiography, 3–20,
    22–35
  artifacts, 309–314
    acoustic shadowing, 311, 311*f*
    electronic noise, 314
    lateral resolution, 311
    reverberation, 313, 313*f*
    side lobe and beam width, 311–312, 312*f*
    suboptimal image quality, 309–311
  beam formation, 9–15
  creating two-dimensional image, 18–19
  display formats, 16–17, 17*f*
  goals, 27
  imaging planes and orientation, 22–24
    multiplane imaging angle, 24
  of mitral regurgitation severity, 136
  signal reception and processing, 15–16
  sound tissue interaction, 5–6, 5*f*
  sound waves
    physical properties of, 3–9
  stepwise examination, 27–34
  transducer design, 9–15
  two-dimensional scan systems, 17–18

Two-dimensional image
  vs. Doppler flow measurement,
    83*f*–84*f*
  normal anatomic variants in, 305–308
    Coumadin ridge, 306, 307*f*
    crista terminalis, 305, 306*f*
    eustachian valve, 305
    Lambl excrescences, 307, 308*f*
    lipomatous hypertrophy of atrial
      septum, 305–306
    moderator band, 307, 308*f*
    pericardial sinuses, 306–307
    pleural effusion, 308, 309*f*
  quality and dynamic motion, 19
  sector imaging, 18–19
Two-dimensional planimetry
  of aortic stenosis, 188–190
Two-dimensional scan systems, 17–18
Type A aortic aneurysms
  morphology of, 253*f*
Type III (Stanford B) dissections
  TEE, 264–265

U
Ultrasound, 4–5
  beam
    electronic focusing, 12
    focusing, 11
    three-dimensional, 12*f*
  frequency
    red cell motion effects on, 78*f*
    frequency graph, 8*f*
  waves
    formation, 10
Univentricular heart, 298–299
  anatomy of, 298
  intraoperative TEE of, 298–299
  physiology of, 298

V
Valve area, 101
  calculation of, 100*f*, 150
Valve gradient area, 205
Valve surgery
  ischemia during, 69–70
Valvular disease
  Bernoulli equation, 102
Valvular function
  TEE assessment
    ICU, 277
Vascular cannulation
  TEE, 242–244
    antegrade cardioplegia, 242–243
    aortic atheromatous disease, 242
    ascending aorta, 242
    femoral arterial cannulation, 243–244
    femoral venous cannulation, 243
    retrograde cardioplegia, 243
Vena contracta
  mapping, 181
  measurement of, 138*f*
  width of, 137–138

Ventricular aneurysm
   partial midesophageal four-chamber view,
     49*f*
Ventricular diastolic function
   evaluation, 110–126
   physiology, 110–112
Ventricular function
   global right
     assessment of, 218–222
     TEE assessment of, 236–238
     in ICU, 276
Ventricular pathology, 47–53
   dilated cardiomyopathy, 49–50
   hypertrophic cardiomyopathy, 50–53
   left ventricular hypertrophy, 47
   left ventricular pseudoaneurysm, 48
   left ventricular true aneurysm, 47–48
Ventricular relaxation
   impaired left
     transmitral color M-mode propagation
      velocity, 123*f*
Ventricular rupture
   TEE assessment of, 172
Ventricular septal defect, 289–291
   anatomy of, 289–291
   atrioventricular canal-type defects, 290
   color flow Doppler examination, 291
   double committed outlet defects, 290, 291*f*
   inlet defects, 290
   intraoperative TEAE, 291
   muscular defects, 290

   perimembranous defects, 290
   physiology of, 290–291
   repair of
     examination after, 291
     two-dimensional examination, 291
Ventricular septum
   components of, 290*f*
Ventricular size
   two-dimensional measurements of,
     236–238
Ventricular systolic performance, 37–47
   ejection fraction, 38
   fractional shortening, 37–38
   isovolemic rate of pressure rise, 42–44
   left ventricular function assessment,
     37
   left ventricular quantitative
     measurements, 38–41
   left ventricular volumes, 38
   optimizing, 44–47
   stroke volume and cardiac output, 42
Venturi effect, 51
Vibrations, 3
   ultrasound transducer, 4*f*
Volumetric flow calculations, 94–101
V-wave, 124*f*

W
Wall motion score index, 64
Wavelength, 3
   soft tissue, 5*f*